"Laurie and I cannot recommend this brain-changing, life-changing book enough, and we pray you'll benefit as much as we have from reading it!"

**Matt and Laurie Crouch**, TBN

"In a well-researched look at our food system, Dr. Leaf serves us a wake-up call to declining physical health if we continue on our current path. But there is hope. In this insightful book, Dr. Leaf helps us understand that each time we eat, we are choosing. With an informative combination of scientific research and scriptural principles, Dr. Leaf shows that healthy eating may not be quick or cheap, but it is something we all can do. Thanks to this book I am motivated to make healthier food choices and help others do the same."

**David I. Levy, MD**, clinical professor of neurosurgery, University of California, San Diego; author of *Gray Matter: A Neurosurgeon Discovers the Power of Prayer . . . One Patient at a Time*

"Betty and I were introduced to Dr. Caroline Leaf by Peter and Ann Pretorius, our missionary partners in Africa. They were excited because she was having such a profound impact on people throughout South Africa. We invited her to be a guest on *LIFE Today*, and she has continued to have a powerful impact—not only in her own country but here in the United States. A neuroscientist, Dr. Leaf shows the connection between our brain and food. The fact is, many people are killing themselves because of what they eat—or don't eat. The pointers Dr. Leaf provides in these pages will surely make us think twice before we take the next bite and equip us to be better stewards of the bodies God has given us."

**James Robison**, founder and president of LIFE Outreach International; founder and publisher of *The Stream*

"This book is unique. There are books about nutrition and there are books about the mind—however, we cannot think of any book that links the mind and nutrition in the detail Dr. Caroline Leaf does. We definitely never learned this information when we were in medical school. The information in this book has changed the way our family eats. We are healthier, fitter, slimmer, and smarter. Dr. Leaf is the real deal. She talks the talk and walks the walk. We know her lifestyle; we know what is in her pantry and fridge and what she eats at her table. Her whole family lives out what she has written in this book. It will change your life."

**Peter Amua-Quarshie, MD, MPH, MS, and Mercy Amua-Quarshie, MD, MPH, FACOG**

"There is a difference between desiring to be well and being tired of being sick. Those who truly desire to be well will confess healing Scriptures every day. They would not dare miss taking their vitamin supplements. They would not eat anything or in any way other than God's way, under any circumstance. Caroline Leaf's new book, *Think and Eat Yourself Smart*, will help anyone who has the desire to be well and who will change their ways and lifestyle to God's ways. It will help you, and here I quote Dr. Leaf, 'Admit it, quit it, and beat it!' Get it! Read it! Do it! And with long life, God will satisfy you and show you his salvation!"

**Kenneth Copeland**, Kenneth Copeland Ministries

"This timely and essential new book from Dr. Caroline Leaf promises to be exactly the resource I need both for myself personally and as a recommended resource that could dramatically benefit all of my patients and their families, as well as my own family and friends. I am eager to faithfully implement its life-integrating principles and important paradigm changes, to recommend it to patients and colleagues, and to reap the benefits of healthier thinking and healthier food choices. With continued estimations that perhaps 80 percent of today's diseases and disorders are directly related to chosen lifestyle issues, Dr. Leaf's challenging call toward deep, long-term, and sustainable changes in our lives—spirit, soul, and body—is a truly life-giving message that can help save us from further devastation of preventable disease, dysfunction, and death. Thank you so much, Dr. Leaf, for applying your neuroscientifically sound perspectives to this important issue!"

**Dr. Robert Turner**, neurologist

"I am so excited about the release of this book from a woman who truly knows what she is talking about *and* lives it out every single day. My last season in life was the most challenging one I've ever faced health-wise, and even though I've always been quite focused on good nutrition and exercise, my body was obviously needing more. I know this book will be a life-changing and life-saving tool in your hand, and with all my heart I say thanks to Dr. Caroline for putting into our hands a book filled with practical answers and a way forward, so that each one of us can live out God's perfect plan for our lives."

**Darlene Zschech**, composer, worship leader, and pastor; author of *Worship Changes Everything*

"It is my honor and pleasure to endorse Dr. Caroline and her new book, *Think and Eat Yourself Smart*. Her passion for the well-being of others is genuine, and I know the lights will go on for many as they absorb the truth and perspective within these pages. We live in a world consumed with so many things—including food and the pursuit of health, beauty, opportunity, and influence. I am confident this book will be life-changing for many and will fuel foundational truths that make for a blessed, effective, and fruitful life."

**Bobbie Houston**, Hillsong Church

"Admit it! Quit it! Beat it! These are the main ingredients to this tasty dish of a book. The brainy truths and guidelines presented in *Think and Eat Yourself Smart* are a welcome addition to Dr. Leaf's prior works. We need to be more *mindful* of how we think about and practice the art of eating. I am sure this work will awaken minds with simple truths that will lead to sharper thoughts and healthier lives!"

Dr. Avery Jackson III, neurosurgeon

"Did you know your body is the temple of the Holy Spirit, and God created us to glorify him? Have you ever thought about the fact that God can't move through you if you're not able physically to do what he wants you to do? In her new book, *Think and Eat Yourself Smart*, Dr. Caroline Leaf reveals how to have a healthier lifestyle and a sharper mind. She is a member of Gateway Church and has spoken during our weekend services and conferences. Her medical knowledge, combined with her revelatory wisdom, will completely change your life."

Robert Morris, founding senior pastor, Gateway Church;
bestselling author of *The Blessed Life*

"My friend Dr. Caroline Leaf has the uncanny ability to explain complex topics in a way that is practical and attainable. Her insights in acquiring health, both physically and mentally, are beautifully penned in every page of this book. I'm grateful for her hard-hitting advice. I've seen it transform the lives of many—including many people close to me. This book will change your thinking and your life."

Priscilla Shirer, teacher and author

"In *Think and Eat Yourself Smart*, Caroline shows how increasing your awareness of emotional responses to food enhances your ability to make wise and mindful choices about what you actually eat. In turn, you enhance not only your physical health but also, more importantly, your mental health and your capacity to use mindfulness in all your daily choices. I wholeheartedly endorse Caroline's program of thinking and eating wisely."

Dr. Jeff Shwartz, psychiatrist and author

"It is my joy to endorse this latest book by Dr. Caroline. She is a marvelous vision of health, vitality, and energy! If what she is recommending to *eat* is testament to her gorgeous mind, body, soul, and spirit—well, in the famous words of the character in *When Harry Met Sally*, 'I'll have what she's having' (on my food plate, please!). We live in a world of 'fast foods' where some children don't even know that milk comes from an animal, not a carton. There is a hunger to get back to basics and actually experience the freshness of an apple, the scent of homegrown herbs, and the zest of a freshly squeezed orange. I'll be the first to experiment with Dr. Caroline's recipes and food combinations—so to all who desire to live a long life filled with energy, joy, and the goodness of fresh, yummy, seasonal foods (as I surely do!), bon appétit!"

Pastor Chris Pringle, senior minister of C3 Church, Sydney

"Have you ever wondered why you eat the way you do? Well, answers to this question and more are in *Think and Eat Yourself Smart*. Dr. Caroline

Leaf seamlessly weaves science and biblical insights together to explain how our thinking relates to our eating habits. Read it and gain the wisdom you need to improve your health!"

**John and Lisa Bevere**, bestselling authors; ministers; cofounders of Messenger International

"Today millions of people are suffering from the health effects of bad eating patterns, while countless individuals are enslaved so that we can have a plethora of cheap food. In *Think and Eat Yourself Smart*, Dr. Caroline Leaf shows us how we can use our minds not only to choose to establish a healthier, integrated lifestyle but also to improve the lives of those suffering injustice within the global food industry."

**Christine Caine**, author of *Unstoppable*

"Think beyond the fork! Dr. Caroline compels us to increase our gastronomical intelligence. Her findings will shock you, and her solutions will inspire you to take back control of the dinner table. If you wouldn't settle for a fake diamond, why settle for fake food? Learn from a trusted source what real food is and enjoy the vibrant life awaiting you when you choose to follow in her footsteps."

**Pastor Colleen Rouse**, Victory World Church, Atlanta

"As a physician and a pastor's wife, I've seen countless individuals suffer unnecessarily from diet-related illnesses. I highly recommend this book to anyone desiring to experience victory in the areas of weight management and wellness."

**Dr. Lillian Robertson, MD, FACOG**, Emmanuel Ministries

"My dear friend Dr. Caroline Leaf is the real deal. She lives out the words in her books and shares with us how we too can eat ourselves smart. God has gifted her with a brilliant mind and the ability to communicate a fascinating message to the world. Be smart and buy this engaging book."

**Shelene Bryan**, author of *Love, Skip, Jump*; founder of Skip1.org

"We always appreciate Dr. Leaf's clear, concise, and helpful point of view on matters of the mind."

**Gabe and Rebekah Lyons**, founders of Q

"Dr. Caroline Leaf has done it again! Dr. Leaf delves into a systemic problem in our individual lives and reveals a systemic solution. *Think and Eat Yourself Smart* is divinely inspired and supported by sound scientific facts regarding how we think and how our thoughts affect our eating choices. This transforming book is a must-have for everyone on planet earth. This book supports 2 Timothy 1:7, which reminds us that God has given us, through the incredible *power* in our *sound* minds, the ability to act on these choices and transform our world."

**Dr. Edith Davis, PhD**, first African-American female geophysicist; author of *How We Really Learn*

# THINK AND EAT
## YOURSELF
# SMART

## A NEUROSCIENTIFIC APPROACH
## TO A SHARPER MIND AND HEALTHIER LIFE

# DR. CAROLINE LEAF

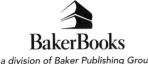

**BakerBooks**
*a division of Baker Publishing Group*
Grand Rapids, Michigan

Published by Baker Books
a division of Baker Publishing Group
P.O. Box 6287, Grand Rapids, MI 49516-6287
www.bakerbooks.com

Printed in the United States of America

Library of Congress Cataloging-in-Publication Data
Names: Leaf, Caroline, 1963– author.
Title: Think and eat yourself smart : a neuroscientific approach to a sharper mind and healthier life / Caroline Leaf.
Description: Grand Rapids, MI : Baker Books, 2016. | Includes bibliographical references.
Identifiers: LCCN 2015037194| ISBN 9780801015717 (cloth) | ISBN 9780801019197 (pbk.)
Subjects: LCSH: Health—Popular works. | Health—Psychological aspects. | Diet—Psychological aspects. | Behavior modification. | Food preferences.
Classification: LCC RA776.5 .L383 2016 | DDC 613--dc23 LC record available at http://lccn.loc.gov/2015037194

16  17  18  19  20  21  22        8  7  6  5  4  3  2

In keeping with biblical principles of creation stewardship, Baker Publishing Group advocates the responsible use of our natural resources. As a member of the Green Press Initiative, our company uses recycled paper when possible. The text paper of this book is composed in part of post-consumer waste.

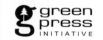

To all of you who want to live a healthy, integrated life, spirit, soul, and body, and who recognize the power of the mind—this book is dedicated to you.

To all of you who recognize the responsibility of stewardship of this beautiful earth God has so graciously given us—this book is dedicated to you.

# Contents

# Acknowledgments

The hours that go into a scientific book of this nature are endless. And as information is conceptualized and formed into ideas that can be expressed logically—an endeavor that never has an end because of the nature of science being a continual cycle of discovery—a highly skilled research assistant becomes imperative to the success of a project of this nature. To this end, I acknowledge Jessica, who not only became such an assistant but did so with excellent skill, professionalism, and brilliance. She helped me read through, evaluate, and think through the minefield that food and eating have become in the world today—a struggle we really had to target. We had so many discussions as she tirelessly helped research and make sense of a plethora of conflicting information. She helped connect multiple complex concepts and edited my writing with excellence and wisdom. She spent hours in the kitchen helping create and prepare our family's favorite recipes to put in this book. She encouraged me when I felt overloaded trying to finish a book in record time in the midst of my challenging travel schedule. In all, she went over and above and beyond the call of duty, burning the midnight oil throughout. And not only did

Jessica play a huge role in helping shape this book with her brilliant mind, but I am proud to say she is also my daughter. Thank you, Jess; your contribution was more than invaluable. I could not have done this book without you.

And my whole family climbed into this creative process: my dearest husband, Mac, who never seems to get tired of listening to me teach, who is consistently excited about the messages I share, and who gave up a flourishing business to run our organization. He unconditionally looks after my every need—he is outstanding and exceptional as a husband, father, and businessman. I love you endlessly, Mac. Dominique, my second daughter, would encourage me over the phone in the midst of her busy studies at university. With her passion for healthy, quality food, she became a great sounding board for my ideas. She also climbed into the kitchen to help develop delicious recipes. Jeffrey, my son, kept us all grounded and amused with his calm, philosophical nature as passionate discussions of ending hunger and resisting big food corporations arose during mealtimes. Alexy, my youngest daughter, literally stretched my mind as she challenged me to explain the neuro-scientific concepts I propose in this book—and adequately so, as this is her field of interest. She came up with the concept of "the mindset behind the meal."

I acknowledge Dr. Peter Amua-Quarshie, who for seven years has been my scientific advisor, patiently listening as I have challenged scientific paradigms in memory and thinking, all while keeping an eye on my scientific accuracy. He also spent weeks combing through the 1,500-plus citations I worked from for this book.

Finally, I wish acknowledge the exceptional Baker Books publishing team—I could not wish for a better one. They have given me the freedom to explore and express my research and have been professional and supportive and enthusiastic. Chad Allen, Karen Lee-Thorp, Brianna DeWitt, Mark Rice, Lindsey Spoolstra, Hannah Brinks, and the whole team—thank you. You are wonderful.

# Prologue

You may have heard that our global food production system is deeply flawed. You're right. In fact, it's probably worse than you imagine. Fortunately, there's hope. It is possible for us to vote with our forks for better practices that respect our health and the health of the planet.

To begin voting for a better way, we need to increase our knowledge about food and food practices. We need to improve our shopping and cooking skills. And, most importantly, we need to change our attitudes toward food, health, healing, and nutrition. Once we have opened our minds to a new, healthy way of approaching food, and have started removing unhealthy foods and habits from our everyday lives, we will have entered a culinary world bursting with magnificent smells, tastes, sights, sounds, and feelings that will bring joy to both our mouths and our stomachs.

Yet such changes will require more than a bit of effort. This book is not a feel-good-quick-fix-magic-solution-pop-a-pill-latest-food-fad-I-have-the-only-solution diet. It is a *long-term, sustainable* challenge to a big problem: what to eat in our world today. It is an attempt to reintroduce a culture of *thinking and effort* back into eating, one based on diligently stewarding the body and world God has entrusted to us. In the spirit of renewing the mind, it is a lifestyle book that seeks to reimagine what we eat within an integrated spirit, mind, and body framework (Rom. 12:2; 1 Thess. 5:23).

The mind is a key factor throughout this book. Thinking, as you will see, plays a dominant role in eating. Toxic thoughts can negate the positive effects of good nutrition. Healthy thoughts can enhance the effects of good nutrition and mitigate the effects of bad nutrition—to a degree. In fact, healthy thoughts lead to better food choices. Eating and thinking are so intertwined that what you are thinking about before, during, and after eating will impact every single one of the 75–100 trillion cells in your body, including the cells of your digestive system. Your state of mind will have a negative or positive influence on your digestive health, and your digestive health will also have a negative or positive influence on your state of mind.

One reason I felt convicted to write this book is because of the plethora of complicated and conflicting messages about food we are all exposed to. There is always someone new telling us they have the solution to everyone's dietary and/or exercise habits, suggesting that if we don't follow their advice we will surely drop dead. Even a lot of nutritional advice from so-called experts is often based on overblown correlations and inaccurate interpretations. And that is not even mentioning the $50 billion supplement industry. I worked out that if I had to follow the advice of just one company, I would be taking up to sixty-five different tablets, three times a day!

The fact is we are all unique, which means that a way of eating, exercising, and sleeping that works for you may not work for me, even if it is a healthy lifestyle and a *real* food diet, which I will discuss in part 1. Let's take juicing as an example. This has spiraled in popularity and for good reason; it is a great way of getting all those necessary fruits and veggies into your daily intake. But I personally get very lethargic and uncomfortable after drinking any type of juice (and I have pretty much tried every combination). I prefer to get my daily intake of veggies in other ways. So this book will not give you the solution but rather teach you how to be your own solution, with the help and guidance of the Holy Spirit.

Rather than getting caught up in whether we should go paleo, vegan, vegetarian, gluten-free, plant-based, raw vegan, or follow the blood type diet or even genetic typing (to mention just a few diets that are popular today), it would be much better to understand the fundamentals of eating, the completely entangled relationship between thinking and food, and how our uniqueness spreads throughout our spirit, soul, and body.

---

The book is divided into three parts that will help you begin approaching these issues with a renewed mindset. Part 1, "Admit It!" deals with the dysfunctional state of our current food system, and how far it has become removed from the concept of *real* food—the *real* food system God gave us. Part 2, "Quit It!" focuses on the power of the mind and the impact of toxic thinking and toxic food choices on the brain and body. Part 3, "Beat It!" deals with lifestyle changes that can help you begin the task of thinking and eating yourself smart. It includes twenty-one of my family's favorite recipes, which can help you apply these lifestyle changes in your kitchen and your tummy!

I am not a dietician, nutritionist, or medical doctor. My area of expertise is the mind, and I have approached eating from this perspective. After extensive research for years in aspects related to mind, brain, and body health from a scientific perspective, I personally do not think you have to have a degree in nutritional science to know what you should put in your mouth. I think the fact that we feel we cannot even make our own food choices anymore without the help of an "expert" is a sign of just how broken our food system has become. Indeed, the field of nutrition is massive, and the research is so extensive that it is not possible in a book of this size or nature to present all sides of every argument. To this end, I have had to be selective and have included as many original sources as possible to encourage and empower you to make your own choices—to encourage and empower *you* to think and eat yourself smart in every area of your life.

God has given us a choice: life or death, blessings or curses (Deut. 30:19). He has also given us, through the incredible *power* in our *sound* minds, the ability to act on these choices and transform our world (2 Tim. 1:7).

And the world we live in desperately needs transformation. Today, nearly a billion people are hungry and almost two billion people are overweight or obese.[1] Indeed, for the first time in our recorded history, millions of people across the world are both overweight and starving: dying of lifestyle diseases that are preventable.[2] The exploitation and waste of the earth's natural resources, partnered with a dramatically expanding world population and increasing levels of chronic diseases, have led many to question what we should eat, how people will eat, and the way in which our current food production system has contributed to these issues.

Despite all our advances—and there are many to be proud of—millions of people are condemned to live out their days in doctors' offices or dying of extreme hunger; the rest of us are confounded by the latest nutritional advice, marketing campaigns, and calorie-dense foods of a global food industry. What exactly is stopping us from avoiding illnesses and premature deaths that are largely preventable? How have our choices led us down this destructive road, away from God's perfect plan for our lives (Jer. 29:11)?

These tragic facts compel us to question the way we *think* about our food. As the stewards of God's creation (Gen. 1–2), we are not only responsible for our own wellbeing—spirit, soul, and body—but that of the entire world: a world that God so loved that he was willing to send his one and only Son to save it (John 3:16).[3]

We can change nothing until we fully comprehend what needs to be changed. Just as every action first begins with a thought, we, as the children of the Creator of this beautiful universe, first have to understand the broken food system we face (Col. 1:15–20). We have to take these thoughts captive unto Christ Jesus, asking him to guide our minds and show us the way forward (2 Cor. 10:5). And, as we renew the way we think about what we eat and how we eat it, we take the first step to renewing our health and the health of God's wonderful planet (Rom. 12:2).

Only after we admit it can we quit it and beat it.

The choice is ours.

# PART 1

# ADMIT IT!

# 1

## *Real* Food and the
## MAD Way of Eating

Today, the McDonald's logo is more recognizable than the Christian cross.[1] And just as the cross represents Christianity, the McDonald's *M* can be seen as the image of what has come to be known as the Western Diet, appropriately referred to by its acronym MAD: the Modern American Diet.[2]

### The Diversity of Diet

Throughout our history, human beings have survived, and thrived, on a diversity of diets.[3] The early Hawaiian peoples, for example, ate a diet that could be called "high carb" in today's nutritional language, with the majority of their calorie intake derived from the foods traditionally grown on the island.[4] The African Maasai tribe's traditional diet, one that my own husband Mac grew up on, largely consists of grass-fed beef and dairy products, including

21

cow's blood. The people that inhabit the Japanese island of Okinawa have customarily eaten a largely vegetarian diet, with limited amounts of fish and meat products.[5] Traditional cuisines are as diverse as they are delicious.

Human beings are also able to adapt to different ways of eating over time. The original researchers who examined the Mediterranean diet, for instance, found that it took several weeks for foreigners on Crete to adapt to the diet, and in particular the olive oil consumption, of the native islanders. Indeed, after suffering quite a bit of initial gastric discomfort, these foreigners reported an improvement to their overall eating habits and health after several weeks.[6] Similarly, over time certain populations have become better adapted at digesting starch, resulting in a greater number of AMY 1 copies of the enzyme amylase in their genes, which enable these individuals to break down carbohydrates more easily.[7]

Indeed, differences in diet are found not only between communities but within them as well. In my family alone, we have had to learn how to navigate a diverse range of foods. I can only tolerate bland meals and get ill from fungi, gluten, avocado, and tree nuts. My husband and three daughters, however, adore avocados, mushrooms, and nuts, and eat rich, spicy foods. Yet my two eldest daughters cannot digest lactose well, while my youngest daughter has a love affair with cheese. My son, on the other hand, can eat anything, including gluten and dairy. Trying to decide what we are going to have for dinner is quite a challenge, as I am sure you can imagine!

A consistent theme across dietary research is that there is no *one* way of eating that works perfectly for everyone. God created fats, carbohydrates, proteins, and all the other important nutritional building blocks that make up the food we eat—all perfectly and intricately balanced within *real*, whole foods. Essentially, we all have to safely experiment within the context of our unique situations, and, like Daniel in the Babylonian court, find a way of eating that is God-centered, enabling us to thrive and carry out

God's will (Dan. 1). We are fearfully and wonderfully made, and our uniqueness pervades every part of our lives, including what we eat (Ps. 139:14). We, like Daniel and his companions, have to find a way of eating that suits us, so that we can run the race that God has set before us (Heb. 12:1).

## *Real* Food Is Wired for Love

Yet there is one thing the cultures discussed above have in common: *they eat real food.*[8] This may sound obvious at first. What else can we eat, besides real food? Unfortunately, this is where the MAD is unique. Despite the apparent diversity of foodstuffs in our grocery stores, restaurants, and homes, many of the products available for purchase today are industrially manufactured "food-like products," as journalist and activist Michael Pollan calls them.[9] They contain unfamiliar substances that extend shelf life and flavor, and are often derived from just three highly processed commodities: corn, soy, and wheat.[10]

*Real* food is food grown the way God intended: fresh and nutritious, predominantly local, seasonal, grass-fed, as wild as possible, free of synthetic chemicals, whole or minimally processed, and ecologically diverse. It is grown according to God's multifaceted genius, transfused throughout interconnected ecosystems, because he created our ecosystems.

If there has been one consistent theme across the research I have done for this book, it is that our food systems are *wired for love*: when we care about the way our food is produced, and care about "what the animals we eat, eat," we consume foods that are the most nourishing for us.[11] For instance, humans (like many other species) are most attracted to fruits when they are fresh, ripe, and succulent, which also happens to be when these fruits are incredibly nutritious.[12] Similarly, animals that have been treated humanely and allowed to roam in an ecologically rich environment are more nutritious for us to consume, with a higher omega-3 fatty acid content, to mention just one of the many benefits.[13] *Seasonal*, *natural*, and *local* are not just trendy bywords. These words actually indicate food choices based on a growing body of evidence on the benefits of locally produced foods grown in strong, diverse ecosystems and eaten as fresh as is possible in a world where not everyone is a farmer. Indeed, many of the best chefs source local, organically grown foods not necessarily for their nutritional benefit but for their wholesome and rich flavor—good nutrition and good flavor are inseparable.[14]

### Organic versus Conventional Agriculture

To understand what *real food* means, we need to examine a hot topic: organic agriculture. The terms *organic* and *conventional* are controversial and have many interpretations. Essentially, organic farming is mainly based on biology, or "using living organisms rather than synthetic chemicals," while conventional farming is mainly based on chemistry, using synthetic substances such as pesticides and growth hormones.[15]

Over the past several decades, conventional agriculture has come to dominate global food production. This dominance has helped to produce the modern food industry, with its large supermarkets and fast-food establishments, through increased yields at lower prices.[16] Organic farming, because it rarely uses chemicals, has to adapt to the local environment. This adaptation promotes biodiversity through smaller and more varied yields.[17] Organic farms are therefore generally considered more ecologically sustainable; they use roughly 30 percent less energy than conventional agriculture and are less toxic to living organisms.[18]

The synthetic chemicals used on conventional farms are, of course, tested for safety before application. Yet they are examined individually and in laboratories, not in the complexity of the real world. For instance, one pesticide in residual amounts may be certified as safe for human consumption, but what of the combination of all the chemicals used?[19] With an estimated 516 million pounds of pesticides sprayed on conventional crops each year in the United States alone, this question should deeply concern us.[20] What is the cumulative effect of these artificial substances, particularly in our chemically laden world, where over a hundred synthetic substances are in our bodies at any given moment?[21] And what of the estimated two hundred million pounds of toxic substances that industrial agriculture leeches into American water systems per year?[22] As biologist and Berkley professor Dr. Tyrone Hayes notes, it is akin to your doctor giving you potentially harmful pills without asking you what other medication you are taking.[23] Additionally, more and more research suggests that even residual, "safe" amounts of chemicals may in fact be more damaging than larger amounts, particularly on the endocrine system.[24]

We also have to ask ourselves how applicable these laboratory studies, mainly carried out on animals, are in terms of human health. We cannot subject humans to similar laboratory testing for ethical reasons (although I certainly agree that there are serious considerations concerning animal testing as well). Yet results from studies done on animals *do not* prove beyond all doubt that such chemicals are safe for human ingestion.[25] Animal studies are ultimately just that: *animal* studies. We cannot copy and paste results from these experiments onto real-life scenarios involving humans. Indeed, in science the absence of harm does not necessarily equal the presence of safety, since it is not a system of absolute certainty.[26]

Unfortunately, synthetic substances are used not only in conventional agriculture but also in conventional feedlots, which is why organic animal products have several particular stipulations. For instance, the USDA requires that organic animals are raised on certified organic land, fed organic grasses or grains, never given antibiotics or growth hormones, and have outdoor access.[27] There is, however, room to interpret these regulations, regardless of how happy the hens may look on the packaging.[28] For instance, "out-door access" could be just a small patch of dirt in some large-scale certified organic farms, with limited opportunities for the animals to graze.[29]

## The Organic-Industrial Complex

When we start to talk about large-scale organic operations, some of the benefits of organic farming mentioned above become clouded. As Pollan points out in *The Omnivore's Dilemma: A Natural History of Four Meals*, how environmentally friendly is the mass transportation of organic products across states, and indeed, across countries? What about the environmental impact of large-scale organic farming operations? And what of the occasional application of organic pesticides, sometimes applied in greater quantities than their synthetic equivalents for the same effect?[30]

Since one of the founding ideals of the organic movement is the restoration of the relationship between consumer and producer, thereby restoring trust and mutual obligations in the arena of food production, the rise of an organic industry is perplexing.[31] How can I know that my food is farmed, as far as possible, in an organic manner if I am so removed from the farmers who grow it? How fresh, nutritious, and "sustainable" is such a system, particularly when my vegetables are picked, shipped, and packaged many days, and sometimes even weeks, before I consume them?[32] Thus, in choosing *real* food, we need to think about the spirit of organic agriculture rather than blindly accept the label "organic."

## *Real* Food and the Modern Supermarket

Now that we have a definition of *real* food and some idea of the difference between conventional and organic agriculture, we can take a look at our local supermarket and assess how *real* the food sold there is.

Let's start with organic foods. The word *organic* has taken on an almost religious significance with consumers, yet here is a subtle trap: organic foods can also be refined, preserved, and highly processed. Organic cookies after your organic microwave TV dinner, anyone? The terms *organic* and *healthy* are not interchangeable.[33] We have seen that *real* food is "whole" food: unprocessed fruits and vegetables, meats, dairy products, nuts, seeds, and grains. *Real* food should, by and large, be processed in a kitchen, not a factory.

Foods that are packaged and transported hundreds of miles should come under our scrutiny, since this is another food industry snare. Organically farmed kiwi fruit from New Zealand, when you live in New Zealand, is a great option, yet the same cannot be said if you live in Texas. Why? Well, in order to maintain the shelf life and further improve the sight, smell, taste, and texture of these long-distance products—both organic and conventional—something has to be done to them to prevent them from rotting. These foods have to be processed in some way, even if the "processing" means picking the produce when it is unripe and adding gases to the packaging so that it withstands long-distance shipping.[34]

Shipping foods over long distances drains the ability of these foods to truly nourish us. Broccoli, for instance, loses many of its nutrients two to three days after being picked, and most of its nutrients after a week.[35] Similarly, many citrus fruits are picked before they are ripe and sprayed with ethylene gas, so that you can buy a nice-colored fruit—a fruit that is not necessarily any more ripe and nutritious than its former green self.[36] "Fresh" in a supermarket does not necessarily mean that the fruit or vegetables were picked that day or week or even month.[37] In most cases, "fresh" just means that these foods rot sooner than the highly processed, sugary products found in the middle aisles of the store.[38] Indeed, how "fresh" can your vegetables truly be if they have traveled fifteen hundred miles to get to the supermarket—the average distance that "food-like products" travel in the United States alone?[39]

As much as it may sound logical to preserve our foods from rotting so we don't get ill, we ought to first ask ourselves the simple question: Why do *real*, whole foods spoil in the first place? The answer is we are supposed to eat food that is as fresh as possible, much like manna given to the Israelites in the desert (Exod. 16). As Pollan discusses in *Food Rules*, the nutrients in most foods (with the exception of some foods such as honey) attract not only us, but also other living organisms, including the microbes that cause food to rot and make us ill.[40] To create foods that can last for days, weeks, or even months on the shelf, and can be transported across states and countries, food corporations have to reduce the nutrient content, while adding preservatives and additives to maintain freshness, flavor, and texture.[41]

The snare of "long-life" foods can directly affect our health. Take the average loaf of bread available today. To adapt the production of bread to the food industry's goal of a large market for cheaply and efficiently produced foodstuffs, the wheat germ, which contains the natural oils that give bread its true, wholesome flavor and make it nutritious, has to be removed, since it causes bread to rot within a day. To make up for this loss of flavor and texture, the wheat, after it is heavily processed into white flour, is made into a bread-like product that contains preservatives and additives such as the infamous high fructose corn syrup (HFCS).[42] Or, in the case of many organic packaged breads that last for days, organic sugars and other strange-sounding ingredients are added.

These preservatives and additives have serious side effects.[43] For instance, azodicarbonamide, a synthetic chemical used to manufacture rubber and plastic, is used in the United States as the food additive E927 to bleach flour and condition dough in industrial bread production.[44] This same chemical may cause respiratory problems, such as asthma and allergies, in the workers who come into contact with it, while there are no conclusive studies that show the additive is safe for large-scale human consumption.[45] As a result, the World Health Organization (WHO) recommends that people should avoid this chemical as far as possible, since the risk of ingesting it is largely unknown, and a number of countries (such as the European Union and Singapore) have made its usage illegal.[46]

Efficiency and affordability are often traps in themselves, with costs that are not apparent in the purchasing price of many modern foods. A major part of that hidden price is reduced nutritional content, the loss of wholesome flavor, and the impact these foods have on our physical health, in exchange for convenient meals with an extended shelf life in our pantries. Instead of taking the wheat germ out of the bread for our convenience, we should ask ourselves why God created wheat like that in the first place.

Yet even if we avoid the bread aisle, the architectural layout of the modern supermarket, designed to influence our food choices, poses a threat to our health. Grocery stores, for example, deliberately place candy and chocolate bars by the checkout counter in order to promote "impulse buying." The less time we spend thinking about the health effects of consuming too much sugar, the more likely we will buy the candy.[47] Likewise, healthier products are often put close to the bottom on the shelves, while processed, sugary foods with bright packaging are put at eye level, socially conditioning us to buy more of them.[48]

How *real*, then, is the food in our supermarkets? *Real* food, again, is fresh and nutritious, predominantly local, seasonal, grass fed, as wild as possible, free of synthetic chemicals, whole or minimally processed, and ecologically diverse. We have seen that in our supermarkets, even the fresh produce isn't very fresh. Foods are no longer whole, but processed to extend shelf life. They travel long distances. And synthetic chemicals are used freely. Even this quick snapshot is looking bleak.

## A Better Approach: Let's Get "Agro-Ecological"

But if our nearest supermarket isn't a good source of *real* food, what other options do we have? We'll explore that question in more detail in part 3, but here I will give you just a sketch of the solutions my family has found.

To ensure that the food we eat is as fresh, nutritionally dense, and whole as possible, we buy local, organically produced food as much as we can. Although "buying local" has become a trend over the past several years, both organic and conventional farming practices can, indeed, be local; there is no official definition.[49] We understand it as merely knowing the faces and facts behind our dinner plates—particularly because these foods are more expensive. In order to achieve this goal, we have planted an herb garden in our backyard with a few hanging fruits (it is a work in progress), and we are part of a community-supported agriculture (CSA) system: a co-op where we purchase meat, egg, and produce shares from local, organically operated farms that are delivered on a biweekly basis. If necessary, we supplement our CSA foods with items bought from local farmstead stores and grocers. Most of our meals are home cooked, and occasionally we will treat ourselves to a delicious dinner at a local organic farm-to-table restaurant.

If we are going to pay more for the food we purchase or grow ourselves, we intend to steward our money wisely, since we view our money, and indeed the whole of creation, as a gift from God, one that we will be held accountable for (Matt. 25:14–30). When we purchase local, sustainably, and organically grown produce or garden items from the local farmers' market or grocery store, for example, we not only build a relationship with the individuals who produce and sell our food but we also have firsthand access to the knowledge of how our food was grown, as well as access to fresher and thereby more nutritious produce.[50] In turn, this knowledge increases our appreciation for the wonderful gift of *real* food. It also enables us to support the wonderful people in our community who work hard to grow this food, care for our local environment, and worship our wonderful Creator (Matt. 14:19). It is easy to believe in God when you see his majestic work in nature, including cow manure, earthworms, and zucchini shrubs!

We use an "agro-ecological" measuring stick to define *real* food. This is a fancy way of saying that, out of love for God's creation and our fellow man, we would like to respect and understand the whole environment our food is grown in, the people who grow it, and the people who eat it. Agro-ecological farming methods essentially imitate, adapt to, and work with nature.[51]

I am not, however, against purchasing any foods grown in different regions of the world. We are a family of coffee, tea, dark chocolate, banana, mango, and quinoa lovers—all of which have to be sourced from outside the United States. Yet we continue to apply an agro-ecological measuring stick to these foods as well: we only purchase items that are fairly traded, sustainable, and organically produced. Not only do these foods help developing regions "grow themselves out of poverty" by supporting local economies, ecosystems, and independent farmers but they are also far more delicious than their chemically laden counterparts and more nutritious.[52] I do believe that a local, sustainable food system can incorporate many global aspects, just as the Slow Food movement (which began in Italy as a response to the industrialization of our food system) is dominated by a global appreciation of *real*, slowly prepared, and naturally produced local foods.[53]

Ultimately, our food choices first begin as thoughts, and taking *every* thought captive unto Christ Jesus includes our thoughts about food. It is essential that we strive for perfection in every area of our lives, including the food we buy and eat, just as our heavenly Father is perfect (Matt. 5:48). As a family we therefore practice, to the best of our abilities, what is known as conscious consumerism: *think before we buy.*[54] As the apostle Paul declares, "Whether you eat or drink or whatever you do, do it all for the glory of God" (1 Cor. 10:31 NIV). Over time we have developed the love-based habit of thinking about how our food was produced—a habit I will be talking more about in parts 2 and 3 of this book.

Before we spend more time on solutions, however, we need to look more deeply at the flaws in our modern food industry. We will turn next to the problems caused by the mass production of crops and animals.

# 2

## The Trouble with Mass Production

God created a natural world that is characterized by incredible diversity (Gen. 1). This ecological variety helps to prevent disease through the special functions, or what I like to call the "I-factors," unique to each species within the ecosystem, just as each of us is uniquely made in the image of God with a specific, love-based purpose in his plan. From the thousands of species of bees that pollinate our world to the millions of tiny microorganisms that enrich our soils, the world is wired for love and life.

In contrast to this rich diversity within each ecosystem, imagine an ecosystem in which a single species of a single plant dominates. This is what we have on many massive farms today. Picture wheat or corn—one species—as far as the eye can see in every direction. This is called monoculture, the mass production of single ("mono") crops.

Food monocultures, such as corn, soy, or wheat, and the factory farming of animals both focus on the mass production of a single species and are removing the delicate ecological balance found in diversity.[1] In 1904, for instance, there were over seven thousand varieties of apples grown in the United States. Today, we have lost roughly 86 percent of these varieties.[2] Certainly, God has given us the freedom to choose, but we are not free from the *consequences* of our choices. And the consequences of a monoculture-style food system are the necessary use of artificial substances such as pesticides to merely keep crops alive, the loss of diversity and thereby health, and the destruction of our planet.[3]

Indeed, the majority of us today consume foods that essentially come from plants kept alive on an IV of synthetic substances.[4] These plants survive our manipulation of the natural diversity found in nature, but they do not thrive in such conditions. And, with the alarming loss of 75 percent of our natural agricultural diversity, seed banks (such as the well-known Svalbard Global Seed Vault in Norway) are being established across the globe to urgently save as many varieties of produce and grains as possible.[5]

Is this a healthy situation? What happens if the crop of that one particular species is infected with some kind of fungus, for instance? The mid-nineteenth-century Irish potato famine, although it happened in a different time in history, with its own unique origins and results, can still serve as a warning for us today. All of Ireland was crippled because it had put its faith in one variety of one crop, the Lumper potato. When these potatoes were infected with fungus, an unknown strain of *Phytophthora infestans*, they turned into a revolting mush. Around a million people starved to death, while countless others were compelled to leave their homeland.[6] With our continued reliance on monocultures such as corn, soy, and wheat, there is the very real danger that our global food production is at risk of failing in a similar manner.[7]

## Corn and Soy: Our "Golden" Crops?

Why have corn and soy in particular become the dominant monocultures today? Although the changes in American agriculture over the past several decades are manifold and complex, one of the turning points was the Farm Bill of 1933, which was a response to the need for an adequate food supply during the Great Depression. A great and admirable goal: millions of Americans were starving, and the individuals behind this bill were passionately driven to help them. However, this same bill, which is reintroduced every five years, continues to promote the large-scale government subsidization of corn and soy production in the United States, despite the fact that the times, and the issues we face, have changed dramatically.[8]

However, the overproduction of corn and soy only began around forty-five years ago. Previously, the Farm Bill paid farmers not to overproduce grains that no one could afford to buy. In the 1970s, the US government shifted its farm policy toward the support of large, consolidated, one-crop farming operations rather than traditional, diverse family farms, since large operations could produce far more food at lower prices. It was the time of US Secretary of Agriculture Earl Butz's "get big or get out": no longer would the US government pay farmers not to overproduce corn. Now the motto of the day was "fence row to fence row": produce as much of these single crops as possible by employing as much scientific and technological help as humans could provide.[9]

Joining the US government's "get big" support with its own, the oil industry further consolidated this trend toward large monoculture farms. Big farms, with their big technologies, require a big bit of oil: the global food industry is largely run on fossil fuels, while it supports the petroleum industry through the development of corn ethanol. Now, at the average gas station in the United States, you can find corn-based nourishment for not only yourself, at the small convenience store, but your car as well: the corn sources of both "foods" are often one and the same. It therefore should not surprise us that agribusiness's special interest lobbying power in Washington is second only to the oil industry's, while members of the US government are often supported by Big Agriculture's dollars during election campaigns.[10] This monetary influence is particularly alarming in light of the fact that many economists consider the use of food for fuel as a major contributor to the high price of food today, further exacerbating our global food crisis.[11]

And there certainly is a lot of corn and soy to go around. These two crops account for roughly half of the three hundred million acres of farmland in production in the United States, while just fourteen million acres produce "specialty crops" such as vegetables and fruit (the other major staple produced in the United States is wheat). This large-scale subsidization has, in turn, allowed food companies to manufacture cheap corn-, soy- and wheat-based products in equally large numbers and to provide us with what appears to be an unlimited variety of foodstuffs. Indeed, it is estimated that the modern American food industry produces an average of six thousand calories per person per day, while more than seventeen thousand new industrial food products are introduced each year.[12] Of these products, a startling 77 percent come from corn, soy, and wheat.[13]

## Great Yields at Great Cost: Mass Animal Production

Without these farm subsidies, the shelves of our grocery stores would not be filled with meat and dairy products, and a burger would not cost a dollar.[14] What do corn and soy have to do with meat and dairy? Today, animal feed is made up largely of corn and soy.

The modern food industry has taken animals off the farm and placed them in industrial facilities called CAFOs, Concentrated Animal Feeding Operations. These facilities are often located in different states and are specifically geared toward feeding, slaughtering, or packaging meat on an industrial scale.[15] Indeed, you need look no further than the average supermarket: rows and rows of neatly packaged pieces of meat overwhelm the customer with choices. It is estimated that these industrial feedlots have doubled meat production in the United States alone over the last fifty years.[16]

Within these operations, it is both cheaper and less time-consuming to feed the animals corn and soy in confined spaces, even though these grain-based, immobile diets are not well adapted to the way God created these animals. For example, cattle have rumens, which are designed to digest various grasses and plants, not massive amounts of grain, and as a result these cattle are more prone to disease and general ill health, such as stomach ulcers, while they are less nutritious to consume. God designed cattle as animals that graze over stretches of grass, but these industrial operations work on economies of time and scale: confined cattle eat all day, getting fatter in a much shorter space of time, while a single operation can hold far more cattle in a smaller space.[17]

In the feces-covered facilities of many industrial operations, these grain-based diets necessitate the large-scale use of antibiotics (80 percent of all antibiotics in the United States alone) to simply prevent the animals from dying. This has significantly contributed to the global antibiotic-resistance crisis. Many animals are also given growth hormones to further speed up the fattening process.[18] These hormones are associated with a number of health risks in both animals and humans, including a possible correlation with cancer, which is why many countries no longer permit the use of hormones in industrial meat production.[19]

Yet the animals are not just fed corn and soy. Expired cookies, candy, and even other animals are often turned into feed, including feed for large-scale dairy operations. We have turned herbivores like cattle into carnivores, often with fatal side effects. Perhaps the most infamous example of this is the recent epidemic of mad cow disease, a variant of bovine spongiform encephalopathy that leads to Creutzfeldt-Jakob disease (vCJD) in humans.[20] In the United Kingdom, cows that were fed the remains of other cows in meat and bone meal contracted this disease, killing over a hundred people in 1996. Although this major incident shows the dangers of feeding animals to other animals, it is often still considered an economically viable practice for industrial operations. Many feedlots in the United States, for instance, feed their cows chicken meat, while some companies even consider it "sustainable" to feed chicken to farmed fish.[21]

Unfortunately, these cruelties have not subsided over time. If you live in America, your tax dollars are currently being used to fund research on the immunocastration of male pigs (boars) to improve the flavor of the animals and make them easier to handle inside the CAFOs.[22] In fact, pigs' tails are already cut off inside these confined facilities, since when the animals are stressed they tend to chew them off.[23] Similarly, chickens have part of their beaks sawed off, since they too are destructive when stressed.[24] Are we being good stewards of God's magnificent creation?

## Animals, Workers, and the Environment: All Are Affected

These industrial meat operations are sources of cruelty not only to the animals they intend to slaughter but often to their employees as well. In *Fast Food Nation*, Schlosser highlights the disturbing abuse of workers, in particular migrant and nonlegal peoples, within the American meat and fast-food industries.[25] The poignant 2014 documentary *Food Chains* further highlights the injustice faced by many of the people who produce the food we consume today.[26] Indeed, human trafficking is a dominant issue in agriculture, both within the United States and globally. Slaves are used to pick fruit and vegetables on a number of commercial farms, in meat-packing factories, and in food-service establishments, while the trafficking of women for sexual purposes often accompanies the development of large commodity farms with many laborers.[27] In some cases it is impossible for these industrial operations to even find people willing to work, compelling these companies to use prisoners to slaughter the animals. In light of these circumstances, where injury and death are ever-present, is it any wonder that many employees in slaughterhouses develop pathological disorders?[28]

In fact, within the often-merciless logic of the industry, the abuse of not only labor but also the environment is often hidden behind the abundance of "cheap" food. In CAFOs, for instance, lakes of sewage can often be found nearby the facilities, releasing toxic gases into the air (such as ammonia and methane) that contribute to our current global climate crisis, while polluting the surrounding land and waterways. One CAFO can in fact produce as much waste as a large city. Likewise, the transportation of animals from the farms where they spend the first few months of their lives, to the feedlots where they are fattened, to the slaughterhouses where they are killed, to the packaging facilities where they are transformed into neat commodities, to the various food establishments that sell these products further contributes to global warming. Overall, the global meat industry contributes more to global warming than cars, trains, and planes—an alarming 18 percent of all emissions.[29]

This environmental pollution is just another example of the danger and narrow logic of monoculture production today. On smaller and more diverse farms, the waste from animals was often used to fertilize the crops: nature worked in tandem. By contrast, in industrial agriculture today we have created two major issues where once we had one solution. As Pollan notes, we took the animals off the farm to plant more crops and created a fertility problem that requires the large-scale use of artificial fertilizer, while we placed the animals in industrial operations and created a waste problem that is contributing to the destruction of God's beautiful planet.[30]

### What Is the *Real* Price Tag?

Yes, more people certainly can afford to purchase meat today than ever before in our recorded history. However, the monetary cost of cheap meat, like that of mass-produced bread and other foodstuffs, does not reflect the true price paid to bring it to our plates: the effect it has on the lives of the people who work in these facilities, the damage it does to local environments, the 38.4 billion dollars a year of taxpayer money given to the meat industry in subsidies, and the strain it puts on our own health as we overconsume meat that is less nutritious and potentially contaminated with deadly microbes from the process of mass production. One could include in that price the fact that all the land used to produce animal feed (around two-thirds of arable farmland), could otherwise be used to feed the millions of starving people in the world today, including the estimated forty-nine million Americans who suffer from food insecurity and hunger.[31]

Finally, we can't appreciate the real price of cheap food until we consider its effects on our health. We'll take a brief look at that next and explore it more fully in part 2.

# 3

## The MAD Diseases

The MAD is aptly named, since it is high in refined sugar, salt, and saturated fat, which are added to make the processed foodstuffs edible and attractive.[1] A diet high in added sugars correlates with a greater risk of obesity, dementia, stroke, cancer, tooth decay, insulin resistance related to diabetes and metabolic syndrome, heart disease, an overload of both unhealthy triglycerides and oxidized LDL cholesterol—the list can go on and on. (For more on sugar, see chapter 17.) Excessive consumption of the high amounts of sodium in processed, salty foods can lead to high blood pressure and heart disease, stroke, kidney damage, cancer, weight gain, osteoporosis, and overeating—this list is equally long and alarming.[2]

Processed, heated, and refined fats, as well as "trans fats" (hydrogenated fats), are the bad fats commonly found in foods such as margarine, shortening, your average American pizza, and the processed cheese so widely available in grocery stores. These bad fats have been linked to a higher risk of heart disease, macular degeneration, multiple sclerosis, certain cancers, diabetes, obesity, osteoporosis, infertility and endometriosis, and depression.[3] (For more on fats, see chapter 16.)

## A Slice of Pizza a Day Keeps the Doctor Away?

With one-third of American vegetable consumption consisting of French fries, iceberg lettuce, and potato chips, and the US Congress having classified pizza as a vegetable, these diet-related diseases are a daily reality for millions of people.[4] Indeed, the average American consumes around 130 pounds (60 kilograms) of sugar per year, including 53 gallons (201 liters) of soft drinks.[5] Fifty million Americans eat at fast-food restaurants daily.[6] A mere 10 percent of grocery purchases are fresh vegetables and fruit.[7]

In fact, recently the American School Nutrition Association (ASNA), which is heavily funded by food corporations and claims that its purpose is "to better serve the nation's children," published a rather disturbing position paper. In order to "prevent waste," fresh fruits, vegetables, whole grains, and low-sodium options are no longer required with every school meal, while junk food is a part of the reimbursable food system in place in these schools and can even be sold as an alternative to school meals.[8] As a mother of four children, I am beyond shocked that the health of our future generations is compromised by corporate money in an institution where they should be protected.

## The Other O Word: Today's Obesity Pandemic

The MAD is not just an American problem. It is one of the United States' most successful, and ubiquitous, exports. More and more of us are eating this way, which is leading to what the United Nations calls a "global public health disaster."[9] In truth, food corporations that manufacture vast amounts of raw materials and processed foodstuffs (that can be transported over thousands of miles without rotting, of course) have come to dominate global food production, while the emerging world is one of their fastest growing markets. Traditional food systems are increasingly being replaced with the preserved, processed, and packaged Western foods that already flood our eating establishments.[10] Now, for example, you can readily find soda, chips, cakes, cookies, breakfast cereals, and candy in small convenience stores in African villages, Guatemalan towns, and Asian cities.[11] Is it any wonder, then, that soft drinks are more readily available than clean water in many public schools in California and many villages in Africa?[12]

In the past thirty-five years, the world's obesity rate has doubled.[13] According to the 2013 Global Burden of Disease Study, around 2.1 billion individuals worldwide were overweight or obese, while obesity-related illnesses were responsible for 3.4 million deaths, with a 3.9 percent reduction of average life expectancy. In fact, emerging nations have a 30 percent higher rate of obesity than developed countries, and are particularly at risk of diet-related illness since malnutrition and starvation early in life contribute to an increased risk of obesity and diet-related chronic diseases later on.[14]

Many obesity researchers predict that these statistics will only take a turn for the worse. By 2030, it is estimated that over two billion people will be overweight, while half this number will be dangerously obese.[15] In the United States alone, diet- and exercise-related chronic diseases, which are largely preventable through lifestyle choices, are one of the principal causes of premature death, while 50 percent of the population will be overweight by 2030.[16] More people die now from obesity-related illnesses than cigarettes. If this trend in rising obesity does not improve, future generations may live shorter lives, and lives more prone to disability, than their predecessors. Indeed, nation members of the World Health Organization (WHO) have called for a 2025 goal to end the rising epidemic of weight gain—this is unquestionably a global issue with profound consequences on global health.[17]

## The Butterfly Effect

Clearly, in the globalized world we live in today, what we buy for dinner has international repercussions—there is a definite "butterfly effect" associated with our food choices.[18] Perhaps one of the most well-known, and indeed controversial, examples of the global impact of food production is the 1994 North American Free Trade Agreement (NAFTA). NAFTA opened the trade borders between the United States and Mexico, making American corn, subsidized by the US government, cheaper to purchase. Subsequently, many Mexican farmers lost their farms (since they could not compete with the low price of corn grown in the United States), compelling these individuals to find work elsewhere and contributing to the rise of illegal immigrants in the United States.[19]

Likewise, labels such as "Fair Trade" or "Whole Trade" on many foods today highlight the fact that what we choose to eat can and does impact the people and communities that produce our foods. Within the globalized context of our food industry, we cannot immediately justify our food purchases by claiming that we do not hurt anyone else when we buy them.[20] It just takes one person to make a difference: read the book of Esther and consider Esther's impact in the Persian court of King Ahasuerus.

## Food Aid That Does Not Aid

Unfortunately, the highly processed, nutritionally wanting foods of the MAD also make their way into emerging countries through American food aid policies. Regardless of the good intentions behind these policies, the United States' emphasis on sending its surplus food to developing nations around the globe has stifled local economic development and food production and led to many of the same diet-related diseases that Americans face.[21] At one recent international Slow Food convivium in Italy, the African delegates put this threat to local food production and health starkly: "We have plenty of resources. We have plenty of knowledge. We have plenty of workers. If you Westerners . . . would just stay out and quit displacing our indigenous economy and food systems with poor-quality commodities, we can feed ourselves, thank you."[22]

# 4

## The Mad Truth about the MAD

If the MAD is so dangerous for our health and the health of our planet, why do we continue to eat this way? Part of the strong allure of our industrial food system is its *convenience*, a factor that has greatly contributed to its global success.[1] In the twentieth century, as more and more women went to work outside the home, foods that required the least amount of time to prepare found a ready and willing market.[2] Many of us today lead incredibly busy lives, and food preparation is often the first part of our schedules that is sacrificed in light of other demands on our time. Buying your food at a farmers' market and coming home to prepare a meal does take significantly longer than heating up a prepackaged box meal in the microwave.

This mealtime expediency has allowed many of us to advance other aspects of our lives. As sustainable food activist Oran B. Hesterman of the Fair Food Network explains, by placing food production in the hands of roughly 2 percent of the population, the other 98 percent have had the freedom to specialize, which has contributed to the development of fields such as technology, medicine, and education.[3]

Nevertheless, the convenience generated by the industrialization of our food system comes at a great cost: our physical and mental health as well as the health of our planet. In 1937, George Orwell said, "We may find in the long run that tinned food is a deadlier weapon than the machine-gun."[4] Unfortunately, as chronic, diet-related illnesses such as type 2 diabetes and cardiovascular disease have become two of the leading causes of death in our world today, Orwell's words seem prophetic.

## Cheap Food: A Modern Mirage

The price tag on real, whole foods such as pasture-raised chickens and organically grown fruit and vegetables is in many cases higher than the artificial foods that characterize the Western Diet. However, the truth is that none of us can afford the true price of following the MAD: its low cost is a dangerous illusion.[5] When I walk down the aisle in my neighborhood grocery store, I do not see cheap breakfast cereals, meats, dairy products, chips, and snacks of all shapes and sizes. I see the annual health care costs, now estimated to be over $100 billion, of obesity-related illness, which is predicted to rise to over $283 billion by 2020. I see the annual $245 million cost of diabetes in America, which is steadily increasing. I see the billions of dollars of food and water waste across the globe. I see the environmental costs of industrial food production, which costs taxpayers billions of dollars each year.[6] I see the cost to many farmers who can no longer compete in such an industrial system of food production, compelling them to sell their farms to meet their debts, while some farmers have even decided to end their lives.[7] I see the cost imposed on future generations, who will inherit a broken food system and an unhealthy planet. I see the cost to our integrity as human beings, indeed as Christians, as we support a food system that allows millions of people to die of obesity, malnutrition, or starvation while we misuse God's earth. There is no such thing as cheap food.[8]

## Fighting for a Better Meal

I do understand and fully appreciate that millions of people cannot afford real, whole foods, which is one of the principal tragedies of our dysfunctional food system—a system that has "forgotten to feed people well."[9] There certainly are a number of amazing individuals out there, fighting for the right of all people to have access to real, whole foods. In New York, a teacher in the Bronx named Stephen Ritz began growing healthy foods in his classroom, teaching low-income children from broken neighborhoods the skills to create "new green graffiti."[10] Ron Finley, who calls himself the "guerrilla gardener," started growing organic foods for his South Central Los Angeles neighborhood, which is a federally recognized "food desert"—there is no fresh produce available in the immediate vicinity.[11] My eldest daughter volunteers in a food desert in the Dallas–Fort Worth metroplex, where a dilapidated football field has been transformed into an organic farm (after supermarket vendors refused to establish a grocery store in the area, since they would not be able to earn enough money) under the management of Elizabeth Hernandez.[12] Indeed, the farm supplies vegetables to local farmers' markets and restaurants, including one of our favorite places to eat in Dallas: Café Momentum. The restaurant's executive chef, Chad Houser, takes former juvenile offenders and trains them to become chefs, truly embodying the spirit of their motto: "Eat. Drink. Change Lives."[13] On alternate Saturdays, my daughter also volunteers at a farm that supplies both Café Momentum and our own CSA, Happy Trails Farm, which is run by Fina Longoria-Johnson, her husband Larry, and her daughter-in-law Jessica Longoria.[14] Stephen Ritz, Ron Finley,

Elizabeth Hernandez, Chad Houser, Fina Longoria-Johnson, Larry Johnson, and Jessica Longoria: these are the true, everyday heroes of the sustainable food movement. And you can be one too.

In the end, unless we *all* collectively participate in re-creating the way we grow and eat our food, we will have a system that continues to choose disease and death over life (Deut. 30:19). We all have to fight, in whatever way we can, for a better meal, since we all deserve to eat *real* food that nourishes us. The United Nations' Universal Declaration of Human Rights (UDHR) states that "everyone ought to have the ability to choose a healthy, wholesome way of eating insofar as they have a right to a healthy, wholesome life."[15] If God feeds the "birds of the air," how much more does he care for our nourishment as his children (Matt. 6:26)? This right should not be denied by large corporations eager to maintain the goodwill of their shareholders, nor should it be denied by government officials eager to maintain the goodwill and financial support of large corporations.[16] Our food crisis is principally a matter of the dignity of each human being on this planet—of every member of God's creation.

Many of us *can* afford to purchase more real, whole foods from local producers who are truly attempting to create a sustainable food system. In the United States in particular, people spend less money on food than the rest of the developed world (around 13.2 percent of their income), while it is estimated that 90 percent of the average American food budget is spent on highly refined and processed foodstuffs. In 2011 Americans spent $117 billion on fast food, $65 billion on soft drinks, $17 billion on video games, $5 billion on ringtones, and $310 million on pet Halloween costumes, just to name a few categories.[17] These statistics are shocking eye-openers, calling for us all to take personal responsibility.

And according to the Centers for Disease Control, income status is *not* a determinant of fast-food purchases in the United States: people do not just buy fast food because that is all they can afford.[18] If we value our health and the health of our beautiful planet and all its inhabitants, why are we not willing to pay a little more for nutritionally dense, wholesome foods by budgeting elsewhere?[19] Is our wellbeing, and the wellbeing of future generations, not worth giving up that large soda and cheeseburger, or dressing up our dog as a fairy on October 31?

## Vote with Your Forks and Votes

It is essential that we not only "vote with our votes" to demand official changes in food policy and support government officials who are trying to change our current food system but also "vote with our forks."[20] Every time we buy food, we support the system that produced it, contributing to its perpetuation. As sustainable food activist Ellen Gustafson highlights in *We the Eaters: If We Change Dinner, We Can Change the World*, as consumers we have the ability to demand better food production, both for ourselves and for the rest of the planet, through refusing to buy products that are destructive to our health and the health of the communities that produce them. When we buy fair trade chocolate, we tell chocolate companies that it is not acceptable to use cocoa beans harvested by child slavery, and that we cannot wait until 2020 to end this travesty. When we buy at farmers' markets that sell local and organically produced foods, we tell food corporations and our government that creating healthy, ecologically friendly communities is more important than convenient, cheap, and unhealthy food; that we, and every other person in the world, should have access to fresh, whole foods, and that we do not support the vast amounts of waste that result from our current food system.[21]

Businesses cannot thrive if we do not purchase their products: as consumers, we can communicate our wishes through our pocketbooks. In fact, this consumer demand for more natural foods is the main reason why Wal-Mart has more and more organic options in their stores, and Whole Foods is continually increasing their number of locally produced items. Our consumer dollars are the main reason that many countries have banned the use of growth hormones in industrial meat production or the use of "pink slime" (meat processed and treated with ammonia). We, collectively, one person at a time, have the power to change the world by changing what we eat, and gradually make healthier foods more accessible for more people.[22] I would go even further: as Christians, it is a way for us to communicate that our God is love, a way for us to be a shining light in this world, by demanding products that respect his beloved creation (Matt. 5:16).

# 5

## Marketing to Children and Other Scandals

Convenience is not the only reason why the MAD dominates our eating habits. We are also manipulated by research and bombarded with marketing messages that encourage this unhealthy way of eating.

Indeed, large corporations spend millions of dollars on research annually, calculating the precise amount of fat, sugar, and salt that will satisfy our taste buds and keep us coming back for more, regardless of the health consequences. For example, one of the leading centers of food research in the United States, Monell Chemical Senses Center, has performed experiments on young children, feeding them various sugary foods to calculate their "bliss point," the level at which their desire for sugar is at its climax. This data is subsequently used to formulate products that can be marketed throughout the globe.[1]

## Is the Health of Our Children for Sale?

Shockingly, children in particular are targeted by the food industry, as the example above indicates. Many youngsters have what corporations call "pester power" over their parents, or the ability to keep demanding certain products until the parents or guardians give in. Since children and adolescents have more and more purchasing power in today's economy, "pestering" is an important source of income for food corporations, which is why they are willing to spend an estimated $1.8 billion annually on marketing to these age groups. Targeting children when they are young is in fact a significant way to establish lasting brand loyalty.[2]

The Rudd Center for Food Policy & Obesity rightly calls this concentrated marketing to children a "crisis in the marketplace."[3] Although the US Children's Food and Beverage Advertising Initiative (CFBAI) was established in 2006 to restrict the advertising of processed foods high in sugar, salt, and fats to children under the age of eleven, these self-regulating efforts have largely proved inadequate. An estimated 86 percent of the food products marketed by CFBAI members to children are still alarmingly high in processed and refined sugars, salt, and fat, while marketing to youth over the age of eleven has increased. Similarly, food corporations have continued to advertise their processed food products through other channels, such as social media, which has led to a 23 percent increase in exposure to children.[4] With the obesity rates among children increasing exponentially, alongside diet-related illnesses such as type 2 diabetes and heart disease, the promotion of these unhealthy food products for the sake of corporate profit is deplorable.[5]

## Gimme, Gimme, Gimme: The Industry Message of "Eat More"

Our current industrial food system has created an environment that essentially floods our senses, adults and children alike, with the message of "eat more" unhealthy, processed foods. Indeed, an estimated 70 percent of all food-related advertising is for highly processed foods and drinks high in sugar, salt, and fat.[6] Children are even exposed to this message at school, where vending machines, snack shops, and lunch bars are often filled with foods high in sugar, salt, and fat.

In a recent visit to a children's hospital in Texas, I found a popular fast-food restaurant on the ground floor, alongside multiple vending machines with sodas, chips, and candy. I watched in horror as "food-like substances," including soda, packaged cookies, and packaged desserts, were served to sick children. I was stunned at the number of obese children and adults walking the floors and sitting in the waiting rooms consuming junk food from the vending machines. And when the doctors and nurses were eating the same things, I had to sit down in shock. In many cases, food corporations make the sale of their products in schools, hospitals, and other institutions attractive by offering financial benefits in exchange for the chance to sell their foodstuffs.[7] It is a tragic state of affairs when dollars can override health—particularly in an institution dedicated to health!

### Do You Want Vitamin C with That?

Some may argue that many of these industrially produced foods are in fact "healthy." Cereals, snacks, and breads are "fortified" with vitamins and minerals, and meat and dairy products have reduced fat content, for instance. Indeed, we are bombarded with phrases like "high in Vitamin C," "full of great antioxidants," "low fat," and a "great source of omega fatty acids," but these are largely marketing devices supported by unhealthy scientific reductionism.[8]

For example, milk in its whole, natural form is full of essential proteins and other nutrients such as vitamins A and E, which are fat-soluble. When we remove the fat from the milk, we lose these fat-soluble nutrients, while the pasteurization process destroys many of the beneficial proteins. The milk, now less nutritious and less flavorful, needs added vitamins and flavor-enhancing ingredients like sugar and even chocolate. Moreover, the sugars in the milk are quickly absorbed into the bloodstream, causing our insulin levels to rise, since there is no longer fat in the milk to slow down the digestion process, while the milk is less filling, possibly leading us to drink more than we ought to.[9] A small glass of *real*, whole, organically produced milk within the context of a balanced lifestyle is therefore a far superior option than a conventional glass of "low fat" milk with "added vitamins," since *real* milk is designed the way God intended it to be consumed—in its *whole* form.[10]

## Reduce Your Fat Intake or Your Sauces?
## The Rise of the Nutritionist Paradox

Nutrition is an incredibly problematic subject. We do not eat carbohydrates, fats, and proteins in a vacuum, for instance. We eat in the complex framework of daily life. How much, when, and why we eat these foods are equally important considerations to take into account. How do they interact with other foods that contain carbohydrates, fats, and proteins? How were these foods grown and prepared? How fresh were the foods? Were we stressed or relaxed when we ate the food? These important considerations will lead to whether we eat *real* foods that will nourish us or food-like products that can make us ill.[11]

As Pollan notes, subscribing to reductionist science, whereby we focus on individual nutrients at the cost of the bigger diet picture, is like losing our keys in a parking lot at night and only searching for them under the streetlight. We know they could be anywhere in that parking lot, but we only look where we are able to see easily. In fact, nutrition science is certainly not at the point where we understand every element of every food, nor what happens to each element when they are separated or isolated.[12] Our vision is incredibly limited, despite all our advances in the science of food. For example, coffee beans have over a thousand phytonutrients (that fight diseases), only a small percentage of which have been identified. The complex yet beneficial interaction between just these hundred phytonutrients we can identify, let alone the other nine hundred or so, is also little understood.[13] Fresh thyme, one of my favorite herbs, has a complex array of antioxidants—from alanine to vanillic acid, the list is as long as it is remarkable.[14] And these are only the antioxidants we have discovered so far, all in a small green sprig! What a wonderful, insightful, and proactive God we serve, indeed.

Yet increasingly, man-made foods have displaced the knowledge of natural cuisine that traditionally originated in our homes and larger cultural heritage, necessitating the advice of nutritionists as we learn to navigate the modern food system. This flood of complex, conflicting, ambiguous, and constantly changing (over time *and* between different nutritional experts, who cannot seem to agree) nutritional information is now available to us on a daily, even hourly, basis.[15] Many of us cannot decide what oil or fat we should cook with, let alone what in the world we should cook. In fact, we cannot even take the word of nutritional professionals at face value. A number of dietitians, for instance, are "sponsored" by Coca-Cola to recommend the soda as part of a balanced diet.[16] How unbiased is their health advice going to be? Since when did something as fundamental as eating become so utterly confusing?

During my travels, countless individuals continue to ask me what they should eat for a healthy mind and body, as if I can, hopefully, solve their "omnivore's dilemma."[17] To use Pollan's popular saying, you should "eat *food*, not too much, mostly plants"—just as your mother and grandmother would have told you in the past.[18] Unfortunately, *real* foods are increasingly hard to come by for many of us and impossible for millions on the lowest rungs of the economic scale, while these "techno foods" befuddle us with their many health claims and odd-sounding ingredients.[19]

## Supplement without Supplements

It is precisely this reductionism that also makes supplements potentially unsafe or ineffective. As professor of nutrition and sustainable food activist Marion Nestle explains in *Food Politics: How the Food Industry Influences Nutrition and Health*, the Dietary Supplement Health and Education Act of 1994 (DSHEA) deregulated the supplement industry and now permits supplement producers to claim health benefits for their products without the oversight of official standards or independent studies. Even when negative health effects of certain supplements are published, the companies that produce these "natural" alternatives do not need to withdraw their products, since the FDA does not regulate the production of these supplements. Unless you habitually read medical journals as a hobby, how will you know what can harm you?[20]

Indeed, who even knows what goes into those capsules, liquids, and powders? The recent herbal remedy scandal involving Wal-Mart, Walgreens, Target, and GNC in the United States should serve as an urgent reminder. According to official court documents, only 4 to 41 percent of the supplements examined actually contained what was written on the labels.[21] Despite the fact that government drug regulations are not perfect (which I will discuss in greater detail in my upcoming book on mental health and wellbeing), allowing the supplement industry to police itself poses an equal threat to public health, particularly when large amounts of profit are involved.[22] The supplement industry, which is often just another arm of the pharmaceutical industry, is worth an estimated 55 billion dollars.[23] Of these billions of dollars, it is difficult to tell what percentage is actually spent on supplements that benefit the consumer.

Medicine is ultimately medicine, whether it is man-made or found in nature, and there are many things in nature that can harm us, such as poisonous plants and fungi. A growing body of research continues to show how even "safe" vitamins can cause damage in excess or out of the context of the foods that naturally contain them.[24] Vitamin C, for example, is an essential cancer-fighting nutrient found in many fresh fruits and vegetables. Studies have shown, however, that vitamin C in its supplement form does *not* reduce the risk of developing cancer, while recent research has indicated that it can in fact increase the risk of developing cancer.[25] Demographic groups who use supplements are generally more educated, have higher incomes, eat better, and exercise more, and thus we cannot say that supplements work and are safe because people who take them are healthier—science is quite a bit more complicated than that.[26] Indeed, official public health organizations will not recommend general supplementation because of the dangers associated with overdosing. Unless supplements are part of a prescribed medical regimen, many of us would be far better off using our income on *real*, whole foods.[27]

### Exercise: The Magic Moving Bullet?

If supplements aren't the solution, what about exercise? According to the WHO, one in three people partake in little or no exercise across the globe, resulting in an estimated 3.2 million deaths annually, which makes physical inactivity one of the leading causes of mortality today.[28] Exercise, however, can never replace an unhealthy diet; it is not a magic bullet that will allow you to eat whatever you feel like without any consequences. Both physical activity and a way of eating that is predominantly characterized by *real*, whole foods are essential for a healthy spirit, mind, and body. The food industry's myopic focus on exercise is in fact a subtle way for corporations to shift attention away from their processed food products, since encouraging people to eat less of their processed food products directly impacts a corporation's revenue—bottom-dollar logic once again.[29]

During the latest Bush administration, for instance, food industry leaders and government officials began a campaign (with Shrek as a figurehead) for healthier lifestyles that focused on physical activity rather than the products these companies sold. It is a sad fact that, around the time of this campaign, Shrek also started appearing on processed food packages such as Oreo cookies, which further contributed to the food industry's confusion of exercise and diet.[30]

With their billions of dollars devoted to research and marketing that harness and shape our food preferences, large food corporations effectively swindle our taste buds. But they do more than that. Through their economic clout and their government connections, they hijack the whole agriculture industry, including farmers. Let's look next at the effect their economic and political clout has on the food that reaches the public.

# 6

# Who Rules the Economic Roost?

By controlling the supply chains, large food corporations rule the economic roost, so they set the economic rules. As the dominant buyers, they put pressure on farmers and other producers in the vertically integrated supply chain, compelling them to produce greater quantities of cheap food—food the corporations want grown. By specializing and controlling the entire process, including the necessary raw materials (such as seeds or young animals), these corporations minimize both risk and expense while establishing uniformity among their products. The individual farmers have to provide the land, facilities, time, and labor needed to produce foodstuffs, while the raw materials remain the same.[1] In fact, the average farmer today earns only 14 cents on every dollar spent on food in the United States, compared to 36 cents in 1974.[2]

With so many calories on the market, the critical issue these companies face is the fact that as humans we can only eat so much in one day—the stomach has a fixed ceiling. How do the companies solve this essentially biological problem? Make portion sizes larger, offer irresistibly cheap deals, tempt you with candy "impulse buys" at the checkout counter, and create foods that leave the consumer with enough room, and the desire, for more—the list of techniques is long, frightening, and subtle.[3]

At the same time, access to healthier foods such as fresh fruit and vegetables is limited by price manipulations generated by government subsidization of foods like corn, soy, and wheat. For the millions of Americans on food stamps, for example, the few dollars a day they have to spend makes it almost impossible for them to choose to eat healthfully. Since the government supports the production of unhealthy processed foods, they are cheaper and more readily available. The US government's artificial support of processed foods makes it impossible for people of low or no income to afford a balanced diet, because a bag of apples is more expensive than sugary breakfast cereal.[4]

### Only Desserts in Food Deserts?

Assuming, that is, that these individuals even *have access* to a bag of apples. Millions of Americans, and particularly people in inner-city neighborhoods, live in "food deserts," areas where local stores within a five-mile radius do not even carry fresh fruit and vegetables.[5] In fact, one recent study has shown that grocery stores are four times more likely to be built in predominantly Caucasian neighborhoods than African-American communities, while African Americans are 30 percent more likely to die from diet-related heart disease.[6] How empowering is the modern supermarket, convenience store, or restaurant to these individuals when the choices are limited to unhealthy, refined, sugary foods that can lead to obesity, chronic illness, and an early death? How empowering, indeed, is the modern food establishment for any of us, when the government's policies intentionally make healthy, *real* foods more expensive by subsidizing the MAD? What, ultimately, is the point of having a food system that does not do what food should do: nourish us?[7]

## The Door That Keeps Revolving

Unfortunately, government officials are as likely to have a relationship with the food industry as they are to police it. Not only do these corporations put pressure on the US government through their lobbying power, but there is also a revolving door between government and industry. Many government officials leave their bureaucratic positions to work for major food corporations, while an equal number have left the corporate world to enter the realm of government.[8]

Former Secretary of Agriculture Ann Veneman, for instance, hired a lobbyist for the meat industry as her chief of staff. On the other hand, Veneman's predecessor left his position as Secretary of Agriculture to work for the food industry (which often has far better pay). These individuals certainly have the knowledge and experience often required to work as a regulator or a corporate employee. Nevertheless, there is always the risk of conflict of interest: How can we be sure they will act in the interest of public health rather than their former colleagues, if there is a conflict between the two?[9]

Even if there is no such relationship in place, the food industry can still influence the US government in favor of its own interests.[10] A disturbing example of this sway is the recent sugar controversy between the US government and the WHO. In 2003 the WHO, concerned about the rising obesity epidemic, recommended that the average individual should limit his or her added sugar consumption to less than 10 percent of daily calories. This percentage was based on a conclusive body of scientific evidence on the dangers of excess sugars in the human diet. Nonetheless, the sugar industry, unhappy with the limit capped on its product sales in the name of health, put pressure on the US government, which subsequently threatened to withdraw funding from the WHO if they did not change their dietary guidelines. A year later, the 10 percent added sugar recommendation disappeared from the WHO's global report on diet.[11]

An article in *BMJ* highlights how the food industry's manipulation of nutritional science continues to pose a threat to our health. Overall, industry-funded research generally favors the products of food corporations.[12] For example, according to a 2013 study published on *PLoS Medicine* (a peer-reviewed online medical journal), papers whose research was supported by Big Agriculture's dollars were five times more likely to say that there was no "positive association" between sugar consumption and weight gain.[13] With companies such as Nestle, Coca-Cola, and Pepsico funding organizations such as the Scientific Advisory Committee on Nutrition (SACN) and Medical Research Council's Human Nutrition Research unit (HNR), how do we ensure that conflicts of interest do not occur? From 2001 to 2012, only thirteen out of the forty scientists at the SACN claimed they had "no interests to declare."[14] What of the other twenty-seven scientists? Whose interests possibly biased their interpretations of their work? The sugar industry? The meat industry? The dairy industry? The list of potential biases can go on and on.

### David versus the Food Goliath

Smaller, more biologically diverse family farms cannot compete with the power of these large food corporations. In terms of bushels per acre, or animals per acre, small family farms do not meet the surface productivity of large farms—large farms supported by the capital of big industry and big government subsidies. At the same time, these smaller farmers lack the financial resources to compete with Big Agriculture for governmental influence, through the large-scale funding of election campaigns, for example.[15] Is it any wonder that the small family farm is slowly disappearing from agriculture, while a mere 8 percent of farms produce 63 percent of our food?[16]

By taking cheaply grown or raised commodities and producing processed foods sold at premium prices, these large corporations are able to expand their profits. Through what farmer and food activist Wendell Berry describes as the logic of short-term economies of scale, these companies aim to keep profits high and expenses low by producing as many goods as possible for the cheapest price possible. "Externalized costs," or the effects of such short-term practices, are left for us as a society to take care of.[17] A percentage of our taxes, for instance, are used for farming subsidies, the treatment of diet-related diseases, and environmental issues such as the dead zone in the Gulf of Mexico (which is related to chemical runoff from conventional agriculture).[18]

Indeed, since many of these externalized costs are long term in nature, such as global warming, chronic illnesses, and water pollution, we are shackling our descendants with the true cost of creating the modern food industry.[19] When I look at our broken food system, one alarming Scripture comes to mind: "The Lord is longsuffering and abundant in mercy, forgiving iniquity and transgression; but He by no means clears the guilty, visiting the iniquity of the fathers on the children to the third and fourth generation" (Num. 14:18). What kind of future are we leaving for our children? How, I ask each one of us, is participating in this dysfunctional food system part of God's commandment to love our neighbors as we love ourselves, including our "neighbors" of the future (Mark 12:31)? Or to love God, through and for whom *all* things (including the world and all the wonderful living organisms in it) were made, with all our hearts, souls, and minds (Mark 12:30; John 1:3–4; Col. 1:16)? Is this bringing heaven—or hell—to earth (Matt. 6:10)? What curses are we leaving on future generations?

## Our Current Food System Is "Wasted"

It is a tragic fact that this short-term logic of exploitation for gain has created an international food system that is characterized not only by vast amounts of convenient, cheap foods but also by what has come to be known as the global waste scandal. Today, we could feed the world's starving with a percentage of the food that is thrown away throughout the world. From bananas left to rot in piles on a farm in Ecuador, where large numbers of people are starving, because they do not meet the supermarket regulations of what a banana should look like, to the thousands of pounds of perfectly edible animal parts that do not please our sensibilities, regardless of the fact that our ancestors ate them, the industrial food system generates more food waste than ever before in human history. In fact, as author and activist Tristram Stuart indicates, in the space of twenty-four hours a supermarket can throw away enough food to feed more than a hundred people.[20] These statistics are truly shocking.

Yet we are all to blame. Industry and households combined waste an estimated 1.3 billion tons of food each year, an alarming figure that excludes the tons of water we also waste. Many sustainable food activists, in fact, see a direct correlation between cheap food and waste.[21] If I only paid $1.99 for my fast-food burger, or for the giant box of cereal I bought at the store yesterday, what does it matter if I throw most of it away? It was so cheap, after all. The less an item costs us, the less we tend to value it.

This scandal is no less than the "theft of the world's natural resources."[22] Indeed, we are essentially stealing from God himself, who commands us to be good stewards of his creation and to care for those less fortunate than ourselves throughout the Old and New Testaments. This abuse of our natural resources is one of the major reasons why close to a billion people are dying of malnutrition and starvation in our world today.

## Good Intentions Should Not Sway Good Decisions

Undoubtedly, not everyone involved in the global food industry is dominated by the logic of corporate capitalism.[23] A number of the pioneers of the industrial food movement, and many of the individuals involved in the industry today, view their work as necessary in light of the world's expanding population, like many of the individuals behind the original Farm Bill did. For example, the 1970 Nobel Peace Prize winner Norman Borlaug, often referred to as the "father of the Green Revolution" in agriculture, was able to feed millions of starving people through his work on the mass production of wheat at the International Maize and Wheat Improvement Center in Mexico.[24] Indeed, my own father was a food technologist in Africa, and his passion was to marry the traditional bakery to modern technology, thereby supporting the development of businesses in impoverished communities.

However, we still have to deal with the consequences of the convenience, efficiency, and productivity of our global food system, no matter how many good intentions support it. As Gustafson points out in *We the Eaters*, we have to adopt Borlaug's innovative *thinking* but not necessarily his methods.[25] The current food system not only leaves almost a billion people starving while billions of dollars of food is wasted but also feeds the rest of us food products that cause disease and death while damaging our health and the rest of God's wonderful creation.[26]

It is imperative that we *renew* the way we imagine global food production and consumption (Rom. 12:2).[27] The huge corporations and industrial farms may dominate in Washington, but if we, the public, vote with our wallets and encourage the innovative thinkers, we can make a substantial difference.

# 7

## The Genetic Elephant in the Room

You may have wondered when I would discuss the genetic elephant in the room. Due to the complexity surrounding the use of genetically modified organisms (otherwise referred to as GMOs or GM foods) in our current food system, I decided to save the worst aspect of the MAD for last.

What exactly are GM foods? Genetically engineered food production, otherwise known as recombinant DNA technology, is based on the science of genetic determinism, which sees mankind, and the world we live in, as essentially materialist or physical. It is based on a "monoculture of the mind," as leading anti-GMO activist Vandana Shiva notes.[1] Indeed, this way of thinking can be traced back to the ancient Greeks, whose philosopher Democritus argued that everything consists of atoms tumbling around in the universe, coming together and breaking apart.[2] We are myopically reduced to our material aspects; in this monoculture of the mind, living organisms act like machines with interconnected pieces, and with the appropriate know-how they can therefore be put together and taken apart like machines.[3] Biotechnologists can, based on this materialist logic, take a specific gene from one organism and place it into the DNA of another organism in order to create a new type of seed with one or more desired traits, such as herbicide-tolerant plants and, most recently, apples that do not go brown after you cut them.[4] This process is known as in vitro DNA modification—and it is somewhat like a complicated genetic game of cut and paste.[5]

Yet where do we draw the line, as Christians, between mimicking creation and thinking we can do better than the Creator by shifting DNA from one species to another, for example? When do we start eating the "forbidden fruit," thinking that God did not quite get it right? The church needs to open a way for a serious discussion of these issues, yet I have never heard a sermon on genetic engineering and Christian bioethics. We are God's stewards, and we will be held accountable for the way we have cared for the world he loves and has entrusted to us (John 3:16). Why are we not talking about how to steward in the real world, with real-world issues?

### Genetically Modified Smoke and Mirrors: What Is Really Fact?

Today the two traits that dominate the market for genetically engineered foods, a market which is concentrated on large-scale soy, corn, cotton, and canola production, are insect resistance (IR) and herbicide tolerance (HT).[6] In the United States, the world leader in industrially produced GMOs, these crops account for half of all agricultural production (169 million acres), which involves an estimated 93 percent of soybean acreage, 85 percent of corn acreage, and 82 percent of cotton acreage.[7] In 2014, farmers using GM seeds accounted for roughly 49 percent of global agriculture usage in the aggregate, most of which is concentrated in a handful of countries, such as the United States, Brazil, South Africa, and Argentina.[8]

While GM crops continue to spread, a number of headlines have recently declared that the debate over the potential risk to our health from GMO consumption is essentially over. This is a premature prediction. Newspaper headlines, and indeed any source of material, cannot be taken at face value. There is potential publication bias, especially considering the biotechnology industry's influence in GM food science.[9] In a 2011 study, for example, Portuguese researchers found that there was a "strong association" between industry-related GMO research and positive outcomes for GM foods in these scientific studies.[10] Merely because a study was published in a journal, and sounds intellectually intimidating, does not mean this study is necessarily true—look at who funded the research.

Essentially, we should always apply the principles of "asking, answering, and discussing" to any piece of information we come across.[11] As the apostle Paul would have said, we need to take every thought (including our examination of GMOs!) captive unto Christ's wisdom. In the case of scientific information, many media outlets are sensationalist at best. Any facts garnered from these sources are essentially the result of the author's interpretation of the scientist's interpretation of their work—very much like the telephone game my four children played growing up.

### GM Science versus GM Certainty

Proponents of GM foods often state that the disapproval surrounding this new agricultural technology is irrational, since science has "proven" that it is safe. Yet, as I discussed above, science is not a system of absolute certainty. The scientific method is a phenomenal tool that enables us to discover and comprehend, within our limited human understanding, God's incredible universe.[12] But it does not replace God.

To argue that GM foods are completely safe is to deny that there are many things we have yet to learn about genes, let alone the way genes react in an organism within our multifaceted ecosystems.[13]

Indeed, we are only beginning to realize that our so-called "junk" DNA is really not junk at all, and how the science of epigenetics (the study of how the environment controls gene activity) is far more complicated and far-reaching than imagined. Who is to say what will happen when we take one gene from an insect and insert it into a plant? The absence of harm in scientific papers does not immediately equal safety in real life; it only means that as far as we can tell, as we look under the streetlight in the parking lot (to once again use Pollan's analogy), we cannot see any immediate health hazards.

The true pursuit of this science has to be as unbiased as is humanly possible. This is an especially hard task when an industry that is heavily invested in a technology controls the research on this technology.[14] International biotech companies such as Monsanto and Syngenta, who dominate the global GM commercial market, publish the majority of the studies available on GM foods. The relationship between these biotech companies and researchers can be either direct (such as employing their own researchers) or indirect (by funding university studies through large grants, for instance). Potential publication bias cannot be overlooked in these instances, since these companies have the most to lose, in terms of billions of dollars of annual revenue, from findings that question the safety of genetically engineered foods.[15]

There are a number of other factors to consider. Researchers cannot access the GM seeds and their particular isogenic lines, that is, any seeds with similar genotypes, without permission from these companies. Furthermore, independent scholars have limited financial support compared to industry-funded research. Even many regulatory bodies, such as the American Food and Drug Administration (FDA), can only access industry information on GM foods if the companies in question give their permission. How can we rely on the "proven" safety of these studies if the biotech companies restrict access to the information necessary to carry out completely independent trials?[16]

In fact, most of the available studies on GM foods do not thoroughly examine long-term and multigenerational health effects.[17] As biochemist and nutritionist Dr. Árpád Pusztai (widely known for his work on GM potatoes) indicates, "the main danger is that we *do not know* what the main danger is."[18]

Although a recent paper by French plant geneticist Agnès Ricroch and her colleagues has argued that these short-term trials, which are usually three months or less in duration, are acceptable measures of GM food safety, the paper itself contains several contradictions. Most notably, while the study indicates that GM foods are safe, according to both the long- and short-term studies carried out over the past several decades, it claims that there are no long-term rodent studies available for one of the main GM crops produced today: corn.[19] According to an academic review of the studies on GM foods and health published that same year by José L. Domingo, a professor of toxicology and environmental health, there are in fact an equal number of scientific papers on both sides of the GMO safety debate, while the vast majority of these studies were industry-funded and therefore at strong risk of bias.[20] Likewise, *Environmental Science Europe* published a paper at the beginning of 2015 noting how there is no global scientific "consensus on GM food safety," no global "epidemiological studies investigating potential effects of GM food consumption on human health," and no global "consensus on the environmental risks of GM crops" by the global scientific community. Indeed, this journal also notes how a "list of several hundred studies does not show GM food safety," while the "EU research project provides no evidence for sweeping claims about the safety of any single GM food or of GM crops in general."[21] Exactly what is "certain"?

As the scientific community still argues over GM foods, the number of studies strikes a disquieting note. GM foods have been associated with autism,[22] allergies,[23] and infertility,[24] to name just a few potential long- and short-term health effects.[25] Most recently, the WHO released a report on Monsanto's Roundup Ready seeds (a herbicide-resistant GM crop), noting that they have potential carcinogenic effects.[26] At the very least, GMO products should have labels, so that the consumer can freely make their own informed decision on the risk that these foods pose to themselves, their loved ones, and the planet.[27]

## I Smell a Rat

One of the few available long-term rodent studies on GM corn is the 2012 Séralini paper on Roundup (also known as glyphosate, the leading herbicide used today) and Roundup-tolerant GM corn. French professor of molecular biology Gilles-Eric Séralini and his team of scientists found that, compared with control groups, rats exposed to both this herbicide and corn over two years suffered from a number of health issues such as tumors, necrosis, kidney disease, and early death related to the additive POE-15. Since POE-15 is not considered an active ingredient, regulators did not assess its safety in the same way that glyphosate was tested.

After a firestorm of both criticism and support for the findings, the *Food and Chemical Toxicology* journal retracted the peer-reviewed paper in 2013. This withdrawal elicited even more international criticism and detailed responses from the authors, while a global petition was signed against the journal's actions. At the same time, the European Food Safety Authority (EFSA) argued that the Séralini et al. paper had not followed its guidelines for three-month-long rodent studies. This announcement was particularly troubling in light of the fact that Monsanto's long-term trials also failed to meet the EFSA's recommendations, yet the biotech giant was not subject to the same criticism. In the summer of 2014 the paper was republished in another journal, *Environmental Sciences Europe*, further adding to the controversy surrounding the study.

This Séralini affair, whether or not you agree with the methodology and findings of the paper, still underscores both the inadequacy of our current methods to examine the safety of GM food production and the convoluted nature of a public debate that is far from over. What other potentially toxic ingredients, inactive or otherwise, are in these chemicals and seeds? Is the uncertain risk associated with commercial GM food production worth the purported benefits of the technology? Indeed, is it possible to have a reasonable scientific debate on a technology that industry and government have already invested billions of dollars in? Or in an environment where the scientists who examine this technology are both personally and professionally condemned?[28]

## The Myth of the Environmental Vacuum

The potential risks of GM food production are not limited to human health. GM crops are monoculture crops and are therefore prone to the issues this type of agricultural production causes, including a dramatic decrease in the environmental diversity essential to a balanced ecosystem. In fact, a growing body of research on the ecological impact of GM food production, for example, indicates that over time both weeds and insects can develop resistance to these new chemicals and crops, thereby necessitating the use of more and more pesticides (chemicals that have been linked to cancer and birth defects) for the same desired effect.[29] For instance, in Iowa many farmers now have to deal with rootworms that have developed a resistance to the genetically modified corn (that contains insect genes), compelling many of them to increase their use of insecticides to combat this infestation.[30] Indeed, some researchers have estimated that GM foods have increased the rate of overall pesticide use in the United States alone by 122 million pounds in the years 1996 to 2011.[31]

Although a recent German meta-analysis, or a detailed survey of the scientific studies available on a particular subject, has argued that GM food production decreases pesticide usage by 37 percent, over half of the studies used in this meta-analysis were *short term* (mainly one farming season). Since insect and weed resistance occur over an extended period of time, this meta-analysis is not an accurate survey of the long-term effect of GM foods on pesticide usage. Also, the data analyzed in this meta-analysis focused primarily on insect-resistant, genetically engineered crops. Herbicide-tolerant crops, however, account for the greater percentage of GM agricultural production today. This meta-analysis is not a suitable account of GM agriculture in general, even though the authors claim that it provides "robust evidence" in favor of GMOs, which will "greatly improve public trust in this technology." In fact, that data collected was restricted to just three crops (soybeans, corn, and cotton) in predominantly three countries (South Africa, India, and the United States) and was based largely on farmer surveys (which are less dependable than fixed measurements). This is by no means "robust evidence" that all GM food production in the world is safe and beneficial. Likewise, correlation in science does not imply causation, and there are other variables, such as different types of farms, that can also account for the findings of this analysis.[32]

GMO agricultural production never occurs in an environmental vacuum. In a research laboratory these genes can be controlled to a degree, although we are only beginning to understand the way genes function.[33] Once GMOs are incorporated into complex ecosystems, however, their effect on the interconnected nature of these systems is little understood. If scientists do not even know 98 percent of the organisms in the soil used to grow the crops, how can we suitably measure the effect of GMOs on intricate ecosystems over time?[34] This risk is particularly alarming in light of the fact that genetically engineered seeds contaminate non-GMO crops through natural processes such as pollination and the weather.[35]

Ultimately, we have introduced artificial organisms into an environment we cannot control. Whether or not we choose to eat GM foods, we are all part of these ecosystems—we are all affected by the agricultural production of GMOs.[36]

Even if genetically engineered food increases agricultural yield, as the German meta-analysis discussed above argues, more processed foodstuffs and grain-based animal feed will not fix our broken food system. Fundamentally, the goal of a food system is not just to feed people but to feed them in a way that nourishes and sustains life. In the sections above we have already seen the result of too many empty calories: these unhealthy foods can lead to disease and early death, just as lack of food leads to disease and early death.[37] GM corn and soy are solutions that stay within the framework of a global food industry that emphasizes quantity over quality.[38]

We have to step out of this pattern of thinking.[39] As Hesterman notes, "The system we have in place is still largely based on this outdated concept that agriculture is part of the manufacturing sector." Food is not the same as food-like products. Ultimately, we need to *renew* the way we think about our meals, and not conform to the way the world thinks about our meals (Rom. 12:2).[40]

## We Have Enough Food to Feed the World

Indeed, hunger is not an issue of food production. *Today, we have enough food to feed the world.*[41] The system that delivers this food, however, is one where millions and millions of pounds of food go to waste on a daily basis, millions of pounds are turned into animal feed and gasoline for our cars, almost a billion people are starving, and 30 percent of the world population does not get enough micronutrients.[42] As celebrated economist and 1998 Nobel Prize winner Amartya Sen notes, "Starvation is the characteristic of some people not having enough food to eat. It is not the characteristic of there being not enough food to eat."[43] GM foods are an oversimplified (and inherently indeterminate) solution to the complexities of hunger, where there is enough food for everyone but not everyone can access this food. We need to change the political, social, and economic forces that do not allow people to alleviate their hunger.[44] Growing more and more corn or soy is merely taking the easy way out and does not solve the underlying issues that lead to food insecurity and starvation. The industrial production of corn and soy are Band-Aids on a gaping wound.

Even the potential of increased yields from GM crops is in question.[45] For instance, Monsanto's genetically engineered soybeans have a "yield drag" (or reduced yield) of 5 to 10 percent compared to conventional soybeans.[46] Indeed, a recent United Nations and World Bank long-term review, known as the International Assessment of Agricultural Science and Technology for Development (IAASTD), analyzed data from 110 countries and 900 participants and noted that GM crops *cannot meet* the food needs of the world's population.[47] In terms of consistent, intrinsic yield increases, or the "amount of food that crops can produce under ideal circumstances," GM crops, as opposed to conventional agriculture, have not lived up to the promises of their defenders.[48] Indeed, the current food industry has failed at meeting its promise of more and more yields: overall crop *losses* have actually increased since the mid-twentieth century in the United States alone.[49]

Thus far, the biotech companies who often promise "better food to save the world" in response to their many critics have not yet lived up to the hype of their marketing campaigns.[50] For example, "golden rice," which was featured on *Time* magazine's front cover as a solution to the tragic levels of vitamin A deficiency that affects millions of children globally, failed to overcome the cultural norms of rice color in Asia in the absence of social programs educating the communities in question.[51] And scientists still debate just how much of this rice (with vitamin A engineered into it, which is responsible for the "golden" color of the grain) will have to be consumed to meet children's nutritional needs. Some estimates note that up to fifty bowls of golden rice a day would have to be eaten to meet the recommended daily allowance of vitamin A.[52]

In light of the potential dangers of vitamin supplements we discussed in chapter 5, it is even more imperative that these nutritional findings are thoroughly and independently tested before they are offered as solutions that can "save a million kids."[53] We should not embrace these new technologies based on future promises that have not yet materialized, in the same way that you would not purchase my products if I only promised to help you in the future.

## Is There a "Seed" of Hope Anywhere?

Is it even possible, however, to create a food system that focuses on both quantity and quality, while stewarding God's planet with integrity and compassion? The growing body of research on agro-ecological farming methods offers some exciting possibilities. Across forty-four projects in over twenty sub-Saharan African nations, for example, agro-ecological yields have been significantly higher than conventional or GM farming methods, with an increased yield of 214 percent within a ten-year period.[54] Similarly, the Rodale Institute's thirty-year-long Farming Systems Trial (FST) has shown how organic farming methods can equal conventional yields, while remaining more resilient during seasons of inclement weather.[55] In a number of cases, organic farming has actually been shown to be as effective in terms of yield as conventional methods.[56]

Additionally, a 2014 meta-analysis on organic versus conventional agriculture found that the previous estimates of low yields for organic farms had been overemphasized due to the views of the scientific community at the time. In fact, both multi-cropping and crop rotations on organic farms significantly reduced the assumed yield disparity between organic and conventional farming methods.[57] We should urgently consider investing our dollars in technologies that promote ecological diversity and resilience.[58]

The search for alternative food systems is indeed urgent, since the production of GM crops has left us with a global issue of food sovereignty—who governs our food supply? Biotech companies and food corporations are continually increasing their control over what we eat, while public institutions for agricultural development, such as Borlaug's International Maize and Wheat Improvement Center in Mexico, suffer under a lack of available funding.[59] Since these companies can patent their GM seed technology, farmers can no longer save their seeds and plant them in subsequent seasons—a time-honored practice that has continued since the beginning of agriculture. Yet God created seeds in such a way that they can sustain a regular food supply by being replanted—this is part of his "wired for love" foundation of our world. Now, however, GM farmers have to purchase new seeds, and new chemicals, each year, often increasing their debts in the process.[60] And according to the USDA's Economic Research Service, giving control of seeds to private companies has in fact led to a significant overall decrease in the amount of funding given to agricultural research and development.[61] We know less, but we are allowing these companies to earn more.

This expansion of the private sector's control over our seed supplies is essentially a monopoly on the "genetic resources on which all of humanity depends."[62] We can survive without a lot of things, but food is indubitably not one of them. Indeed, in countries such as India the fight against GM foods is not predominantly concerned with the human and environmental health effects of these crops but rather campaigners focus on food security and sovereignty, and the freedom for local communities to control and determine their own food sources.[63]

The patenting of GM seeds involves significant amounts of money. Monsanto can gain millions of dollars per annum by abolishing all the seed-saving habits of farmers in the United States alone, while its earnings from court cases against farmers who have purportedly saved their seeds is equally high. An alarming pattern has emerged over the past several years whereby some farmers are prosecuted by these multibillion-dollar companies for the use of GM seeds, even if they argue that their lands were, unbeknownst to them, contaminated by these genetically engineered crops. The private investigating teams hired by these biotech companies, which search the countryside for patent infringements, have discovered many of these purported cases.[64]

## *Real* Food and Real Scientific Advances

I am, of course, in no way antiscience. As someone who has spent the last thirty years researching the mind and brain, I have a great appreciation for the scientific method as an exciting tool that enables us to discover more and more about our God by examining his magnificent creation. I do believe that genetically engineered biotechnology has significant research potential within a laboratory, enabling us to identify particular genes in isolation (as was done with "snorkel rice," which failed to create a flood-resistant rice variety but provided scientists with an important body of information nonetheless).[65] And there certainly are many pro-GMO scientists and organizations, such as the Center for the Application of Molecular Biology to International Agriculture (CAMBIA), that are challenging private corporate control of GM food technology.[66] Yet, as an uncertain technology that enables large corporations to gain control of our food supply, the process of science, and even politics, GM foods pose an imminent threat to us all.

---

Rather than *trying to change* what God has given us in nature, a far better use of science in our food system is science that devises ingenious solutions that *imitate God's creation*. Over the past several years, the science of "biomimicry" has sought to do just this: to mimic the genius found in nature while at the same time respecting the intricate complexity of our world's ecosystems.[67] Essentially, this exciting field is focused on "innovation inspired by nature," or what I like to call innovation inspired by God's design.[68] Farmers, inventors, and researchers are continually making incredible advances in sustainable and natural food production, from the use of fish tanks and water-grown vegetables in greenhouses (known as aquaponics), to practices that use cows to imitate wild animal grazing patterns to reverse desertification by fertilizing the soil, and to multifaceted organic farming methods and animal husbandry used to sequestrate excess carbon in the land, thereby helping to combat global warming.[69] For example, Will Allen, a Milwaukee-based organic farmer and the founder of Growing Power, "provides safe, healthy, affordable" produce for communities using an astonishing array of natural, scientific techniques: "acid-digestion, anaerobic digestion for food waste, bio-phyto remediation and soil health, aquaculture closed-loop systems, vermiculture, small and large scale composting, urban agriculture, and permaculture."[70] Allen, whose farms are incredibly productive per acre, has rightly received an honorary PhD for his incredible contribution to the field of biomimicry.[71] The genius of these sustainable farmers and food producers can easily be compared to that found in the offices, practices, and laboratories of individuals with many degrees behind their names.

### It Is Time to Quit the System

The MAD way of eating is the product of human *choices*. Many of us are not compelled to eat its highly processed foods, nor should we accept its many chronic diseases and starving millions. By opting out of this system we collectively make it more possible for others less fortunate than ourselves to access *real*, whole foods and rewire our food system toward health again. Yet before we plant a garden in our backyard, we have to plant a healthy garden in our head. In the following chapters I will show you how *thinking* is the key to a healthier you and a healthier world. Admitting there is a problem with our global food system is the first step. Now it is time to quit the system and beat it at its own game.

# PART 2

# QUIT IT!

# 8

# Mindset and Meal

By now you have a detailed picture of a global food system that has gone devastatingly wrong. Some might say you have all you need to know to start making better choices as a shopper, eater, and voting citizen. But unless you are able to identify and change your mindset about food, all of this information will be useless.

Suppose, for example, that your mindset includes beliefs like *What Dr. Leaf calls* real *food will be hard to find, is expensive, and tastes like sawdust. Cheeseburgers make me feel good.* These deeply rooted beliefs will cause you to disregard much of what I've said. Or suppose you feel discouraged and believe that *There's nothing I can do about the global food business. It's too big and I'm too small.* That emotion and belief can also short-circuit your willingness to take action.

Because mindset is so important to what we actually do, part 2 is devoted to the mindset behind the meal and the meal behind the mindset. How does thinking affect eating, and how does eating affect thinking?

## The Mindset behind the Meal

Research shows that 75–98 percent of current mental, physical, emotional, and behavioral illnesses and issues come from our thought life; only 2–25 percent come from a combination of genetics *and* what enters our bodies through food, medications, pollution, chemicals, and so on.[1] These statistics show that the mindset behind the meal—the *thinking* behind the meal—plays a dominant role in the process of human food-related health issues, approximately 80 percent. Hence the title of this book: you have to *think* and eat yourself smart, happy, and healthy.

God has given us a "sound mind" (2 Tim. 1:7). We have the mind of Christ that enables us to think well (1 Cor. 2:16). You will learn about the enormous impact thinking has on your brain and body as you *choose* and eat food. Indeed, the power in our mind to think and choose is incredible. Since God gave us this powerful ability to think, feel, and choose, we therefore have a responsibility to understand this power and use it well in every aspect of our lives, including what we choose to eat and how we eat (1 Cor. 10:31).

If we do not have a healthy mind, then nothing else in our life will be healthy, including our eating habits. This discussion of the impact of *thinking* on eating incorporates the elements of choice and its consequences (Deut. 30:19), bringing all thoughts into captivity to Christ (2 Cor. 10:5), renewing the mind (Rom. 12:2), being led by the Holy Spirit (Rom. 8:5–6), respecting the temple God has given us (Ps. 139:14; 1 Cor. 3:16–17; 6:19–20; 2 Cor. 6:14–18; 1 Pet. 2:5), and respecting the earth and animals God has entrusted to us (Gen. 1:26; Lev. 25:23; Ps. 24:1–2; 50:9–12; John 1:3; 3:16–17; Col. 1:16–17).

## The Meal behind the Mindset

Although your brain is only 2 percent of the weight of your body, it consumes 20 percent of the total energy (oxygen) and 65 percent of the glucose—what you eat will directly affect the brain's ability to function on a significant scale.[2] Your brain has "first dibs" on everything you eat. I call this the "20 percent factor," or the eating behind the thinking, and it underscores the fact that how and what we eat affects our mind, brain, and body.

Even though this factor is only 20 percent of the story, you can't just eat whatever you feel like and expect your life to improve if you think good thoughts. On the contrary, God wants us healthy in our spirits, souls, *and* bodies (1 Cor. 6:19–20; 1 Thess. 5:23; 3 John 1:2). All three are important and are supposed to work in an integrated way, influencing and feeding into each other in a cyclical fashion.

Thinking is fundamentally intertwined with our mental and physical health. In fact, one of the things you will learn in part 2 is that if you eat while emotional, your body does not digest your food correctly. If you think right, you will eat right, and if you eat right, you will think right.

I hope you have begun to see the reasoning behind eating and our spiritual and physical responsibility to eat a healthy diet. Many people ask me, "If our minds are so powerful, why does it matter what I eat?" Some individuals have even declared passionately that "I can eat whatever I want and pray God will bless it to my body even though I know it isn't healthy." Certainly, you are free to choose, but you are not free from the consequences of your choices.

Those of us who can afford to purchase better quality food, once we understand how dysfunctional our current food system is, have a responsibility to change the way we eat. Turning a blind eye for the sake of convenience is not worshiping Christ in everything we do (1 Cor. 10:31). To make this choice indicates a lack of respect and stewardship for our own body and the blessings of the earth God has graciously provided. We cannot pray God will turn our cake into kale. This may sound hard, but the reality of what we eat is truly a matter of life and death. We cannot survive, let alone thrive, without proper nourishment.

And the situation is urgent. As we saw in part 1, the MAD diet has morphed into the global industrial diet. Even though people in other countries disapprove of American fast food and TV culture, this MAD diet has invaded virtually every country. As mentioned earlier, it is, unfortunately, one of the largest US exports.[3] On a daily basis, more and more of us are consuming foods that destroy rather than nourish our bodies and our planet. Changing our mindset behind the meal, and the meal behind the mindset, is a *global* issue.

Yet in this book I am not going to give you a list of what to eat and what not to eat to improve brain and body health. I am going to teach you how to *think about what and how you eat*. The thought of writing yet another diet book that you may read and use for just a few weeks, with minimal long-term changes in your life, does not interest me. As a clinical therapist and scientist, I want to help you make lasting changes in *all* areas of your life by teaching you to use your incredible mind. You do not have to be a nutritionist to know how to eat. You have to learn how to *think* before you eat.

### Renew Your Mind, Renew Your Plate

As a culture, we have become so accustomed to our current, global MAD food system that it has become a part of our nonconscious minds. When was the last time you thought about what the chicken who laid your eggs ate? Or how the sugary breakfast cereal in your pantry was made? Or how long ago your neatly shredded and packaged lettuce was picked? It is a learned and habituated food system.

Most of us do not even stop and *think* about the principles of cheap, easy, and fast that this system is founded on. The MAD establishment, from supermarkets to fast-food restaurants, did not dominate the food landscape fifty years ago, yet in just a few decades it has taken away the most important part of eating: *think-ing has been supplanted by convenience.*[4]

We saw in part 1 that with the large-scale industrialization of our food system came big agribusinesses dominated by the logic of short-term economics and extensive food marketing campaigns to keep profits high. One thing we will see in these next several chapters is that research on the mind shows how marketing has changed our thinking both about what food is and how, when, and where to eat it.[5] We have been subtly shaped by a culture of convenience.

Yet we are not doomed to follow the ways of the MAD. God has designed our minds to control our brains—our biology does not control us![6] When we change our mind, we change our brain, and our body follows suit. We can undo the effects of marketing.

# 9

## Taking Responsibility

Our first step in undoing the effects of a lifetime of marketing is to face the fact that it has happened to us and decide in our minds to take responsibility for what we eat. The brain does the bidding of the mind—where the mind goes, the brain follows.[1] What you think affects what you eat, and what you eat affects what you think.

There are countless research studies in journals, online, in the media, and in bookstores highlighting the impact of both *thinking* and *diet* on the brain and body. We can now say with certainty that consuming highly processed, sugar-, salt-, and fat-laden MAD foods contributes to increased levels of obesity, cardiovascular disease, diabetes, Alzheimer's, stroke, allergies, autism, learning disabilities, and autoimmune disorders. The list can go on and on.

Although we are seeing an ever-increasing public awareness of the effects of lifestyle choices on our health, fast-food establishments and supermarkets are continually being built across the globe.[2] Within my own neighborhood, four new chain grocery stores have opened in the last several months!

## A Mental Blank Wall

Many individuals do not know, or do not want to acknowledge, how dysfunctional our food system actually is. While writing this book, I often had discussions on food and healthy eating with the pastors, leaders, drivers, and other incredible people I have had the opportunity to meet during my travels. These people are compassionate and loving, yet most of them had no clue that our food system was so far removed from their own belief systems and values.

Even when I speak of these issues from the podium, I often come face-to-face with a mental blank wall. It never ceases to amaze me, for instance, that when I speak on the dangers of soda, which creates structural damage in the brain, several people in the audience always visit the vending machine and buy cans of soda during the lunch break. Indeed, the green room is usually filled with such drinks: many of the visitors grab one and joke, "Don't let Caroline see you with that!" After drinking soda not only will you have a distended colon and an insulin rush but you will also reduce your IQ level, invite brain fog, throw your body into toxic stress, and contribute to the destruction of the earth's natural resources. How is this respecting our bodies as God's living temples? Are we being good biblical stewards?

Ultimately, the MAD industrial food system dominates our world. Parents take their children to fast-food restaurants between school and their next sporting activity. People fill up their grocery carts with foods containing strange ingredients no one can pronounce, or no ordinary kitchen has ever heard of. Many restaurants do not even know how their chickens were raised or how their vegetables were grown. Church functions are hotbeds of fast, convenient, and highly processed foods. Charities and food aid still cripple local, healthy food production in developing nations with imported processed foods, good intentions notwithstanding.[3]

## The Only Balanced Meal

We need to take *personal responsibility* for what we put on our plates. If we eat the MAD diet on the very, very odd occasion, we can rest assured knowing that God, in his gracious and loving way, has built backup systems into our brain and body that will pull us out of potential danger. After all, stressing about our food is as bad for our health as eating unwholesome foods! But if we *knowingly* continue down a path of eating food-like products instead of *real* food, merely because we would rather use our money to buy that new iPhone, we should not be surprised when the consequences are far from what we desire.

It is foolhardy to believe that we can live our lives however we choose and, when medical problems arise, run to our doctors and dietitians for a quick fix, ask God why this is happening to us, and tell everyone we are under spiritual attack. We are *always* under spiritual attack on *every* front. Paul says we are *in* a war, not going to war (Rom. 7:23; Eph. 6:11–13; 2 Thess. 1:4). We are part of this battle of restoration: we are called to be God's heirs, soldiers, and high priests, extending his love and forgiveness in the world; this is what it means to be true followers of Christ, who extended God's love and mercy into the world by conquering sin and death (John 14:12–14; Heb. 4:14; 1 Pet. 2:9). We are called to bring heaven to earth, and this does not happen without a fight (Matt. 6:9–13).[4]

In fact, I think a frightening mentality among many Christians today is a pervasive view of the world as fallen and hopeless, despite the fact that Christ has already made all things new (2 Cor. 5:17; Rev. 21:5). We have the God-given responsibility to care for the earth—the whole world is waiting for Christians to fully appropriate their identity as God's heirs and take responsibility for creation (Rom. 8:19–22).

The world is *being restored*—a restoration that began with Christ and will be completed with Christ, and through us as his heirs.[5] We were not created to stand by, complaining about the evil things we witness or hear about and exclaiming that we cannot wait to go to heaven and leave this wretched earth behind. We are supposed to bring heaven to earth, to apply God's love to the terrible things that make us want to duck our head in the ground like spiritual ostriches—terrible things like our corrupt food system. Once we know, we have a responsibility to act (James 4:17). As Christians we cannot say that it is impossible to escape or change the MAD diet—while hoping that saying grace over our food will make it healthy. Real grace is not just said before a meal; real grace *is the meal.*

I am not trying to make you feel guilty. Negative emotions will just make things worse, and give you terrible indigestion to boot. I write these words with a spirit of conviction, not condemnation, for we "are destroyed for lack of knowledge" (Hos. 4:6). Destruction is a final, horrific thing. I am trying to increase your awareness by warning you of the dangers of putting trash in your mind *or in your body.* I know life is challenging, yet I also know God is greater than our struggles—nothing is impossible for him (Matt. 19:26). And Jesus himself said that God cares about what you eat, just as he cares for the nourishment of the birds and all living creatures (Matt. 6:26).

Essentially, *thinking* about the impact of your lifestyle choices will have a profound influence on the health of your spirit, soul, and body. I know I am belaboring this point, yet it truly cannot be said enough: the only balanced meal is one that includes your *thoughts.*


## Lose the Mindset, Lose the Weight

As we take responsibility for the condition of our bodies, the question arises, what is a healthy weight for us? Scientists think about this in terms of body mass index (BMI), a ratio of weight to height. Unfortunately, what exactly is a healthy BMI is still being debated. According to a growing body of research, a healthy BMI can be as high as 35—contrary to the long-held scientific dogmas that have defined what is considered overweight and obese.[6] These findings are perhaps unsurprising in light of artwork from the Renaissance and Baroque periods, for example, where women are frequently portrayed according to standards many of us would consider overweight or obese.

The BMI is an imperfect scale, since it does not take into account many factors associated with our weight, such as body fat percentage.[7] Wearing a size zero does not necessarily mean you are healthy, just as an organic label does not necessarily mean the food is healthy. We are all different, uniquely created in the image of God.

Yet this shift away from popularly held conceptions about BMI is not an excuse to lie on your couch and binge on food-like products such as soda and fast food. There certainly is a point where being obese or overweight is damaging to your health, and a lack of exercise negatively affects both your physical and mental well-being. MAD processed foods have many negative health effects. Our ultimate goals should therefore be a healthy diet and a lifestyle that nourishes and sustains us, not a supermodel body that is defined by superficial cultural standards.

Indeed, you may lose weight on a diet or by taking a pill, yet such weight loss shocks your body while your mind is still entrenched in old patterns of eating.[8] The effect is short term at best. However, when we understand and remove the habits, mindsets, and cues that result in incorrect eating and overeating, we can make truly *sustainable* lifestyle changes based on a balanced, thought-based way of eating.

How, then, do we reshape our mindsets and habits? That's what we need to consider next.

# 10

## The Meeting of the Minds

For many years I researched, developed, and tested a theory that delineates what the mind is, and how we think and build memory in order to learn.[1] I describe this theory, the Geodesic Information Processing Theory, as the science of thought, which I have applied in many ways with my patients and in my research over the past thirty years.[2] Based on this theory, in the following chapters I am going to explain how easy it is for us to get caught up in incorrect thinking patterns when we do not monitor what enters our minds. You will also begin to understand how mindsets become mindsets (which are really entrenched memories with emotions attached, thus the equivalent of an attitude) and influence our perceptions.

If you look at this schematic of the Geodesic Information Processing Theory, you will see that your mind is divided into two parts: the nonconscious metacognitive and the conscious cognitive. You will also see a section that is called the symbolic level, which represents our senses and what we say and do. Across the bottom strip of the model you will see text boxes that represent what is happening in the brain, or the neural correlates, as a result of the mind in action.[3]

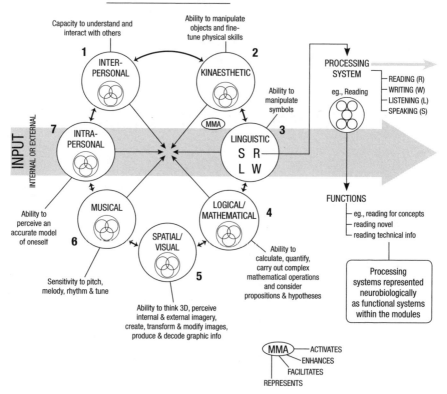

NONCONSCIOUS

## METACOGNITIVE LEVEL

90% of Learning

MMA

Root of Thinking Process
and then structure of the
non-conscious

Automatized
complex higher
cortical functions

1–7 METACOGNITIVE MODULES

Capacity to understand and
interact with others

**1**
INTER-
PERSONAL

Ability to manipulate
objects and fine-
tune physical skills

**2**
KINAESTHETIC

PROCESSING
SYSTEM

eg., Reading

READING (R)
WRITING (W)
LISTENING (L)
SPEAKING (S)

Ability to
manipulate
symbols

**7**
INTRA-
PERSONAL

MMA

**3**
LINGUISTIC
S R
L W

INPUT
INTERNAL OR EXTERNAL

Ability to
perceive an
accurate model
of oneself

MUSICAL

**6**

SPATIAL/
VISUAL

**5**

LOGICAL/
MATHEMATICAL
**4**

FUNCTIONS

eg., reading for concepts
reading novel
reading technical info

Sensitivity to pitch,
melody, rhythm & tune

Ability to
calculate, quantify,
carry out complex
mathematical operations
and consider
propositions & hypotheses

Processing
systems represented
neurobiologically
as functional systems
within the modules

Ability to think 3D, perceive
internal & external imagery,
create, transform & modify images,
produce & decode graphic info

MMA ACTIVATES
ENHANCES
FACILITATES
REPRESENTS

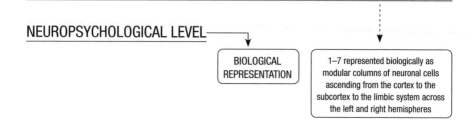

## NEUROPSYCHOLOGICAL LEVEL

BIOLOGICAL
REPRESENTATION

1–7 represented biologically as
modular columns of neuronal cells
ascending from the cortex to the
subcortex to the limbic system across
the left and right hemispheres

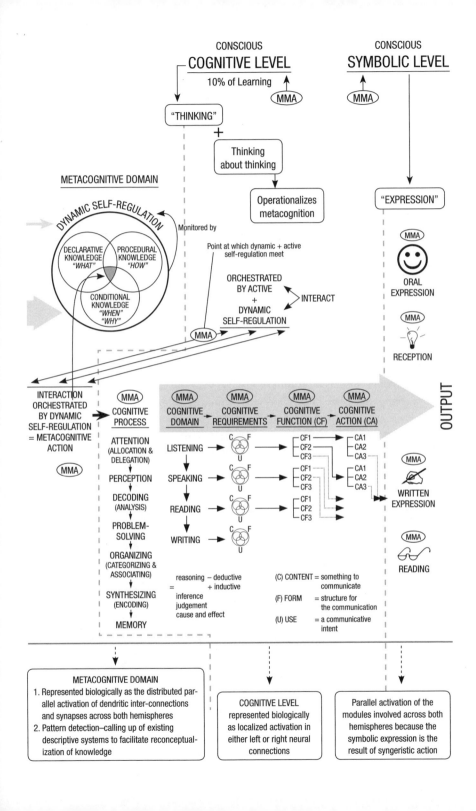

When you are thinking, choosing, and forming thoughts or memories, your mind is "in action."[4] The mind is separate from the brain and changes the biology of the brain.[5] A mind in action changes the physical structure of your brain biology. This process is called *neuroplasticity* and is something I have been studying for the past thirty years. Although the idea of neuroplasticity was rejected in the 1980s, when the prevailing wisdom was that the brain could not change (a damaged brain would always be a damaged brain), it gained validity in the mid-1990s and is now discussed throughout the scientific community.[6]

The brain only changes, however, because of the action going on between the nonconscious and conscious mind. As you think about what you are listening to, smelling, touching, tasting, or looking at, your nonconscious and conscious minds kick into high-energy action and your genes respond by switching on and off, making proteins that form into treelike structures called dendrites, which are memories.[7] You literally wire thoughts into your brain, thereby transforming the biological landscape of your brain.

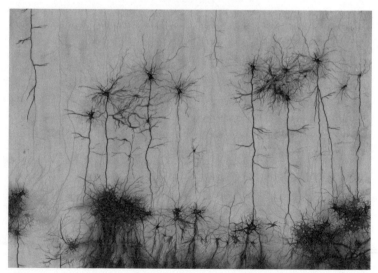

"Magic Trees of the Mind" Golgi Stain

The more you think about something, the more developed your memory concerning this thing becomes. In fact, over a period of twenty-one days, short-term memory becomes long-term memory.[8] It takes another forty-two days (two more twenty-one-day cycles) to automatize that long-term memory and turn it into a *habit*.[9] This means it takes a minimum of sixty-three days to form a habit, not twenty-one as is often quoted.

There is an interesting interplay that takes place between the incredibly fast nonconscious mind, with its trillions of memories, and your slower, more evaluative, but *equally powerful* conscious mind. The conscious mind assesses the incoming information from your five senses, yet it does so through the lens of four to seven embedded thoughts that have moved from your nonconscious into your conscious mind at any one moment.[10] Current events are examined in terms of existing and related memories. What you have already built into your mind determines how you will understand and make decisions about new information.

In the following chapters I will explain my theory in more detail, ending with an analogy that will show you how it applies to the food we choose to eat.

### Nonconscious Metacognitive Level of the Mind

The nonconscious metacognitive level of the mind, which is on the far left of the graphic above, is incredibly extensive. It is beyond the constraints of space and time and operates in a quantum way: unlimited, interrelational, and simultaneous.[11] It is where your stored memories interact in a dynamic fashion, setting up your belief systems and shaping your uniqueness, which I term the I-factor.[12]

Essentially, your I-factor is the perfectly created you. It is your uniqueness as a human being made in God's image (Gen. 1:26) and all the choices you have made, which have created genetic changes, consequently adding layers to the core of *who you are*.

These layers enrich you if they are Holy Spirit–led layers, or they diminish you if you choose to believe the enemy's lies. Who you *choose* to listen to is vitally important in terms of the quality and level of truth you build into your nonconscious mind. Where your mind goes, your brain follows.

The nonconscious mind is responsible for somewhere between 90–99 percent of your mind's activity.[13] For example, out of the 10 million bits per second processed through the eye, only a maximum of 50 bits per second are processed consciously.[14] The nonconscious mind operates twenty-four hours a day, at fantastic speeds, about a quintillion ($10^{18}$) bits per second at a synaptic level and an octillion ($10^{27}$) bits per second at a microtubular level, for the whole brain.[15] Indeed, the mind is truly magnificent. It is the orchestra conductor, operating in the brain in the form of rhythms and frequencies, which communicate among its biological components like a beautiful piece of music.[16]

The nonconscious mind drives and influences the conscious mind, which means it is the dominant part of your mind.[17] Once a thought is planted and becomes a habit in your nonconscious mind, it will shape your perception of anything related to that thought. This interrelated nature of the mind gives a whole new level of meaning to James 1:21: "The implanted word [will] save your souls." What you have stored in your nonconscious mind will shape your perception of reality.

The nonconscious mind is connected into the spiritual part of who you are.[18] What this means is that God has already provided answers to our issues (including what to eat, how to eat, and for any kind of eating disorder). Everything we need for our future is already completed (Isa. 46:10), and it's all good (Gen. 1:31). The answers are already accessible to us through the Holy Spirit (John 16:13).

In fact, the past, present, and future are not fixed variables in your nonconscious mind, which means it is not bound by time. Essentially, the nonconscious mind works on quantum principles, which do not follow the normal rule of time in classical physics. The past, present, and future affect each other—much like what happened with Denzel Washington's character in the movie *Déjà Vu*.[19] By implanting the Word in your soul (mind), you affect your past, present, and future!

Yet we need to *choose* to implant these spiritual realities in our nonconscious minds to "save [our] souls" (James 1:21). Once we begin to do this, we will truly comprehend how the work of the cross created our future: "For I know the thoughts that I think toward you, says the LORD, thoughts of peace and not of evil, to give you a future and a hope" (Jer. 29:11).

## The Conscious Cognitive Level of the Mind

The conscious level of the mind, which is represented in the middle of the schematic above, is responsible for roughly 1–10 percent of our mind's activity.[20] It is much more sedate than the nonconscious mind but equally as powerful. For instance, it operates at only 50 bits per second through the eyes as compared to the total of 10 million bits per second.[21] It is dependent on the nonconscious mind, which is the source of our individual uniqueness, and is therefore influenced by what is stored in the nonconscious mind.[22] The conscious mind only operates when we are awake, and it is the part of us that is *consciously and deliberately* thinking and choosing.[23] We have the ability, with our conscious mind, to change and reconceptualize embedded memories—*this means we can change and overpower toxic eating habits*.[24]

Remember, 2 Timothy 1:7 says that we do not have a spirit of fear but of love and power and a *sound mind*. The core of the design of our conscious and nonconscious levels of mind is based on these latter qualities. We are essentially designed to think and choose well; we are made in the image of a powerful, loving God! This is called "the optimism bias" in science.[25] Because of this bias, memories can be willfully redesigned in a positive direction.[26]

This powerful ability to redesign or reconceptualize our thoughts, however, can only take place when these memories move from the nonconscious mind into the conscious mind—that is, when we become aware of our thoughts. As the Scripture says, we need to bring *all thoughts* into captivity (2 Cor. 10:5).[27] We have to *choose* to change our minds.

Our conscious mind operates on a "one thing at a time" sequential basis, within the context of classical physics principles. The conscious level of mind is therefore bound by space and time. This space-time framework enables us to fully direct our attention, focus our reflections, and apply repeated, diligent, and rigorous effort to a particular issue (including what we eat), which leads to true learning.[28] This is called the Quantum Zeno Effect (QZE) in quantum physics.[29] I know this may sound like a highly complex and strange phenomenon, yet it is essentially what is happening as we repeatedly pay attention to and process information. Constantly thinking about something or listening to something creates genetic change, and learning takes place. This can happen with everything: when we are constantly exposed to messages about fast food, for example. These new thoughts become entrenched and implanted into our minds.

The QZE aligns with Proverbs 4:20–22. In this passage, the author cries out, "My son, give *attention* to my words; Incline your ear to my sayings. Do not let them depart from your eyes; Keep them in the midst of your heart; For they are life to those who find them, and health to all their flesh" (emphasis added). Having a healthy mind, body, and spirit begins in the mind, when we start implanting healthy lifestyle patterns of *thinking* in our nonconscious mind and choose to act on them through our conscious mind. This is a truly hopeful scenario that shows God's loving grace and mercy. When we understand how we wired in an unhealthy mindset, we can wire it out and replace it with a healthy and life-giving mindset. And this ability to change the landscape of our brains goes for all thoughts, not just food thoughts! God really did design us with the amazing ability to renew our minds (Rom. 12:2).

## The Level of the Senses

The symbolic output level, the third section on the schematic of my theory, incorporates the five senses through which we express ourselves and experience the world. These senses are the bridge between the external world that we inhabit and the internal world of our mind.[30] We experience the events and circumstance of our lives through our senses, including what we taste, what food we smell, what food and food marketing commercials we see, what food advertisements we hear, and what foods we touch. Our senses are therefore a food battleground, and we have to *choose* what we will allow inside our mind.

## A Perfect Circle

The Geodesic Information Processing Model operates as a perfect circle. Information from the events and circumstances of life (including marketing messages about food and the latest diet fads) comes in through our five senses and is received by the conscious cognitive level. This incoming information activates the four to seven related memories/mindsets to move from the nonconscious level to the conscious level of the mind. These existing mindsets/ belief systems/clusters of thoughts with their intertwined emotions or attitudes, as I mentioned earlier, shape how you perceive and think about the incoming information. As you pay directed and focused repetitive attention to this thought, a short-term memory is built. Over time (sixty-three days, to be precise, as mentioned earlier) it will become an automatized memory (a habit) and will move into your nonconscious mind, dynamically influencing your conscious mind. And so the perfect circle goes on.

## The Mind versus Big Food

A frightening example of this circle is food marketing. Marketing campaigns firehose information into your conscious mind through your five senses. This sensory information is designed to grab your attention with emotional and visual effects that fire up the senses, which, in turn, excite the brain. This excitement occurs as your mind tells your brain what to do with the incoming information, establishing the ideal conditions for building memory. In addition, the repetition factor in food marketing through various media such as billboards, radio, displays in retail centers, magazines, newspapers, books, and the internet on a continual basis will succeed in planting and automatizing these memories into your nonconscious mind—but only *if you choose to pay attention to them with your conscious mind*. This is precisely because whatever you pay attention to on a regular and continual basis becomes automatized as part of your long-term memory store.

Indeed, because your nonconscious mind drives your conscious mind, whatever you implant in your nonconscious mind influences your conscious mind within the context of the circle discussed above. This circle acts as a continual feedback loop, promoting whatever eating patterns you have planted in your mind. The more the circle focuses on a particular thought, the stronger that thought grows.

## Getting Ads Stuck in Your Head?

What does this look like in real, everyday life? Here is an example: you take your kids to school along the same route each day, you see and hear the same food-related radio advertisements, billboards, and fast-food establishments on a daily basis. Every day, these purposefully designed and emotionally laden food advertisements follow the circle between your nonconscious mind and conscious mind, and their messages are reinforced in a rigorous, disciplined way. By the sixty-third day, these food messages have turned from short-term memories into long-term memories. In other words, this repeated exposure to food marketing causes learning to take place, which eventually becomes part of your long-term memory; it has been automatized into a *habit*. You have actually changed your brain structure, which is neuroplastic, through changing your gene expression with your *thoughts*.[31] This process is the Quantum Zeno Effect (QZE) I discussed earlier. You have built a memory/mindset of *I am hungry now. Fast-food places sell yummy food.* Suddenly you are feeling hungry, or your children are complaining that they want something to eat, and the first thing you think of is that cheeseburger that was advertised on the radio!

Yet we *can consciously* override these food habits embedded in the conscious mind and rewire them, as I discussed earlier. Many individuals in the scientific community and business world tell us that we cannot change who we are or overcome bad habits, that we are essentially victims who have brain diseases. However, if we line up science with God's written Word and our scientific interpretations are led by the Holy Spirit, we will be able to see a glorious world where we *can* change and *can* overcome whatever is thrown our way. By our choices, we are more than conquerors through Jesus Christ (Rom. 8:37). Each time we make a choice, we collapse probability into a reality. We make something that has not yet happened into a real physical thought, which in turn impacts every one of our approximately 75–100 trillion cells. This collapsing of probabilities through our choices is called the *observer effect* in quantum physics; it is happening all day long as we are doing life.[32]

The example above highlights the *potential* power of food marketing, and the need for us to constantly be on our guard (1 Cor.

16:13). If we are not aware of the impact of our environment, we will unintentionally be collapsing probabilities into realities—realities that have very real consequences. That cheap fast-food hamburger you are eating was a probability that collapsed into an actuality on the first bite.

We must continually monitor what passes through our five senses. Whatever you think about will grow, and what you grow is what you do (Prov. 23:7). Essentially, whatever you are paying attention to and thinking about becomes part of the memories/mindsets in your nonconscious mind, influencing the choices made by your conscious mind. Indeed, the real tragedy of the food marketing example is that this disciplined and repeated memory-building process should be applied to our thinking, our schoolwork, our jobs, and other healthy pastimes—not the consumption of processed, MAD, food-like products.

Unfortunately, one of the most stubborn mindsets we have to contend with tells us that we are too busy to do the mental work to change our eating habits and too busy to prepare meals at home. We will explore this hurry sickness next, with a view to uprooting it from our minds. We will also look at the link between hurry sickness and television viewing and explore the effects that television has on our food mindsets.

# 11

## Toxic Schedules and Television: Twin Enemies of Our Minds

### Hurry Sickness

I do understand that many of us live incredibly busy lives. Indeed, I would go so far as to say that many of us have what I call toxic schedules: rest is a luxury we frequently yearn for. And, when it comes to food, our fast-paced modern lifestyles have produced the mindset of *I am too busy to cook, and convenient foods at least give me a little bit of time to do what I want. I just need a break.* Sticking that TV dinner in the microwave, and getting our comfy chair ready in front of the TV to watch the latest celebrity show, seems to be a far better deal than fussing about in the kitchen trying to prepare something edible, knowing we will have to clean all those pans later. After a long, hard day's work in our cubicle, even the idea of preparing quinoa and chopping some fresh cucumber and tomatoes seems as if we have just been handed one of those twenty-page-paper topics we were assigned in college.

Although modern technology has made our lives easier in many respects, thereby saving time for the things we like to do, it is nevertheless a two-edged sword.[1] As James Gleick notes in *Faster: The Acceleration of Just About Everything*, these advances have in fact made it easier for us to work *all the time*.[2] We essentially live under the Directorate of Time: the clock has become our master.[3] Indeed, we can fall into the trap of living under an unnecessary sense of urgency, which can put us in chronic toxic stress and make us ill—and give us terrible indigestion.[4] Is it any wonder more and more of us suffer from discomforting stomach ailments?

This hurry sickness now drives a significant part of our daily lives, challenging the value of a good, homemade meal with fresh, *real food* ingredients.[5] Sitting in front of the television and watching in-depth discussions on famous break-ups with our microwave meal in hand now seems like a much better deal for many of us. Certainly, I am taking some liberty with my caricature, yet if we are honest with ourselves there is more than a little bit of truth in the picture I have painted. It never ceases to amaze me that more people know about the latest hair color of a celebrity than where their food comes from. And yet healthy food is essential for life!

The rise of what journalist and activist Eric Schlosser calls a "fast-food nation" has in fact contributed to our hurry sickness.[6] According to Gleick, fast-food establishments "have created whole new segments of the economy by understanding, capitalizing on, and in their own ways *fostering our haste*."[7] The more we patronize such institutions with our hard-earned money, the more we build a mindset (through the QZE and the perfect circle between the conscious and nonconscious mind) that food should be cheap, fast, and prepared with little effort or time.

Under this Directorate of Time, we can become nutritionally starved even though we are surrounded by what appears to be an abundance of food. As I mentioned in part 1, today we have a new health threat: more and more people suffer from both obesity *and* malnutrition.[8] Our current food system is overloaded with empty calories that do not sufficiently meet our nutritional requirements, and an increasing number of us are suffering, both mentally and physically, as a result.[9]

## Eat Less from a Box, Eat Less in Front of a Box: Toxic TV Schedules

Talking about the effect of food marketing on our nonconscious and conscious mind leads us to a discussion about television and how it plays into poor food habits. First, I am in no way against television in general. I have my own television show, and my son Jeffrey loves film production and screenwriting. I myself watch television (yes, I am a *Downton Abbey* fan!), and I believe that all forms of media can be wonderful sources of relaxation, cultural communication, and learning.

Yet *excessive* television viewing is one of the defining features of our modern culture and correlates with mental and bodily ill health.[10] For example, a study of more than two thousand toddlers showed that watching TV between the ages of one and three was linked to attention span issues and a decreased ability to control impulses later on in childhood. Every hour spent watching TV increased toddlers' chance of focus and attention problems by a frightening 10 percent.[11] A 2015 study published in the journal *Infant Behavior and Development* supports the findings of this earlier paper, putting this correlation in startling terms: "cognitive, language, and motor *delays* in young children were significantly associated with how much time they spent viewing television."[12] Similar correlations between viewing time and mental and physical wellbeing have been found for both adolescents and adults.[13]

How is this risk related to our eating habits in particular? Because governmental bodies and food conglomerates use the television to market their food-like products to both adults and children, the MAD food diet is being wired into the nonconscious minds of every individual who is not aware of its influence, including toddlers. We merge with our environments because of the plasticity of our brains, and environmental influences can become our new norm if we are not guarding our thoughts.[14] Wired-in mindsets are *learned* mindsets and may feel normal because of familiarity, even if the mindset or habit is essentially unhealthy and toxic.[15]

## Toxic Targets: Are Our Children for Sale?

As a society, we should be especially concerned about the impact of food marketing on our children. A growing body of research shows that a greater familiarity with fast-food restaurant advertising is linked to an increased chance of obesity among children and young adults and is associated with the consumption of high-calorie snacks, drinks, and fast food, and a lower consumption of fruit and vegetables.[16] For instance, in one study individuals who were surrounded on a daily basis by images of predominantly MAD foods via TV advertisements, billboards, magazines, and other forms of media were more likely to overindulge when they ate a meal.[17] Constant exposure to food cues within our environment impacts eating habits. This impact in turn suggests that the advertising does indeed make us think more about food.[18] Likewise, several research projects indicate that children are far more likely to eat unhealthy, calorie-dense foods when they drink sugar-sweetened beverages (SSBs) *and* if they watch excessive amounts of television.[19] Another study showed that each additional hour in front of the television increased the likelihood of regular consumption of sugary beverages by an alarming 50 percent.[20]

And children are constantly surrounded by these MAD food images. The average child will be exposed to approximately thirteen food commercials every day, or 4,700 a year, while teenagers see more than sixteen food advertisements per day, or 5,900 a year.[21] These statistics are related to television viewing only and exclude food commercials in other mediums of advertising such as magazines, shopping malls, *schools*, social media, and so on.[22] What is the cost to their health? The "eat-more-processed-foods" message is wired into their nonconscious minds through repetition and automatized learning. These learned habits or mindsets will shape their conscious thoughts about food, and thereby their food choices. Is it any wonder then that exposure to MAD food advertising is associated with higher consumption of fast food by children?[23]

Unfortunately, food marketing campaigns directed at young people are a global phenomenon. MAD food and drink advertisements are common during children's TV programs in the United Kingdom, Ireland, and across the Americas, to name just a few regions.[24] The food industry spends $1.8 billion per year in the United States alone on food marketing targeted to young people.[25] The overwhelming majority of these ads are for unhealthy products high in empty calories, sugar, unhealthy fats, and/or salt.[26]

Although policies and regulations have been introduced to control food marketing, they are often flawed. Statutory legislation to control children's exposure to highly processed and sugar-laden foods on television was introduced in the United Kingdom in 2007, and similar regulations have recently been established in Ireland.[27] However, these regulations are not applied to program content, while the American food industry remains largely, and unsuccessfully, self-regulated.[28]

With an estimated two hundred million school-aged children overweight or obese globally, the impact of food marketing is truly a *global* health issue.[29] As the MAD food industry continues to insufficiently self-regulate its marketing agendas, more and more youth are crippled with lifestyle diseases that can affect their future development, spirit, soul, and body.[30] Is this not a form of child abuse?[31] Is it not our responsibility as the guardians of future generations to do all we can to create a healthy environment for them to develop in? Is it not our task to love, care for, and protect our children (Ps. 127:3; Matt. 19:14; 1 Tim. 3:12)? With children as young as two years of age being treated for obesity, and official bodies such as The Obesity Society (TOS) concluding that SSBs contribute to the US obesity epidemic, especially among children, we need to start asking ourselves these difficult questions.[32]

## This Is Your Brain on "Speed"

Up to now we have been speaking of television's influence. Now let's consider social media too. It turns out that TV and social media actually increase our hurry sickness because media outlets flow at a much faster pace than real life.[33] Indeed, new forms of media are getting faster as technology advances. A Twitter post, for example, has an estimated life span of roughly a second, if your followers subscribe to a lot of other profiles.[34] Again, I am not against these forms of media per se. I do have a Twitter account, as well as a Facebook page and an Instagram profile. Yet as we become saturated in a high-paced media culture, we tend to develop an increased desire for these whirlwind transitions because they satisfy the processing speeds of the brain ($10^{27}$ bits per second).[35] We are essentially designed to do busy well.[36]

Television in particular, with its cuts, edits, zooms, pans, and sudden noises, changes the brain by triggering the release of dopamine and various other transmitters related to neuroplasticity, and therefore learning.[37] Indeed, your entire body responds to fast-paced media forms. As Norman Doidge explains in *The Brain That Changes Itself: Stories of Personal Triumph from the Frontiers of Brain Science*:

> The response is physiological: the heart rate decreases for four to six seconds. Television triggers this response at a far more rapid rate than we experience it in life, which is why we can't keep our eyes off the TV screen, even in the middle of an intimate conversation,

and why people watch TV a lot longer than they intend. Because typical music videos, action sequences, and commercials trigger orienting responses at a rate of one per second, watching them puts us into continuous orienting response with no recovery. No wonder people report feeling drained from watching TV. *Yet we acquire a taste for it and find slower changes boring.*[38]

Even your heart and entire body get accustomed to the speed of modern life! Thus, you have to remember that what your brain and body will be learning is based on *your choices*. The more you choose to watch television and/or participate in fast-paced social media outlets, or allow your children to do so, the more your brain will change, and the more you will desire the "speedy" rush. Ultimately, there is a fine balance between being intellectually stimulated through conversation, learning, and understanding and becoming negatively addicted to these swift forms of media as one picture or video or piece of information after another floods your senses.[39]

## Following the Leader: You Control the Circle

Despite the fact that we feel the pull of the sensory information coming into our conscious minds through the media commercials, we *can control* how we process this information. Indeed, one of my favorite advertisements is for a fast-food establishment in South Africa—it makes me laugh every time I watch it on YouTube! Yet the message behind this particular commercial has no effect whatsoever on me, since my nonconscious mind is embedded with information on how the fast food was produced and what effect it will have on me if I consume it. These memories/mindsets are immediately brought up from my nonconscious mind into my conscious mind when I view this commercial. When this happens, I do not crave the fast food, or think I should go to a fast-food establishment when I am hungry—I just laugh because the advertisement

111

is genuinely funny. I have *learned* to control my reactions to the sensory information I receive through *directing my mind*.

Yet what will happen if you do not plant healthy mindsets into your nonconscious mind? You feel thirsty, so you think *soda*, and choose to go out and purchase a soda because you associate that soda with the happiness of the marketing campaign you saw on television. You may not believe that you will be transplanted to a gorgeous beach with happy individuals drinking soda, while dolphins leap excitedly in the background, but the positive emotions associated with the idea of fun, relaxation, and friendship imbue that sugary drink with a strong appeal. The perfect circle has built a mindset that says, *I am thirsty. And if I drink this soda I will quench my thirst . . . and be happier.*

Now you may say that the scenario I have painted is ridiculous, and that you do not think like that at all. Ultimately, however, we each live out of what we have built into our nonconscious minds. The reason fast-food corporations spend millions of dollars associating soda with contentment is because these commercials make soda attractive *in your mind*.[40] When you think of that soda, your nonconscious mind will bring up the four to seven happy memories that the advertisement promised, or the short-term satisfaction associated with a past experience involving soda. These corporations do not hold a gun to your head, compelling you to drink the soda. Ultimately, *the choice is yours*. And your choices are based on what you have built into your minds.

How could you redesign this mindset? You need to learn how to *think* about soda again. First, you need to bring that thought about soda *into captivity* (2 Cor. 10:5). Remember that journal article about the relationship between added sugar consumption and lifestyle-related diseases like diabetes. Remember that documentary on today's obesity pandemic, and how our children may end up living lives that are more disease-prone and shorter than our own generation. Remember that newspaper article on sugar production and slavery in the Dominican Republic. Remember that book on the sugar industry's manipulation of scientific data. Remember the damage to our world's water supplies associated with the large-scale production of soda. Remember the information in *this* book!

Begin *asking* yourself hard questions and accept that there will be some hard answers. Are there not roughly ten teaspoons of sugar in a can of soda?[41] This added sugar can cause your insulin to spike, and the enteric nervous system of your gut (or "gut brain," as we will see in chapter 12) to secrete an abnormal amount of amyloid protein, which will start destroying the blood-brain barrier and can contribute to the formation of the amyloid plaques of Alzheimer's disease.[42] This sugar will bind to the proteins in your blood, and your hemoglobin AC1 can rise in a frightening process called *glycation*, which contributes to neurodegeneration.[43] Excess sugar can be stored as triglycerides in your body, making you gain weight, while your normal stress response has been activated into protect mode, which may cause unhealthy physical responses in your brain and body if it carries on in the long term.[44] And these are just a few of the negative effects excess added sugar consumption may have on your own body. What of the destruction of our planet's natural resources, or the cost in human lives associated with sugar production?[45] Are we being righteous stewards of God's creation? Of our own temples? Are we loving our neighbors, or ourselves?

Now, does that soda actually live up to its commercial promises? If you examine the facts behind soda production and consumption, think critically about the impact of the soda industry and your own choices in terms of both your own life and the world, and plant these thoughts in your nonconscious mind through this process of "asking, answering, and discussing,"[46] the next time you watch that TV advertisement your reaction will be determined by an entirely different set of memories. Memories that *you have chosen to implant in your mind*; memories that will determine whether or not *you choose* to drink the soda. You choose life or death with your food thoughts and food choices (Deut. 30:19–20).

## The Choice Is Yours

Yet why do so many people acknowledge that soda is unhealthy—and continue to drink it? I have emphasized choice in the passage above, since information is only as powerful an influence as we allow it to be. We have to *choose* to *process* this information, or create a mindset/habit in our nonconscious minds based on the information we receive on a daily basis through our five senses.

The true cost of soda, and our MAD food system in general, can be frightening. Do we really *want* to acknowledge this cost? Is it not more convenient, and more comforting, to ignore it? And it is certainly difficult to rewire our habits, although it is not impossible. It is easier to continue following old patterns of thinking. And if we have spent sixty-three days or more (which establishes habituated thoughts in our nonconscious minds as discussed above) processing the sensory information we receive from drinking a soda (such as the smell, taste, and touch of soda) in the context of the "good life," reading just one article on the dangers of excess sugar consumption will not necessarily convert us to a healthier lifestyle overnight. The positive marketing of soda, perhaps married to your own happy experiences drinking soda, has (insidiously I would add) become an established memory in your nonconscious mind. Now, "soda = good life" is packing that 90–95 percent punch in terms of influencing how you perceive the information in the article on the dangers of soda consumption. Soda and its association with the good life has been automatized into a powerful nonconscious force in your conscious mind—and thus a powerful force on your choices. And, as the health article fades from your short-term memory within the space of twenty-four to forty-eight hours, the "soda = good life" emerges with a renewed vigor.[47]

After all, you may think to yourself, *How bad can soda really be? Everyone drinks soda. If it were so bad for us, why would the shops and restaurants still sell it? Even my own doctor drinks it! Many hospitals even give Coke to patients as part of their meals. Anyway, nutritionists are always telling us something is bad, then it is good, then it is bad. Not even they know what they are talking about.*

My soda example may sound like a food industry conspiracy theory, but ultimately the choice is yours. On a daily basis, we are all bombarded with sensory information, from all walks of life. Yet we have the ability *to choose how to process* this information. We allow this information to affect our choices. I certainly do not believe the marketing of all products should be completely forbidden (although I find fault with unrestricted marketing of food products to young children), nor do I think we need legislation against diet gurus or individuals who promise that certain foods or ways of eating will heal all our ailments and help us live to a hundred and five. But I do believe we should be taught how to process all the food-related information we come across, and indeed all information we receive through our five senses; we should be taught how to *think critically and develop wisdom*. Once we recognize that we do have this ability to think and choose—to truly think and truly choose for ourselves—we will become empowered to make healthy, life-promoting decisions, not just in terms of what we eat but in every area of our life.

As I keep repeating, the only balanced diet is one that *includes your thoughts.* We need to be selective, indeed "fussy," about what we allow into our heads and what we put on our plates. God has designed the body to work together perfectly. As the apostle Paul noted, "Each part does its own special work, it helps the other parts grow, so that the whole body is healthy and growing and full of love" (Eph. 4:16 NLT). This Scripture not only applies to the church as the body of Christ but to the whole of creation, since we all came from God (Gen. 1:1–31; John 1:3).

Critical thinking is vital, because our choices determine our mindsets. And as we'll learn next, those mindsets aren't just locked away in our brains, far from our stomachs. The truth is that physically there is a tight connection between the mind and the gut. They communicate in ways that scientists have been astonished to discover.

115

# 12

## What's Eating You?

The act of eating is not just a biological function for survival. The consumption of food, as normal as it is, is in fact a highly emotional and metacognitive event. Indeed, this should come as no surprise to us: throughout human history, gathering around a table and eating food has been a way for us to celebrate or commemorate notable seasons, individuals, and events.[1] Meals are a focal point for social gatherings, and sharing food is a powerful medium of communication both within and between cultures. I certainly believe that the joy of preparing a meal and sharing it with people is incredibly powerful and therapeutic. As my daughter likes to say, one seasoning every cook should use is the pleasure of a hearty gathering, which should be sprinkled generously on every plate. Who needs a handful of digestive supplements when you have good, *real* food and good, real company?

Yet meals can have either positive or negative emotional "seasonings," both of which affect the way our bodies digest food. Our gastrointestinal (GI) tract is very sensitive to our emotions, since it is connected to our brain's hypothalamus, which controls the feelings of satiety and hunger and deals with our emotional state of mind. Our mind and gut are acutely interconnected, and thus happiness, joy, and pleasure, as well as anger, anxiety, sadness, and bitterness, for example, trigger physical reactions in our digestive systems. Our large and small intestines are densely lined with neurons, neuropeptides, and receptors (the "doorways" into cells), which are all rapidly exchanging information laden with emotional content. Indeed, we have all experienced this gurgling emotional activity in our guts, colloquially known as being "sick to your stomach," having a "gut feeling," or having "butterflies in your stomach."[2]

Indeed, unless we are aware of what our digestive system is telling us, we may fall into the trap of overeating. The pancreas releases at least twenty different emotionally laden peptides, which regulate the assimilation and storage of nutrients and carry information about satiety and hunger.[3] Do not ignore the information these peptides provide. Just as eating when we are angry or when we are trying to bury another unpleasant emotion will affect the way we assimilate the nutrients in our food, eating when we are not hungry will upset our digestive system.[4] Overeating will make the food we eat or drink less beneficial, since the emotions generated by toxic thinking interfere with the proper workings of our body.

Eating when we are in a distressed emotional state, or not hungry, is essentially like adding every spice and herb in the cupboard to the meal. All these seasonings will destroy the balance of flavors among the meal's components. Emotionally driven food consumption literally adds a flood of chemical, emotional "seasonings" to our food; our digestive system, like our palate, will not know how to interpret such a conflicting range of signals.[5]

When we react incorrectly to the events and circumstances of life, we move into toxic stress, or stages two and three of stress.[6] Toxic stress keeps our "fight or flight" response activated, which inhibits gastrointestinal secretion and reduces blood flow to the gut, thereby decreasing metabolism and affecting our body's ability to digest food.[7] In fact, toxic thinking and emotions, which lead to toxic stress, can affect the movement and contractions of the GI tract, cause inflammation, make us more susceptible to infection, decrease nutrient absorption and enzymatic output, upset the regenerative capacity of gastrointestinal mucosa and mucosal blood flow, irritate intestinal microflora, cause our esophagus to go into spasms, give us indigestion and heartburn by increasing the acid in our stomach, make us feel nauseous, cause existing digestive issues such as stomach ulcers to worsen, and agitate our colon in a way that gives us diarrhea, constipation, and/or extreme bloating.[8] To say that we should not eat food because we are stressed, unhappy, angry, or any other negative emotion is most certainly an understatement.

## A Healthy Gut Is a Happy Mind

Yet thinking good thoughts cannot excuse an unhealthy diet. The digestive system itself is a rich source of neurotransmitters, which carry signals inside the brain and body.[9] In fact, 95 percent of the serotonin and half the dopamine in the body are produced in the gut.[10] Considering these neurotransmitters are famous for their mood-calming and reward effects, respectively, we should be paying a lot more attention to what we are putting in our gut—what we eat affects the way these neurotransmitters function. Indeed, beneficial symbiotic gut bacteria produce benzodiazepine-like substances, which are naturally occurring antianxiety neurochemicals.[11] A healthy gut promotes a calm, satisfied, and happy mind.

## Sweet Dreams Are Made of Cheese

Digestive functioning even affects our sleeping patterns. Researchers have found that people with Irritable Bowel Syndrome (IBS) tend to have enhanced Rapid Eye Movement (REM) sleep.[12] REM sleep is one of the stages of sleep, and we cycle through these stages in specific time periods in order to obtain optimal memory consolidation and restoration of the mind.[13] Since dreaming occurs during REM sleep, disturbed digestion is associated with excess dreaming—so-called "pizza dreams" actually do occur.

The "gut-brain link" is highly influential, two-way communication, affecting everything from our digestion to our sleeping patterns.[14] The "gut brain" and "brain brain" need to engage and talk, and these conversations are controlled by our thought lives. This is why it is so important to make sure our minds are implanted with the Word of God, since our minds affect every part of our bodies.

## Sick to Your Stomach:
## A Brief History of the Mind-Gut Connection

The gut-brain link is not a new discovery. In 1833, American army surgeon William Beaumont treated Alexis St. Martin, a French-Canadian traveler who had been shot in the stomach.[15] The wound left an opening in the skin that allowed Beaumont to observe the pumping, to-and-fro motion of the stomach and also to see what happened when his patient expressed different emotions.[16] St. Martin's stomach, for instance, produced less acid (acid necessary for the proper functioning of the digestive system) when he was fearful, angry, or impatient.[17] In the French-Canadian's stomach, upset thinking led to upset digestion!

Over a century later, Michael Gershon, known as the father of the gut-brain connection, researched and wrote extensively on the effect of thinking and the enteric nervous system (ENS). His work highlighted the GI system's sensitivity to emotions.[18] Anger, anxiety, sadness, elation, pleasure—all of these feelings (and others) trigger symptoms in the gut.[19] Moreover, Gershon showed how the gut-brain connection is a two-way street: the gut feeds back into the brain, thereby affecting the mind.[20] His work has since been supported by numerous studies, and many researchers today continue to probe the complex relationship between thinking and the GI system.[21] The new science of neurogastroenterology was born, which includes the examination of psychosomatic upsets that have a gastrointestinal expression and their relationship to the central nervous system (CNS).[22]

## The Enteric Nervous System

The gastrointestinal (GI) system is controlled by the enteric nervous system (ENS), often called the "second brain."[23] The ENS consists of about 200–600 million nerve cells, which control every aspect of digestion—a considerably higher number of neurons than in the spinal cord.[24] The ENS communicates with the central nervous system (CNS) through the nerve pathways; in fact the ENS originates from the same tissues as the CNS during fetal development. It also contains a number of structural and chemical counterparts to the brain.[25] Indeed, researchers have found that the ENS uses many of the same neurotransmitters, or chemical messengers, as the CNS.[26]

As food makes its thirty-foot journey through the digestive tract, there is ongoing dialogue between the ENS and the brain via the autonomic nervous system (ANS), which controls the body's vital functions.[27] These two systems are connected via the vagus nerve: the tenth cranial nerve that runs from your brain stem down to your abdomen.[28] This back-and-forth communication is why, in normal circumstances, you stop eating when you are full. Sensory neurons in your GI system inform your brain when your stomach is distended and full.[29] Likewise, this communication between these nervous systems also explains why being anxious about something can ruin your appetite or make you feel bloated: the entire gut-brain connection is saturated with our emotions.[30]

## If You're Happy and You Know It, Go and Shop

Our emotions impact not only the way our body digests food but also our choices—before our meal even enters our mouths! As obesity and diet-related statistics continue to rise at an alarming rate, a growing number of officials, organizations, and individuals are demanding better labeling and improved nutritional knowledge.[31] Yet this approach may do little to alleviate our "global eating disorder," since it does not place enough emphasis on thinking and emotional awareness. What is the point of knowledge, including nutritional information, if we do not know how to apply it or if our nonconscious mind is already filled with toxic thoughts about food?

A number of studies indicate that training people to pay attention to their emotions is a far more effective approach to developing a balanced diet than nutritional labeling.[32] People have a tendency to not think about their food choices and the attached emotions when shopping for, preparing, and eating food.[33] Yet some researchers have found that as emotional awareness develops, food choices can be improved with an approach that is geared toward *deep thinking*. In one study, for instance, participants who had received training in recognizing their emotions shed, on average, excess weight over time, whereas the individuals who received no emotional training tended to gain weight.[34] Similarly, a review of thirteen separate studies showed that people with functional gastrointestinal illness who tried psychologically based approaches found greater relief from their symptoms than those who received conventional treatment alone.[35]

When we eat *reactively*, that is, without deliberately examining the mindsets embedded in our nonconscious minds, we increase our risk for making unhealthy food choices. These mindsets may have been shaped by the latest food marketing campaign or by the need to bury our sorrow in a tub of ice cream, but unless we are aware of these memories and their power to influence our choices, how useful is knowing the number of calories per serving or the warnings of health professionals?

If we are honest with ourselves, we understand this "willful blindness" all too well.[36] How many times have we had a bad day and grabbed that tub of ice cream, knowing that it is bad for our health? And how many times have we eaten the whole thing anyway? The nonconscious mindsets of *I have had a bad day; I deserve ice cream* and *Ice cream tastes so good* override the temporary memories of *I know I should not eat this ice cream because I want to be healthy* and *I know that I will regret eating it later* in our conscious mind. Of course, no one has strapped us to a chair and is forcing spoonfuls of ice cream down our throat. We have *selected*, or *chosen*, to suppress our knowledge of the health facts of excessive refined sugar and fat consumption; we have *chosen* to eat the ice cream. However, if we are not aware of how we are selecting certain food-related thoughts, and selecting to ignore other food-related thoughts, how can we truly make the right food choices—food choices that are *sustainable* in the long run because they are built on unyielding, healthy memories? Truly, we are destroyed for a *lack* of knowledge; many of us lack the knowledge of how to apply our knowledge.

It is perhaps not surprising, even if it is troubling, that people still drink soda after I talk on the health dangers of consuming sugary beverages. These members of the audience have chosen to suppress the temporary memory of my talk in their conscious minds in light of the mindsets associated with drinking soda that *they have chosen to implant* in their nonconscious level of mind. Although it saddens me to see people drink soda, it is their choice nonetheless.

Indeed, what we are thinking about when we choose the food we are going to eat influences how we enjoy that meal, and the value we place on that meal. If we believe a certain food is expensive and exclusive, for instance, we will enjoy it more—even if the food is not really any better than its cheaper counterpart.[37]

If we think a certain food is cheap, on the other hand, we place less value on it and enjoy it less, even if it is exactly the same as a more expensive substitute.[38]

Likewise, a number of studies show how individuals, when they are not aware of their eating behavior, will consume food regardless of their hunger level. Paul Rozin, professor of psychology at the University of Pennsylvania, showed that amnesiac patients who were told it was dinnertime ate a second complete meal within ten to thirty minutes after having eaten the first meal, and a third meal ten to thirty minutes after the second meal, even though they could not have been physically hungry. Just *thinking* it was time to have a meal or a snack was enough to make them want to eat![39]

## All You Need Is Love

All the structures of our brains and bodies are *wired for love*. We are made in the image of a perfect God, a God who is love (Gen. 1:26; 1 John 4:8). We are wired to think good thoughts and make good choices. We are designed to wire in healthy, beautiful thoughts and eat healthy, beautiful food. Yet we also have free will, and can choose to do the opposite—but not without *consequences* (Deut. 30:19; Eccles. 7:29).

Emotional awareness in terms of your food choices is so important that I would in all honesty recommend putting "positive attitude" on your shopping list! Feelings rooted in love, such as peace, hope, joy, and compassion, inspire food choices *rooted in love*. According to one study in the *Journal of Consumer Research*, for example, when people are hopeful, they think about the future, and they tend to be aware of eating for the future: a healthy diet is a hopeful diet. On the other hand, when people tend to ruminate on negative things from the past, they are less inclined to purchase food products that promote longevity: if things are so bad anyway, why bother buying that local, organically grown kale?[40] Emotions,

123

choices, and actions cannot be separated since they are part of the perfect circle in your mind, which in turn impacts your entire body. Your thoughts, with their associated emotions, determine what you choose to eat: you are what you eat, *and what you think*.

## The Real "Balanced Meal": Eating for the Spirit, Soul, and Body

The relationship between the gut and the brain, and the relationship between our feelings and shopping habits, are just two examples of the multifaceted, interconnected lives we all lead—a concept often at odds with modernity. We live in a world that tends toward intellectual *reductionism*. Globally, we have become accustomed to a parts-rather-than-whole approach, including the way we approach food. Why else would doctors, as our go-to health figures, have negligible training in nutrition, even at Harvard's medical school?[41] To say that what we eat affects our health is certainly redundant. So how can such a basic, fundamental fact be overlooked when dealing with matters of health and illness?

It is imperative that we shift the way we *think* about health. Our brain is not an input-output machine. Our body is not an input-output machine. We are each intrinsically, brilliantly, and intricately designed with a spirit, soul, and body (Gen. 1:26; 1 Thess. 5:23). This is known as our *triune nature*.[42]

Our triune nature is divided into different components. Our spirit is our "true you," or what I call our *perfectly you*.[43] Our spirit has three parts: intuition, conscience, and communion (worship). Our soul, which is our mind, also has three parts: intellect, will, and emotions.[44] Lastly, our body has three parts: the ectoderm, mesoderm, and endoderm, from which the brain and the body form.[45]

Our mind, or soul, has one foot in the door of the spirit and one foot in the door of the body. The mind creates coherence between the spirit and the body, and therefore influences and controls brain/body function and health, and influences spiritual development. Our mind, with its intellectual ability to choose and its emotional authority, controls *all physical aspects*.[46] Thus emotions, as part of the mind, are an intrinsic part of our food choices.

Our brain is designed to respond to our mind, and our mind is designed to respond to our spirit (John 14:26; 16:3; Rom. 8:14; Gal. 5:16). Every thought, feeling, and action begins in the internal activity of our mind, which means that *we choose with our mind*s to listen to our spirits, *we choose with our minds* to listen to the Holy Spirit speaking truth into our spirit, *we choose with our minds* to act, *we choose with our minds* to speak, and *we choose with our minds* to eat. And all these mind-based choices impact our physical brain and body as well as our spiritual development and mental health. The ultimate question is, what have we implanted in our mind? What mindsets will be shaping our choices? Remember, "as he *thinks* in his heart [*mind*], so is he" (Prov. 23:7, emphasis added).

### Fasting for the Spirit, Soul, and Body

One aid to disciplining the mind is fasting. Whether it involves skipping one meal or more or excluding certain foods from the diet, fasting has played an important role in human history—spiritually and physically. In today's world, however, eating three meals a day is generally understood as healthy, although there is actually no conclusive scientific basis for not skipping breakfast, lunch, or dinner, or even all three occasionally.[47]

A growing body of research actually indicates that different types of fasting can improve health and longevity, such as intermittent fasting (eating fewer meals), caloric restriction (eating less per meal), and alternate day fasting.[48] These types of fasting can potentially improve cardiovascular function, increase longevity, increase resistance to age-related diseases, and enhance mental and physical health in general.[49] Intermittent fasting and caloric restriction both affect energy levels and free-radical production from oxygen metabolism, as well as cellular stress response systems, in ways that protect neurons against genetic and environmental factors while enhancing energy production from the mitochondria, which generate chemical energy in the form of ATP (adenosine triphosphate).[50] Likewise, caloric restriction triggers a decrease in inflammatory factors, which contribute to the onset of disease.[51]

Skipping a few meals on a regular basis can even protect against the onset of illness. Fasting has been shown to enhance brain function and reduce the risk factors for coronary artery disease, stroke, insulin sensitivity, and blood pressure.[52] For instance, restricting calories can support the induction of sirtuin-1 (SIRT1), an enzyme that regulates gene expression and enhances learning and memory. Fasting actually has a similar effect on the body as exercise. Skipping a meal or eating less and exercise are both mediated by brain-derived neurotrophic factor (BDNF), suggesting they are underpinned by similar mechanisms in the body.[53] And we definitely want BDNF mediating! This neurotrophic factor helps maintain brain health, prevents cell death, and builds memory.[54]

In fact, intermittent fasting and caloric restriction can aid intra-brain communication by supporting interactive pathways and molecular mechanisms that specifically provide benefits to the neurons. These pathways produce protective protein "chaperones"—neurotrophic factors like BDNF and essential antioxidants, which help our tiny cells cope with stress and resist disease.[55] Similarly, fasting may protect neurons against the onset of Alzheimer's disease by preventing amyloid beta and tau pathologies on synaptic function.[56] Overall, research on fasting indicates that skipping a meal or two can promote resistance to stroke and neurodegenerative disease. Our food choices literally change the environment around our cells and the environment within our cells—an incredible support system (one of many) that highlights the goodness and mercy of God.[57] By making the right food choices we can change our brains!

## Triune Fasting

On a spiritual level, fasting is a common practice. For example, Greek Orthodox Christians fast from certain foods 180–200 days per year, prior to Easter, Christmas, and the Assumption. Catholic Christians fast from certain foods for approximately forty days before Easter.[58] The Daniel Fast is very common among Christians, and usually lasts between twenty-one and forty days.[59]

Biblically, the call to fast is found throughout both the Old and New Testaments. It is a way for Jews and Christians to make their beliefs part of their everyday lives, in a sense of bringing heaven to earth (Matt. 6:9–13).[60] It enables us to put God above our earthly pleasures, in the sense that we put God first and appreciate food and drink as a gift from him rather than love food and drink in and of themselves.[61] It enables us to become *addicted to God*. We do not fast merely to get healthy and lose weight.[62] We fast for the spirit, soul, and body: by putting God first, "all these things shall be added to you" (Matt. 6:33). The growing body of fasting research actually confirms the integrated triune nature of man, since as we discipline our mind and choose to reduce our bodily food intake and focus on God, our spirit, soul, and body all develop.

Fasting is a way of asserting our mind's and spirit's control over our body. It's so important for us to understand that we have the freedom to choose our mindsets that chapter 13 will briefly address the opposing view, that our physical brains make us do what we do. We'll see that despite the glamor of brain scans, we are very far from being stuck with the mindsets we currently have.

# 13

## This Is Your Brain on Brain Scans

We have all seen the headlines: "This is your brain on drugs"; "This is your brain on porn"; "This is your brain on YouTube cat videos." All right, perhaps not quite the last headline. Nevertheless, the unscrupulous use of brain imaging by media outlets, companies, university press offices, and many researchers seems to offer us physical proof that everything from obesity to murder originates from a brain that is imbalanced or diseased.[1] These visual pictures are misleading when it comes to where the responsibility lies for our health. Our biology is not our destiny.[2] The damage in the brain that results from incorrect lifestyle choices—including what and how we eat—does constrain an individual's ability to think and choose, but it *does not destroy it*.

Based on my research, experiences, and beliefs, I view the brain and mind as separate and, more importantly, I believe that the mind controls the brain. Over the twenty-five years that I practiced clinically and trained thousands of teachers and students and corporations, I saw countless people overcome biological and societal difficulties, pursue their dreams, and succeed. I have met so many people in the course of my travels teaching this message around the world, and have had the privilege of seeing them overcome impossible circumstances. I have seen, both firsthand and in scientific literature, indeed in history, the power of human choice.[3] And I believe in a God who is love, a God who has given us powerful, sound minds (2 Tim. 1:7; 1 John 4:8).

We cannot get excited when we hear sermons about how powerful God has made us and refuse to hear the other side of the coin—that is, that we can use this power incorrectly. If we believe we are fearfully and wonderfully made, there is a heavy responsibility that comes with bearing God's glorious image (Gen. 1:27). If we believe we are powerful lions of God, then we also have to recognize our ability to kill—an ability that can be used for both good and bad. We have to take personal responsibility for the way we think, speak, act, and eat (Luke 6:46; 12:48; 2 Cor. 5:10; James 4:17). We need to stop being victims of our biology, of what happens to us, and start being victors. Are we not more than conquerors through Christ (Rom. 8:37)? Is anything impossible for our God (Matt. 19:26)? We are not meant to just cope. We are called to conquer. We are called to choose *life* (Deut. 30:19).

### My Brain Made Me Do It

Today, there is a massive split in the world of neuroscience. Many scientists believe that the mind is a result of firing neurons: they see the mind as an *emergent property* of the brain.[4] On the other hand, many scientists (myself included) are mind-body dualists: we argue that the mind changes the brain.[5] The neurocentric perspective of the former argument arises out of humankind's desire to worship the created (brain) instead of the Creator.

Indeed, this neurocentric, brain-focused mindset is, alarmingly, influencing all walks of life. It has become increasingly fashionable to assume that the brain is the most important level of analysis for understanding human behavior, and that the mind is more or less expendable, literally a by-product of the brain.[6] We see the firing of neurons and we assume that this is what love or hatred is. Yet what if love causes the neurons to fire? It is a "chicken and egg" question that ultimately requires us to make a judgment based on our own interpretation of the data. In a secular world, I understand, even if I do not agree with, the mechanistic emphasis on the brain and the belief in matter that can be measured in a quantifiable manner held by many scientists and researchers today.[7] Their beliefs have shaped their interpretations of neuroscience, just as my beliefs in an almighty God, human free will, and the intangible power of the mind shape my interpretations of neuroscience.

Yet why is this neurocentric vein of thought so dangerous? Essentially, the "oversimplification, interpretive license, and premature application of brain science in the legal, commercial, clinical, and philosophical domains" can lead us into murky waters when it comes to taking responsibility for our actions.[8] Are you a murderer, or did the different activity seen in that brain scan make you do it? Are you addicted to food because your brain is wired that way, because you have inherited a genetic disposition from your parents—or because you have made choices?

Someone may say, "My brain scan shows I have an overactive amygdala, so it is hard for me to control my emotions and that is why I cannot control my eating." Once you start down this path, you will ultimately have to question your belief in free will, since a predominant focus on the brain takes the control away from the individual and places the blame squarely on the brain.

I do not deny that very real changes will happen in the brain (how the mind changes the brain is my area of expertise) when we lead a toxic eating and thinking lifestyle, nor do I deny that some individuals do have damaged brains through no fault of their own. Yet for the most part the mind (that is, our thoughts and choices) comes first, which causes problems in the brain and body, which in turn feed back into the mind, making us feel awful if our mind is toxic.

## There Is No Excuse for Excuses

Even if we do feel awful from wrong lifestyle choices, we need to stop looking for excuses and recognize that the mind is more powerful than the brain and body. Where the mind goes, the brain and body follow. In most instances we got there first with our mind, so we can get back to a good place in the same way: with our mind.

The colorfully illuminated brain on an fMRI scan, SPECT, or other imaging technology cannot be trusted to offer an in-depth view of the mind. This phenomenal but developing and limited technology provides a mere glimpse into activity happening in the brain in terms of energy, glucose metabolism, and blood flow.[9] It *does not show our thoughts*. Neuroscientists are very far from determining the exact link between what they see on the scans and the content of our thoughts.[10] Brain-imaging technology cannot read your thoughts, desires, loves, lies, feelings, morals, or the uniqueness of who you are—nor what is going on in your mind when it comes to eating.

To some neuroscientists and philosophers, you may be nothing more than your brain, but to God, you are a spirit, soul, and body—uniquely, fearfully, and wonderfully made—the crowning glory of his creation (Ps. 139:14). This gives us great hope for getting eating right so we can have healthy bodies, brains, and minds. Our brains and bodies have to do what we tell them to do through our minds (our choices, which are real electromagnetic and quantum signals with real chemical effects in the brain and body).

It is not logical to see behavior, including food choices, as beyond a person's control simply because some associated neural activity can be seen in the brain. As psychiatrist Sally Satel and psychologist

Scott O. Lilienfeld explain in *Brainwashed: The Seductive Appeal of Mindless Neuroscience*:

> Scans alone cannot tell us whether a person is a shameless liar, loyal to a product brand, compelled to use cocaine, or incapable of resisting an urge to kill. In fact, brain-derived data currently *add little or nothing* to the more ordinary sources of information we rely on to make those determinations; mostly, they are *neuroredundant*. At worst, neuroscientific information sometimes distorts our ability to distinguish good explanations of psychological phenomena from bad ones.[11]

We know someone is a shameless liar when they lie shamelessly. The same can be said for loyal customers, addicts, and murderers. Viewing their brain activity on a slide is essentially "neuroredundant" in terms of knowing that they have chosen to do these things. If we look for answers on a brain scan, we can fall into the trap of seeking all the solutions to all our problems in an image of glucose metabolism, energy, and blood flow. This is scientific reductionism at its worst, focusing myopically on a sense of "we are what our neurons do."

Brain scans are essentially as accurate as trying to hear the exact conversation in the street below when you are standing on the roof of a skyscraper.[12] You may see the mouths moving, but you will not hear the conversation. By the same token, brain scans see activity but they don't know the actual conversation happening within the depths of the brain as the result of the mind in action. Such an overreliance on information from brain imaging does a great injustice to the beautiful complexity of the scientific method as a means of understanding the beautiful complexity of God's creation.

It's clear, then, that we have both the precious freedom and the awesome responsibility to choose our mindsets. They aren't determined by our brains or our genes. Let's take a closer look at how that responsibility plays itself out with respect to the destructive eating habits in which we or our children can find ourselves ensnared.

# 14

## Confused Emotions, Destructive Behaviors

Many diet plans today are principally based on behavioral changes. They all tell us that we need to exercise more and eat better, often with some elaborate plan that feels like someone has just removed the joy from eating and locked all pleasure in a dark medieval dungeon. But remember, our minds are more powerful than our behavior—our minds direct our behavior. The only way weight will come off, and stay off, is through our minds: when we plant healthy food "trees" in our brains with our minds, we will eat heathy food in reality.

When we discipline, or renew, our minds, we change how we think about eating, thereby changing the framework of our food choices. The nonconscious mind is very influential in our thinking and choosing, as I have discussed earlier, but the equally powerful conscious mind can override the past. Until we build an *awareness mindset* of how and when to eat, with the correct emotions attached to the process of choosing and eating food, *sustainable* weight loss will not occur. We literally have to convince our dominant nonconscious level of mind (95 percent of brain function, remember) by building an automatized, reconceptualized mindset into it, which replaces the reason we have an unhealthy diet, and unhealthy weight, in the first place. We do this convincing; we take charge of our minds. The toxic behaviors of our pasts do not have to take over our future. We are what we think.

Yet this change is not instant. It takes twenty-one days to rewire neural pathways, plus another forty-two days for a full sixty-three days to firmly build these new mindsets into our nonconscious level of mind so that we use them and actual change is evident in our life.[1] Any diet that promises instant results should come under our intellectual radar; real, permanent change always takes time and effort. No amount of positively affirming that *I will not eat that ice cream, even if I had a hard day and feel I deserve it* will succeed single-handedly in the creation of healthy eating patterns. Until the toxic food mindset that dominates our minds is dealt with, we are essentially swimming vigorously against the tide of thoughts in our own heads. We are fighting a battle we do not *believe* we can win.

But we can win. God designed the human mind with an absolutely breathtaking ability to change itself. We can renew our thinking (Rom. 12:2). I will address the techniques for correcting thinking patterns in part 3 of this book, and more information on renewing the mind scientifically and spiritually can be found in my book *Switch On Your Brain.*[2]

## The Apple Never Falls Far from the Tree

What we choose to eat affects not only our health, but our children's health as well. At first glance this statement may sound redundant. Of course, what we choose to cook and eat, our children will eat as well. Yet we are not only giving them a meal. We are teaching them a way of eating—a food mindset that they can carry with them throughout their lives. It is therefore imperative that we as parents and guardians focus on teaching our children about dealing with emotions and healthy eating patterns.

*Children will do what we do, not what we say.* A sedentary lifestyle and poor diet can predispose a child to a toxic, lifestyle-related illness, even in the happiest of families where emotions are balanced.[3] Nourishing lifestyle patterns that foster a healthy response to the need to eat must be established at a young age.[4]

We also need to teach our children about their emotions and how to handle them, even when it is uncomfortable for everyone involved. Confused emotions create disorders in the mind, which in turn will produce behaviors that are equally confused and self-destructive.[5]

## The Elephant in the Dining Room: Eating Disorders

One category of self-destructive food behavior is eating disorders. Much research has focused on how negative, destructive emotions contribute to anorexia nervosa, bulimia, and other eating disorders.[6] These are seen as *emotional eating patterns.* Yet there has been a sore lack of research that could help gain insight into how positive emotions are distorted by those suffering with these life-threatening disorders, which have a death rate up to twelve times higher than all other causes of death combined for females between the ages of fifteen and twenty-four.[7]

One recent study, however, has highlighted the role normal, positive emotions can play in exacerbating eating disorders. The researchers found that the subjects of the study battled with negative emotions such as poor body image, in addition to having a paradoxically positive sense of pride over being able to maintain and exceed their weight-loss goals. Indeed, this study also found

135

that the women who had the most difficulty understanding how to recognize when positive emotions were becoming distorted (through their thinking) engaged in more frequent anorexia-type behaviors such as vomiting, laxative use, restricting calories, excessively exercising, checking body fat, and constantly controlling weight. Many of the participants knew they were damaging their health, yet their sense of pride at their results helped maintain their destructive eating habits.[8]

Yet eating disorders are *disorders*, not *diseases*. Change in these life-threatening patterns of food consumption comes with *choosing to change* based on an awareness of the fundamental *need to change*. The concept of a brain disease is very limiting and almost always gives a sense of hopelessness: the view that you are what your brain does, and there is really nothing you alone can do about it. A brain disorder, on the other hand, brings hope in the sense that although there have been significant biological changes in the brain, the brain can change (neuroplasticity). The mind is more powerful than the brain: it directs the change.

Choosing to change and quit a toxic thinking pattern can in fact result in brain regrowth. A number of psychologists and neuroscientists have found that adult brain volume, which can be reduced by anorexia nervosa and other eating disorders, can also be regained through changing thinking patterns or mindsets.[9] Renewing your mind does not just apply to changing the way you think. By *choosing* to change the way you think, you can literally regain gray matter in the brain! When God said his plans for you are full of hope, he truly meant it (Jer. 29:11).

## Processed Food and Addiction

Eating disorders necessarily bring me to the topic of food addictions. All addictions are similar in that the sufferer craves the feel-good buzz they receive from their chemical neurotransmitters when they binge eat, gamble, smoke, have sex, or take drugs.[10] The term "food addiction" certainly tends to conjure up a vision of obese individuals hiding in a pantry and eating uncontrollably in the dark.

Yet it is more important to consider the concept of food *and* addiction, versus food addiction. In other words, how does something that is biologically necessary for life become an addiction? It is different from an addiction to alcohol or drugs, which are not necessary for survival.[11] Have we altered our foods in such a way as to make them particularly prone to becoming addictive?[12] Why do we not get addicted to kale or tomatoes as easily as potato chips or soda, for example?

Among many food researchers, there is a consensus that the food-like products more and more of us are consuming today can influence brain function in an addictive way by distorting normal thinking pathways.[13] As I discussed in part 1, the three main constituents of processed, preserved, and refined foods in particular—sugar, salt, and fat—can hijack brain function and constrain our ability to choose.[14] I briefly mentioned studies done by major food companies on calculating "bliss points," where taste buds are titillated "scientifically" to determine the point at which foods will literally be irresistible or the point where we will want more and more, thereby giving birth to potential "food addictions."[15] Through this process, damage can occur in the brain.[16]

Walter Willet, chair of Harvard's department of nutrition and also one of the single most cited nutritionists today, points his finger directly at the food companies when it comes to today's food system. Willet regards the transformation of food into an industrial product, which I discussed in part 1, as stripping away most of the nutrition from our foods.[17] Processed sugar, salt, fat, and other components of food have been distorted and made into decontextualized and concentrated forms of their original design.[18] Is it any wonder, then, that these foods impact our brains like drugs?[19]

It gets worse. Although the food industry is well aware of the power of manipulating our taste preferences and reward circuitry in the brain, as we saw in part 1, the government does not regulate their efforts. The food industry "is not required to test its products for addictive effects on the brain or the extent to which constituents of its food provoke overeating."[20] Of course, if someone deliberately designed a product in such a way as to manipulate your biological processes in order to make more money, you would be outraged. Yet why are the food industries allowed to do so without encumbrance?

Indeed, the high amounts of refined and processed sugar, salt, and fat in the majority of MAD foods, and thus the majority of food products many of us consume today, are incredibly alarming from a brain science perspective. These ingredients cause massive abnormal dopamine releases each time they are consumed, in far greater amounts than we have ever before been accustomed to in human history.[21] Dopamine enhances memory formation, so the memories of these foods keep getting stronger, reinforced in our minds with toxic effects. These foods are particularly adept at getting us "hooked."[22] This is called the plastic paradox: our mind changes our brain's wiring in response to external signals.[23]

Why is this a paradox? The signals that change our brains can be good or bad. The same plasticity principles are employed as we wire in a good or a bad habit. Yet if the mind can change the brain, why are unhealthy habits so hard to break? We used plasticity to build these habits over time; we used plasticity to implant them in our souls. As you well know, whatever you think about the most grows. Thus, by the same token, the same kind of effort goes into breaking the habit, but because we are reversing the tide, there is effort involved. Plasticity does not equal effortlessness. Plasticity means change, and true change is never effortless.

Essentially, where our mind goes, our brain follows. As you will recall, our thoughts make up roughly 80 percent of these signals, and other external factors make up the remaining 20 percent.[24]

Good, healthy signals equal good, healthy brain changes, while bad, unhealthy signals equal bad, unhealthy brain changes.

Yes, the process of change is a challenge. Yet remember, we are designed by God to bring all thoughts into captivity (2 Cor. 10:5). Regardless of how subtle and clever the marketing campaigns of the food industry are, and how irresistible the bliss point becomes, we still have the mind of Christ (1 Cor. 2:16). We are not machines running on chemicals, and we are not victims of our biology. We are highly intellectual, thinking and choosing beings made in the image of a perfect God (Gen. 1:27). And we have been given the Holy Spirit to aid us, who is far more powerful than a cheeseburger craving (Rom. 8:26–27).

### Are We Hooked on Being Hooked?

Addiction, including food addiction, is not a chronic, lifelong disease, as the current biomedical model depicts it to be.[25] According to the American Society of Addiction Medicine (ASAM), addiction is "a primary, chronic disease of brain reward, motivation, memory, and related circuitry."[26] However, there is extensive evidence, particularly in population studies, that the vast majority of people who quit addictions do so on their own.[27]

Unfortunately, "food addiction" is being placed into the same brain disease category, which inevitably aims to remove responsibility from the individual.[28] According to this vein of thinking, being overweight or obese becomes something we just have to cope with, "very much like the management of other chronic diseases, such as asthma, hypertension or diabetes," says Dr. Daniel Alford at Boston University Medical Center. "It's hard necessarily to cure people, but you can certainly manage the problem to the point where they are able to function through a combination of pharmaceuticals and therapy."[29] The brain disease model and food addiction language focus predominately on bearing, not healing, lifestyle-related issues.

Of course, God did not say that life would be easy and carefree. But Christ did come to set us free and give us life abundantly (Luke 4:18; John 10:10). He came to heal us (Exod. 15:26; Ps. 30:2; Matt. 9:35; Mark 5:34; Luke 8:43–48; James 5:16). God has made all things new in Christ Jesus (2 Cor. 5:17; Col. 1:20). Jesus has already won the victory (John 16:33; 1 Cor. 15:57; 2 Cor. 2:14). We are more than conquerors through Christ (Rom. 8:37). We were never created to just *cope*.

### We Are Designed to Be Addicted . . . to Love

Our brain's reward circuits fire up a neurophysiological response par excellence when we think and eat in a healthy way. God has given us an incredible variety of foods, and ways of eating, which are exactly what we need specific to where we live. I call this the "wired for love" concept that is operational in our brains and bodies, and in this universe we inhabit. Indeed, God is love, and the whole of his creation is therefore based on the principle of love (1 John 4:8, 16).

When we try to recreate foods in such a way as to go against the design of nature rather than mimic nature, as I discussed in part 1, we interfere with God's plan. Ultimately, science is here to understand God's universe, not to recreate it: science explains the "how" of creation. It enables us to learn "how" to steward God's world in a way that allows it to function optimally within its own created parameters. Indeed, with a sense of awe and humility we are able to learn from nature through biomimicry. Science is not here to improve on a design that is *already* good. The latter is an "eating from the tree of knowledge" approach: we think we can do better than God (Gen. 3:5).

Taking this into the world of addiction, reward circuits in the brain become hijacked by our choices (mind), which change the brain physically. Defunct biology is not to blame.[30] The toxic reward circuits from wrong thoughts and wrong food choices (and other environmental factors) in a circular feedback loop can certainly affect the clarity of the mind. In fact, the foods our parents ate also affect our health epigenetically.[31] Yet the mind is still stronger than the brain: Christ said he would never give us any more temptation than we are able to bear, and he has provided a way for us to bear it (1 Cor. 10:13). The brain will rewire, or renew, in the direction the mind sends it; as discussed above, this is known as the plastic paradox.[32] This is why the vast majority of people can and do quit addictions on a daily basis. Choosing to get out of a toxic addiction is what testimonies, and indeed miracles, are made of.

## Fight Fire with Fire

If the food corporations are deliberately thinking about how to get us to buy their products, it is time for us to be *deliberately thinking about* what this is doing to our life, our loved ones, and our planet—and what we can do to fight back. All of us should be planning how we can fight back in our own unique way. Whether it is growing a garden, raising chickens, lobbying, farming, cooking, blogging, writing, speaking, filming, dancing, or whatever our passion is: we name it, we believe in it, and we do it. We all have an incredible power to think, which enables us to succeed at whatever we "put our minds to"—literally!

Just reading the statement above gives us the power to override the influence of the food industry. Because of neuroplasticity, what we read changes our brain, which can start to change the way we think.[33] We merge with our environments, and if we *choose* not to merge with the current food system, if we choose to opt out of its dysfunctional MAD diet, we will be amazed at how our life can change. Wherever our mind goes, our brain follows.

Awareness and knowledge are powerful tools in the "thinking" fight against the MAD diet. Reading the information in this book should be only the beginning of the journey; there are a number of incredible references in the endnotes to this book that will increase our knowledge arsenal. In fact, just knowing that the grocery store layout is designed to get us to purchase processed and refined food-like products by companies that do not have our health as their bottom-line focus can empower us to make more life-sustaining food choices and dramatically shift our mindset behind the meal.

## What Kind of Addict Do You Want to Become?

We are designed to be addicted to God. Our brains are wired to latch onto something, and that something is God. Any toxic addiction, whether it be to food, drugs, or even a person, is the result of misplaced choice. Yet, as a growing body of research shows, the majority of people can quit addictions.[34] Individuals who stay addicts usually subscribe to the biomedical model and defeatist philosophy of "once an addict, always an addict."[35] Yet God came to set us free, not lock us in (Luke 4:18). As C. S. Lewis said in *The Weight of Glory*, "We are far too easily pleased."[36] Do not make food your idol, nor any other created thing. It will always disappoint you, but God never will.

Never forget that you are more than an addiction. The toxic choices you may have made in the past do not define you. You are defined by your identity in Christ (Gen. 1:27; 1 Cor. 6:17; 12:27; Gal. 3:27–28; Col. 2:9–10). You are his child—you are his heir (John 1:12; Eph. 1:5; 1 Pet. 2:9; 1 John 3:1–2). Let us start acknowledging this divine identity in our food choices as well. This is what it means to "seek first the kingdom of God and His righteousness, and all these things shall be added to you" (Matt. 6:33). Seek Christ first, and the pleasure of *real* food and good health will come as a by-product of being addicted to him.

Let us start this process of change by increasing our knowledge of what *real* food is; let us start changing our attitude toward food;

let us start developing the skills necessary to change. We must *choose* life (Deut. 30:19).

And we can choose. As we'll see in the next chapter, not even our genes are set in stone and beyond the reach of changes. The science of epigenetics is teaching us how environment and choice alter even our genes.

# 15

# Me, Myself, and My Epigenetic Environment

In 1988 John Cairns, a British molecular biologist, produced compelling evidence that our responses to our environment determine the expression of our genes. Cairns, through examining gene mutations, saw that not only does gene expression change in response to internal and external signals but the gene itself also changes.[1] A new field in science was subsequently born: the science of epigenetics, using the term coined by Cairns's predecessor Conrad Waddington (who used the term as a way to describe how an organism adapts over or above how he commonly understood genetics, hence *epi*, which means "upon" or "above" in Greek).[2]

Epigenetics examines how environments regulate gene activity and expression as a response to both internal and external signals. Through these observations, the scientific community has developed a greater understanding of how what we think about, say, and do changes the environments of our cells.[3] For instance, when we think, we learn because we are changing our genes and creating new ones in response to our need to store the new information. To understand how this works, think of the way our bodies produce antibodies in response to viruses like measles or chicken pox. New genes are created by recombination (the process by which genetic material is broken up and joined to other genetic material) in response to the need to express the proteins to make these antibodies and protect our bodies.[4] The same happens with our thoughts—thoughts are real things!

Essentially, people, plants, animals, and other living organisms start with a certain genetic code—the "nature" part of the well-known nature/nurture concept—at conception.[5] Yet, the choice of which genes are "expressed," or activated, is strongly affected by environmental influences in terms of epigenetics.[6] These environmental influences are the "nurture" part of the equation: the social, emotional, cultural, and economic environments we grow up in.[7]

God has set up a complex and beautiful interplay between us, our biology, and our environments. Due to this exchange, the expression of genes can change rapidly over time: genes are influenced by internal and external factors, and those changes can be passed along to our offspring.[8] Yet there is one other factor, the most powerful factor in God's intricate design, which dominates both nature and nurture: our uniqueness or I-factor.

## The I-Factor

We have a love-filled, powerful, and sound mind (2 Tim. 1:7). We are fearfully and wonderfully made (Ps. 139:14). We have a phenomenal I-factor. And we can change our mental and biological environments with the thoughts we choose to think.[9]

The emerging science of epigenetics is beginning to shine a light on how mental and physical health are within our reach, which contradicts the dominant, mechanistic belief that humans are biological machines.[10] Epigenetics highlights our ability to respond to our environment, which includes everything from what we think to what we generally understand by environmental exposure.[11] Thoughts and emotions, alongside exposure to sunlight, exercise, food, and everything we choose to put onto and into our body, directly affect DNA expression.[12]

Epigenetics is therefore the process of *how* the operation of genes changes in response to internal and external signals. Epigenetic changes occur apart from the genes, switching them on and off through processes called methylation and acetylation, respectively. Acetyl and methyl groups are clusters of atoms that attach onto the gene and associated proteins, making them more or less receptive to receive and respond to biochemical and mind signals.[13] An acetyl group switches the gene on and a methyl group switches the gene off.

A growing body of research is highlighting how these methylation and acetylation patterns change in response to *thinking and lifestyle choices*.[14] Thinking toxic thoughts can change gene expression, just as certain diets or exposure to chemicals and pollutants can also result in changes that affect our genes.

We see this power over our circumstances mirrored in Scripture. In Philippians 4:7, the apostle Paul notes how the peace of God can protect our hearts and minds, a powerful truth reflected in Isaiah 26:3: "You [God] will keep him in perfect peace, whose mind is stayed on you, because he trusts in You." Proverbs 4 praises the beauty of God's living words, which "are life to those who find them, and health to all their flesh" (v. 22). When we implant God's Word into our minds through our thinking, we fill our brains with the powerful environmental influence of God's love, which directly impacts our mental and physical health in a positive direction. Talk about a "sound mind"!

## Fat Is in the Fire: The Danger of Toxic Food Environments

Epigenetics is essentially the pathway by which our body takes a signal from the external world (food, events, and circumstances) and internal environments (thoughts) and turns them into a set of chemical, electromagnetic, and quantum instructions for our genes.[15] Thus, through our thought and lifestyle choices, we can create either a very healthy or very toxic environment around our cells.[16] Whatever we eat directly influences the environment around our cells; this biological process is what sustains life.[17] Good, *real* food means a healthy environment in our brain and body, and this allows genetic expression to happen as it should. The proteins, fats, sugars, vitamins, minerals, phytonutrients, and all the other necessary components of food will affect our body in a wired-for-love way—just how God intended. And add a positive, love-based thought life to our menu, and we are set on the pathway to true, sustainable health!

Yet what happens if the environment is toxic? Say we go to the store and buy conventional burger patties, which came from cattle raised on a large-scale feedlot similar to the ones I discussed in part 1. First, the fats such as omega-3 and omega-6 fatty acids in the meat have a different structure from the fats in chemical-free, grass-fed cattle because the animals have been fed grains (many of which were genetically modified). In many cases these cows are even fed animals, and stale cake and candy with wrappers on (not to mention the fact that they eat these foods standing in their own feces).[18] These new types of fats upset our biochemistry in much the same way as dropping crunchy crumbs into the keyboard of a computer upsets the functioning of the buttons. Just as that computer will experience difficulties, our biological processes will not function as they ought to, which can increase our risk of developing heart disease, diabetes, obesity, infertility, and Alzheimer's disease, to name just a few diseases.

Of course, both omega-3 and omega-6 fatty acids are essential for our health, and without them we would die. Omega-6 is necessary to make the epigenetic signals that promote inflammation, while omega-3 develops epigenetic signals that calm inflammation.[19] These two fatty acids work together in cell membranes and share regulatory enzymes, so when omega-3 needs more enzymes, omega-6 will need fewer enzymes.[20] The wired-for-love design, in terms of omega-3 and omega-6 content, is such that we get the correct balance between these two fatty acids in our meat. When we eat foods with this balance of essential fatty acids, we will feel better, have more energy, and be able to think more clearly and quickly. In fact, our blood flow will be smoother and thinner, which prevents inflammation and protects against brain disorders and heart disease.[21]

When we eat conventionally raised beef, however, our omega-6 to omega-3 ratio goes up in favor of omega-6. Traditionally raised cattle fed a 100 percent grass diet have a ratio of omega-6s to omega-3s that averages to about 1.53 to 1. The ratio of these fats in cattle fed grains like soy and corn, however, skews heavily in the direction of omega-6 to 7.65 to 1.[22] A recent study, for example, showed that eating moderate amounts of grass-fed meat for only four weeks can give individuals healthier levels of essential fatty acids. The volunteers who ate grass-fed meat increased their blood levels of omega-3 fatty acids and decreased their levels of the pro-inflammatory omega-6 fatty acids, potentially lowering their risk of cancer, blood clots, cardiovascular disease, cognitive decline, and inflammatory diseases, to name just a few of the health benefits of omega-3s. The individuals in the study who had consumed conventional, grain-fed meat, however, ended up with *lower* levels of omega-3s and *higher* levels of omega-6s than they had at the beginning of the study, suggesting that eating conventional meat can be especially detrimental to one's health over time as omega-6 levels increase.[23] Processed and refined gluten products are not the only foods that cause inflammation, contrary to popular opinion surrounding gluten- and grain-free diets. Conventionally raised animals are also a problem: as omega-6 levels increase, the risk of inflammation increases. Essentially we have to remember it is not the foods per se that are to blame but rather what *humanity has done* to these foods.

## Biting Off More Than We Can Chew?

And it's not just the fat in the fire, as the saying goes. Animals forced to live miserable lives in reprehensible conditions, having hoses forced down their throats when they choke from the diet their rumens cannot handle, have higher levels of stress hormones, as I am sure you can imagine.[24] These hormones toughen the meat since they remove glycogen from the muscles just before death, which leads to decreased levels of the lactic acid needed to make meat tender.[25] These hormones also lower the concentrations of vital B-complex vitamins; zinc; copper; chromium; antioxidants such as glutathione, potassium, iron, and linolenic acid; and vitamins A, E, and C, to name just a few, that make up an essential part of our dietary health.[26] Grass-fed, organically raised, and humanely treated cattle, on the other hand, provide a perfect balance of what we need to both survive and thrive in a wired-for-love way.

Ultimately, we should be concerned about the way these animals are being treated, not only for their sakes but for our own health. As Michael Pollan says, "You are what you eat eats."[27] If we make toxic food choices, they will affect the epigenetically balanced environment in our brain and body, not to mention the effect raising cattle in large confinement facilities has on the intricate balance of our ecosystems. Our health, and the health of our beautiful planet, will suffer as a result. Yet food choices rooted in love will sustain life, since God created the world, and God is love (1 John 4:8).

## An Epigenetic Investment in the Future

In the early twentieth century, Dr. Francis M. Pottenger Jr. researched the dietary patterns of cats to gain a greater awareness of how food consumption and health are related. His findings were extraordinary: dietary choices not only affected the cats eating the food but the health of the next four generations of cats.[28] His findings suggested that diets can alter the way genes function, since the behaviors of the previous generation were passed on through a form of genetic memory inheritance.[29]

Pottenger's research has since been corroborated by a number of animal and human studies.[30] One of the seminal studies done on epigenetics and diet was carried out on agouti mice by the American scientist Dr. Randy Jirtle.[31] The agouti gene is closely related to a human gene that is expressed in obesity and type 2 diabetes.[32] Agouti mice, which have yellow coats, tend to eat ravenously if given the opportunity and have an increased incidence of food-related illness and death as a result.[33] This same pattern of overeating is repeated in their children.[34] Jirtle, however, changed this—epigenetically. He bred agouti mice offspring that were normal, slim, and healthy, simply by changing part of the environmental signal: the diet of the pregnant mothers![35] Jirtle fed the agouti mothers-to-be a diet rich in a chemical known as "methyl groups."[36] These methyl groups are molecule clusters that are able to inhibit the expression of certain genes. This shift in food consumption changed the expression of food consumption genes in the younger agouti mice without making changes to the maternal DNA sequence.[37] Thus a simple change in diet (the 20 percent part of the mind-body connection discussed in chapter 10) in the pregnant mother changed the genetic environment and had a dramatic impact on the gene expression of her baby mice. Epigenetic changes are incredibly important!

According to a growing body of research, the same diet-related epigenetic changes occur in humans. According to one recent study, a mother's diet during pregnancy can alter the DNA of her child and increase her progeny's risk of obesity.[38] Further studies have confirmed that a mother's diet before conception can permanently affect how her child's genes function.[39] These findings suggest pregnant women should follow careful dietary advice, as diet may have a long-term influence on the baby's health after it is born. The maternal diet can affect the environment of both the mother and her child.[40] Indeed, women of reproductive age need to have greater access to nutritional, educational, and lifestyle support to improve the health of the next several generations, since awareness can reduce the risk of diet-related conditions such as diabetes and heart disease.[41]

Yet maternal diet is not the only important factor in terms of epigenetic inheritance and diet. Researchers have found mice with obese fathers, even those mice with no symptoms of obesity or diet-related illness, frequently passed these characteristics on to their daughters.[42] Sons cannot dodge this epigenetic bullet either. Both sons and daughters of obese fathers can inherit an increased risk of developing diet-related metabolic diseases.[43] Scientists have also found that the offspring of obese mothers may be spared health problems linked to obesity but their own children then inherit them, so obesity and its health consequences may skip a generation.[44]

Understanding how epigenetics functions through the generations is particularly critical in terms of malnourishment. When a pregnant mother is undernourished, her child is at a greater risk of developing obesity, type 2 diabetes, and other diet-related chronic diseases, in part due to epigenetic effects. A new study in mice demonstrates that this "memory" of nutrition during pregnancy can be passed through the sperm of male offspring to the next generation, increasing risk of diet-related disease for the grandchildren as well, although it is uncertain at this point in time how long such effects will continue to have a heritable impact.[45]

### Your Children Are What *You* Think

Our food choices are not the only epigenetic legacies we leave to our children. Another study found that the experiences of a parent, *even before conceiving*, markedly influenced both the structure and function of the nervous system of subsequent generations. In particular, this study found that a traumatic event the parent experienced affected the child's DNA, thereby altering the brain and behavior of the next generation.[46] Similarly, when researchers examined the brains of rats that had been nurtured in a loving way by their mothers, they found significant biological differences, especially in a region of the brain called the hippocampus, which plays a significant role in regulating our response to stress. The more nurturing the mother was, the more this gene was activated, and the more the mother's children were able to deal with stress in a healthy way.[47] This is not surprising, since God is love and his entire creation is meant to function in a wired-for-love way. Love heals, since love is the source of all existence.

Studying epigenetics, or how thinking and eating environments impact current and future generations, is essential. With the rise in neuropsychiatric disorders, obesity, diabetes, and metabolic problems, we need to develop a multigenerational approach that looks at the fact that genetic memory can be passed between generations.[48] This science is of course still developing. Researchers are not entirely sure of how the signal works and changes the environment, but change does occur.[49] If we care about the health of our descendants, we cannot ignore our epigenetic impact.[50] God was not merely being vindictive or harsh when he said that the sins of the fathers would be visited on subsequent generations (Exod. 34:7; Deut. 30:19). He wanted us to realize that we have to be careful about what we think, say, and do, since our choices affect not only us but our progeny. Science is catching up to the Bible.

## Planting Healthy "Trees" in the Future

If you eat a healthy diet, you are not only investing in your own health but the health of your progeny. By planting an apple tree in your garden, or by planting a healthy thought "tree" in your mind, you are investing in not only your own physical and mental health but that of your biological legacy. What better way to show love for your neighbor, including your neighbor of the future (Matt. 22:39)? What better way to love selflessly and without limit than to give up a momentary pleasure not only out of care for your own wellbeing but also the wellbeing of your children's children's children?

The pathway through which epigenetic signals change our internal and external environments and affect the expression of genes has many twists and turns. We can literally nurture epigenetic change by directing these twists and turns using our I-factor, or the unique way we think.[51] We can get involved in the process of changing our mental and physical health in either a good or bad direction through our choices.[52]

Indeed, the price of *real*, whole foods is a bargain if it buys not only our own mental and physical health but that of the next four generations after us. By that same token, what is the true price of cheap, processed, and refined MAD foods if they are crippling the health of our progeny?

# 16

## The Whole Beef
## and Nothing but the Beef

What do epigenetic food choices look like in our everyday lives? In this chapter I want to explore protein, fat, and cholesterol. In chapter 17 we'll look at sugar, and in chapter 18 we'll discuss wheat and gluten. And we'll find that the conventional advice is not always supported by science.

Let's begin with protein. As we saw in chapter 15, the right protein choices positively affect the environment around our cells, and thus our health. We all probably learned in school that proteins are the building blocks of our cells: protein's vital role is to build, maintain, and repair all our bodily systems, and it is necessary for growth and development throughout our life. We may also remember that protein is broken down in the body into amino acids and fats, which both our brain and the rest of our body need to thrive.[1] Amino acids are actually the building blocks of proteins.

Everything from our bones to our organs, muscles, arteries and veins, skin, hair, and fingernails is made of protein.[2]

In fact, we have around eight billion ($8 \times 10^9$) proteins per cell.[3] Proteins called hemoglobins help carry the oxygen that reddens our blood.[4] Enzymes that digest our food, synthesize essential substances, and break down waste products for elimination are all proteins.[5] Proteins produce the energy needed for life when fats and carbohydrates are in short supply during times of starvation.[6] Proteins and steroids form hormones, which regulate the delicate chemical changes that constantly take place within the body governed by the endocrine system.[7] Our chromosomes have proteins in their structures. Protein is like a vehicle that "drives" fat and cholesterol throughout the body.[8]

To say that protein is an important nutrient is certainly an understatement. And, as with most nutrients and vitamins, too much, too little, or poor-quality protein in the diet will have detrimental effects on our physical health.[9]

### Your Brain on Protein

Your brain thrives on good-quality protein sources. It needs protein for neurotransmitter activity, since many of your internal chemical messengers consist of amino acids, amino acid derivatives, and small proteins that are built from amino acids, known as peptides.[10] Neurotransmitters enable the brain cells (neurons) to "talk" by relaying information between them.[11] Adrenaline, noradrenaline, and dopamine are made from the amino acid tyrosine.[12] These neurotransmitters make you feel good, stimulate you, motivate you, and help you cope with stress.[13] GABA, derived from the amino acid glutamate, on the other hand, counteracts these neurotransmitters, relaxing you and calming you down after stress.[14] Serotonin is another important neurotransmitter, made from the amino acid tryptophan, that keeps you emotionally balanced.[15]

Melatonin, also derived from the amino acid tryptophan, is crucial in establishing the sleep/wake cycle.[16] Endorphins are peptides (small proteins) and act at opioid receptors and therefore modulate pain.[17]

Neurotransmitters carry electrical signals across synapses, the gaps between nerve cells, thereby delivering chemical messages from one cell to the next.[18] This inter-cell interaction is what it means to build short-term memory.[19] And once a neurotransmitter has delivered a chemical message, it is released back into the synapse, which is like a swimming pool filled with an electrical-chemical cocktail. The neurotransmitter is recycled, reabsorbed, or broken down.[20]

A deficiency in amino acids affects your neurotransmitters' ability to have these meaningful conversations. It can make you feel flat, apathetic, and unable to relax; lacking in motivation, focus, and concentration; and unable to build solid memory.[21] Clearly that is not a desirable situation for your brain!

On the other hand, sufficient amounts of good-quality proteins in your diet, and thus amino acids, help with mental health issues.[22] These amino acids are more effective than prescription drugs—most of the latter have awful side effects.[23] When Hippocrates said "let food be thy medicine," he truly hit the mark, since a healthy, balanced diet of *real* foods can keep both your brain and body in shape by ensuring that you receive an adequate intake of amino acids.

Of the twenty amino acids needed for proper construction of proteins, eight (or nine, for children) are called essential amino acids, since the body cannot synthesize or make these for itself.[24] These essential amino acids must come from our diet.[25] Good-quality animal proteins, such as grass-fed, organically raised beef and eggs from pasture-raised hens, are excellent sources of these amino acids.[26] Many of these essential amino acids are also found in plant-based proteins, such as soybeans, quinoa, seeds, nuts, beans, rice, and legumes. These plant-based proteins are incomplete sources of all the amino acids and need to be eaten in combination with other foods in order to maintain good health.[27] Brown rice and lentils, for example, combine to give us a complete protein source.[28]

Another important point to note about meat is how much muscle meat we consume, and the impact this has on our bodies. Muscle meat has large amounts of the amino acid methionine, which produces the toxic by-product homocysteine.[29] Even though meat is a good source of vitamin $B_{12}$,[30] our body uses up vitamin $B_{12}$, as well as vitamin $B_6$, folate, choline, and betaine, to neutralize the homocysteine. If we consume excess amounts of muscle meat, we can reduce the amount of these vitamins in our body, which are essential to the proper functioning of many biological processes.[31] Indeed, high amounts of methionine can decrease the level of glycine in our body, which is another essential amino acid predominantly found in the skin, bones, cartilage, and organs of the animal. An imbalanced methionine-glycine ratio can have negative health effects on our mental and physical health, potentially increasing our risk for mortality.[32]

Our obsession with muscle meat is actually a recent historical phenomenon. In the past, the sections of animals we prize most today, such as muscle cuts like sirloin steak, were often thrown away or fed to the dogs, while the animal bits we have deemed less culturally pleasing, such as eyes, kidneys, bones, and feet, were treasured for their life-sustaining properties.[33] Even in nature, many carnivores leave behind the muscle meat in favor of the more nutritious parts of their prey.[34] Although eating these parts of the animal may sound unappealing, if you do eat meat, and want to do so in a healthy and balanced way, try slowly incorporating them into your diet in blended soups, bone broths, and stews.

The bottom line with protein: get enough high-quality protein without overdoing your servings of muscle meat. Consider plant proteins, eggs, and organ meat, and look for grass-fed beef and pasture-raised poultry.

## Cholesterol: Scapegoating the Scarecrow

The subject of eggs and meat leads us inevitably to a discussion of cholesterol. It is a rather unfortunate truth that "science advances one funeral at a time."[35] Many individuals today equate the consumption of animal protein sources with cholesterol levels and a higher risk of mortality. Yet, while the cholesterol and heart disease hypothesis has gained much ground culturally, with the low cholesterol and "heart healthy" labels on food in grocery stores around the world, the science of cholesterol has regressed into a game of broken telephone. The original data in this area of nutrition, with its imprecise correlations, has been lost in a sea of interpretations and so-called facts: high cholesterol levels are bad news.[36] How could anyone possibly argue otherwise?

Today the terms *LDL cholesterol* and *HDL cholesterol* are bandied about with such ferocity that it certainly is useful to stop and ask yourself what exactly they mean. LDL and HDL are lipoproteins that carry cholesterol around your body—they are not cholesterol. LDL is the "vehicle" that carries cholesterol to the cells, and HDL takes excess cholesterol away from the cells.[37]

Cholesterol itself is mainly synthesized by the liver. It is essential for the production of hormones, vitamin D, bile acids for food digestion, and cell membranes, to name just a few of its beneficial functions.[38] It even acts as an antioxidant, combating the damage done by free radicals in the body. One of the major flaws in the cholesterol/heart disease hypothesis is the assumption that cholesterol, observed at sites of damage in the body, must somehow have caused that damage. As an antioxidant, however, cholesterol is a vital part of the healing process, not the cause of the damage![39]

Of course, vitamins, antioxidants, and herbs do reduce cholesterol levels in the body. Yet these substances do not fight and destroy cholesterol as a malignant substance—they take over cholesterol's role as an antioxidant.[40] If you decided to take out the garbage at home, instead of your spouse for instance, your husband or wife is not the "bad guy" by default. It is the same with cholesterol: a decreased amount of cholesterol does not mean that cholesterol is unhealthy; it merely means someone else is taking out the trash.

In most cases, the body does a very good job all on its own of balancing cholesterol levels.[41] We have all been led to believe, for example, that eating a piece of steak will raise cholesterol levels. However, this is not necessarily the case. The liver will simply reduce its cholesterol production in response to signals from the digestive system, thereby maintaining the correct cholesterol balance that the body needs.[42]

Similarly, neither LDL nor HDL is intrinsically unhealthy.[43] The problem comes in when you upset the balance of the system. An "accident" in your body keeps LDL in your bloodstream, preventing it from reaching the cells, much like an accident during rush hour will prevent you from getting to work—you are stuck in the resulting traffic jam. During this time, the LDL oxidizes and is now seen as a threat (think of those individuals who get irritated in traffic and develop road rage), which kicks your immune system into action and can contribute to plaque buildup inside the blood vessel walls, which leads to heart disease. Essentially, the biological processes associated with cholesterol are a lot more complicated than merely good and bad cholesterol.[44] Just as there is no magic bullet for health, there is no one "bad guy" to point out in terms of disease.

### Death by Low Cholesterol?

Limiting your cholesterol intake can actually lead to physical and mental ill health, as well as early death.[45] According to a growing body of research, low levels of cholesterol are associated with decreased cognitive performance,[46] increased mortality risk,[47] increased risk of cancer,[48] less emotional stability and control,[49] a greater chance of developing depression,[50] an increased suicide risk for certain parts of the population,[51] a higher risk factor for hemorrhagic stroke,[52] and a decreased ability to fight infection.[53]

The brain, in particular, needs cholesterol. Despite the fact that your brain makes up just 2 percent of your body weight, it uses 25 percent of your free cholesterol.[54] Cholesterol is an essential nutrient for neurons and a building block of the cell membrane.[55] When cholesterol levels are low, the brain does not work very well: adequate cholesterol levels improve mental cognition.[56]

## The Big Fat Myth?

So how exactly did cholesterol become the evil Professor Moriarty of nutrition research? One of the key figures behind the diet-heart hypothesis that dietary cholesterol can lead to cardiovascular disease was Ancel Keys.[57] Building on earlier experiments carried out by Russian scientist Nikolai Anichkov, who researched the dietary patterns of rabbits and concluded that cholesterol in the blood leads to heart disease (otherwise known as the lipid hypothesis), Keys concluded from his own studies that saturated fat consumption leads to increased cholesterol levels, which in turn leads to an increased risk of cardiovascular disease and heart-related mortality.[58]

Keys's research, however, was far from conclusive. The 1950s informal Six Country Analysis,[59] which compared a country's overall amount of saturated fat available for consumption and heart disease levels, began by excluding data from a number of the countries—argued by many to be a classic example of publication bias. What would his results have looked like if he had used the data from all the countries he examined at the start of his research? When he chose to exclude the other countries, what did he mean by their lack of "fully comparable dietary and vital statistics data"?[60]

Yet despite this missing data, Keys's actual observations do not equal causation, regardless of how many times they are repeated in government policy, media sources, clinical offices, scholarly establishments, and academic sources. In fact, when all the data was analyzed by two of Keys's contemporaries, an entirely different observational conclusion emerged: saturated fat consumption *decreased* the risk of overall mortality (in terms of death unrelated to heart disease).[61]

Keys's Seven Country Study, a cohort-based research project that follows groups of individuals over time, began in the late 1950s and continues to this day. Like the Six Country Analysis, this study has its limits. It is based on observational data, and, while there has been a correlation between saturated fat intake and heart disease, it is by no means an unambiguous one. For instance, participants in Italy, Croatia, Serbia, and Japan did not experience an increased risk of heart disease with higher cholesterol levels. On the other hand, the cohorts with the highest levels of cholesterol (American railroad workers) did experience a rise in heart-related disease and mortality. Based on this study, it therefore appears that cholesterol is not always an alarm bell—it depends on the context. Instead of blacklisting cholesterol, researchers should try to determine what makes these populations particularly susceptible to heart disease.[62]

In fact, the cholesterol witch hunt that has taken place over the last several decades has actually hidden a number of important findings in the Seven Country Study. For instance, a 2002 paper noted that lower LDL levels were associated with an increased incidence of depression among the older groups. Moreover, like the Six Country Analysis, individuals with higher cholesterol levels actually lived longer than the cohorts with lower levels of cholesterol, who were actually at a greater risk of developing cancer. Nevertheless, Keys's studies have become the foundation of the diet-heart hypothesis, despite the lack of conclusive clinical evidence to support it.[63]

Indeed, even the renowned Framingham Heart Study, another cohort-based research project that began in the mid-twentieth century to examine the causes of heart disease and continues to this day, does not support the diet-heart hypothesis.[64] According to one of the lead researchers, "There is, in short, no [overall] suggestion of any relation between diet and the subsequent development of coronary heart disease."[65] Indeed, according to a pattern that began to emerge by 1997, limited saturated fat intake may in fact result in an increased risk of cognitive decline and cancer.[66] These findings are similar to the overall mortality results of the Six Country Analysis and Seven Country Study discussed above and highlight the critical need for more research to be carried out on the long-term effects of decreased saturated fat consumption and the relationship between saturated fat intake and cholesterol.[67]

### The Good, the Bad, and the Ugly Fats

Your body needs fat for all its processes, as does your brain.[68] Fats protect you from disease; aid the absorption of fat-soluble nutrients such as vitamins A, D, E, and K; control inflammation; help with blood clotting; balance your mood; make you more focused; and can maximize your intelligence through improving cognitive function, to give just a few examples.[69] In fact, your brain is around 60 percent fat—without fat in your diet you cannot think or build memory correctly.[70]

Fats come in several different forms: saturated fats, monounsaturated fats, polyunsaturated fats, and trans fats.[71] Saturated fats have no double bonds in terms of their chemical makeup and are found predominantly in animal products and tropical oils (such as coconut or palm oil). Monounsaturated fats, which consist of one double bond, are found in nuts, seeds, olive oil, and avocados, for example. Polyunsaturated fats have two double bonds and can be found in animal products, nuts, seeds, and many different kinds of oils. Trans fats, or hydrogenated fats, are mainly found in highly processed and refined foods, such as margarine, fast food, and heated oils. Food sources generally have varying combinations of these types of fats.

A simple internet search of fats will inevitably come up with a list of sites noting the same warnings. Saturated fats are principally associated with trans fats in the scientific "naughty corner" because they are said to raise blood cholesterol levels and lead to heart disease, while mono- and polyunsaturated fats are "good fats" that form an essential part of a balanced diet. Yet, as I discussed above, both unoxidized LDL and HDL cholesterol play a vital homeostatic role in many of the biological functions of our brain and body. Indeed, reduced cholesterol intake has been associated with increased overall mortality, increased risk of stroke, and cognitive decline in the studies mentioned above.[72] It is unclear, based on the evidence pool we currently have, if a diet high in unoxidized LDL and HDL cholesterol and low in saturated fat will achieve the same benefits or be more detrimental.

Yet even if you are especially worried about saturated fat intake, you do not have to give up animal products. Wild game meats like venison have a significantly reduced saturated fat content compared to modern, industrial-based sources of meat, eggs, and dairy, and even compared with domestic grass-fed animals. However, grass-fed domestic animals like lamb and beef have a significantly higher concentration of a particular kind of saturated fat, stearic acid, as opposed to conventionally raised beef. Stearic acid does not raise cholesterol levels (not that we should be particularly concerned with cholesterol per se, as I discussed above, but rather the context of cholesterol) compared with the two other types of saturated fat: palmitic and myristic acid.[73] Animal livers and shellfish (if you are not allergic!) are also low in fat but are excellent, concentrated sources of essential fat-soluble nutrients such as vitamins A and K.[74] Since all these naturally raised meat sources are nutrient dense, a *little* goes a long way in terms of their health benefits.[75]

In fact, animal foods that contain saturated fat play other important roles in human nutrition. For example, some individuals cannot effectively turn beta-carotene, found in vegetables such as sweet potatoes, for instance, to vitamin A (the two are not inter-changeable, contrary to popular opinion) in the body due to their genetic makeup and other environmental factors, such as food allergies.[76] Similarly, there are two types of vitamin K.[77] Vitamin K1 is found in dark green leafy vegetables and other plant-based foods, while vitamin K2 is found in animal products.[78] Due to genetic factors, a large number of people cannot benefit from K1 alone.[79] How will the health of these individuals fare if they reduce or eliminate all animal sources that contain saturated fat from their diet? Indeed, since animal fats are one of our best sources of these essential fat-soluble nutrients, how will the health of mankind in general fare if we remove them entirely from our diets? Not only do these animal fat sources contain essential vitamins but they also increase the absorption of fat-soluble vitamins in other foods, such as vegetables and fruit.[80]

In terms of fat-soluble nutrients, the observations of Weston A. Price, a dentist and researcher who spent years traveling and researching the various diets of populations around the world, are particularly interesting. He noticed that it did not matter what kind of foods the different people he came across consumed, whether they ate what we consider a "low-carb," "high-carb," or "high-fat" diet, as long as they ate a diverse traditional diet based on their respective locations. Yet a similar characteristic of all the healthy populations he observed was the intake of fat-soluble vitamins in animal foods, such as organ meats, eggs, seafood, dairy prod-ucts, and small animals and insects. Ultimately, the exact amount of animal fat the populations ate did not matter as much as the fact that they ate these types of foods, and therefore consumed concentrated sources of the essential fat-soluble vitamins needed for the maintenance of good health.[81] Yet as soon as the native populations made the "nutrition transition" to the current Western diet of unvaried, processed, and refined foods, their health suffered as a result, with an increase in the incidence of chronic illnesses such as diabetes and heart disease.[82]

### Throwing (Polyunsaturated) Fat onto the Fire?

There is also a potential health risk in replacing dietary saturated fats with polyunsaturated fats (PUFAs) for the long term. Most famously, the randomized and double-blind 1969 LA Veterans Heart Study, which followed 846 elderly veterans for up to eight years, found an increased risk of cancer over time among the group that consumed four times more PUFAs than the control group, who ate a typical American diet.[83] Apparently, nutritional science now tells us it is a matter of picking our demise: Would we like a side of heart disease, or cancer, with our fat?

And if this study is not perplexing enough, the several major research projects that are predominantly used to support an increased consumption of PUFAs are subject to a number of scientific difficulties. Although the 1968 Oslo Heart Study found a reduced rate of cholesterol and heart disease in the experimental group, which consumed more PUFAs, they gave this group far more attention compared to the control. For example, the experimental group, unlike the control group, were handed more than just a general multivitamin: they had to decrease their added sugar consumption, decrease their trans fat intake, increase their fish consumption (and therefore omega-3 intake), and exchange white bread for brown bread, among other requirements. [84] All of these changes can have positive health effects! How much of the reduction in cholesterol levels and mortality rates from heart disease in the experimental group can be attributed to saturated fat alone? We don't know; all the other changes made in their lifestyle habits could be equally important.[85] At best, this study shows that lifestyle factors can play an important role in the risk of heart disease, as does the St. Thomas's Atherosclerosis Regression Study (STARS) trial and the Diet and Reinfarction Trial (DART 1), both of which made a number of other changes unrelated to dietary fat (such as an increased consumption of fruit and vegetables) to their participants' diets.[86] The "background noise" of these variables makes it impossible to draw the conclusion that reduced saturated fat intake is healthy.

The 1972 Finnish Mental Hospital Study (1972), however, was particularly shocking for its lack of control.[87] For instance, a number of the participants in the trial were on thorazine, an antipsychotic drug that can cause heart problems such as arrhythmia. Considering the study was attempting to find out if PUFAs were a suitable alternative to saturated fats in terms of heart disease, the presence of an uncontrolled variable with the potential to increase cardiovascular disease and heart-related death is not really a clever idea, to say the least.[88]

What is more, several meta-analyses that have examined the relationship between dietary fat in general and heart disease highlight the lack of certainty in this area of nutrition. A 2009 systematic review of randomized control trials (RCTs), the most rigorous and reliable form of trials in medicine, for instance, noted that there was "insufficient evidence" for a link between saturated fat consumption and cardiovascular disease.[89] Likewise, in 2012 the Cochrane Collaboration, an independent and not-for-profit scientific research organization whose reputation for high-quality and unbiased data is exceptional, noted that there are "no clear effects of dietary fat changes on total mortality . . . or cardiovascular mortality."[90] The 2010 systematic analysis on dietary fat and heart health that did favor a reduced saturated fat intake strangely included trials like STARS, DART 1, the Oslo Heart Study, and the Finnish Mental Hospital Study discussed above, which in all likelihood skewed their data in favor of PUFAs.[91]

Anthropological data also suggests that keeping your PUFA intake to a minimum can be beneficial in terms of heart disease. For example, three Pacific island populations (the Pukapuka, Tokelau, and Kitava) with varying carbohydrate, fat, and protein intakes all had almost no incidence of heart disease, despite the fact that they did not eat the same kinds of diets. Yet regardless of the culinary diversity among these three populations, all of them maintained a fat ratio that predominantly kept PUFA intake to around 2 percent of their fat intake, while saturated fatty acids were their main source of fat. From this observational data, it appears that the amount of fat you consume is not as important (in terms of heart disease) as the ratio of your saturated fat to PUFA intake.[92]

### This Is Your Brain on Saturated Fat?

It is not any more "certain" that saturated fat intake causes cognitive decline. In 2012, the media were quick to sensationalize a study that linked saturated fat to mental issues. The researchers, after examining the dietary fat intake of more than six thousand elderly women over a period of time, noted that higher saturated fat intake was "associated with worse global cognitive and verbal memory trajectories." Yet, once again, this study was observational, and only examined one population group: mature women. Its conclusions cannot be applied to the population in general.[93] Most significantly, the results are *correlational* in nature—this study does *not* indicate cause and effect.[94] You cannot say that it is now a proven fact that eating a steak will give you heart disease and brain damage to boot. It would be nice and simple if science worked this way, but it does not.

Higher fat intake has actually been associated with increased mental wellbeing. For instance, in a recent study carried out by the Mayo Clinic, there was a reduction in the risk of developing dementia among the group that consumed a diet high in saturated fat.[95] And, as I discussed above, lower cholesterol levels have been associated with decreased cognitive performance. Adequate amounts of "good" cholesterol are incredibly important for healthy nerve transmission.[96] Your brain cannot communicate very well without this nutrient, a finding supported by a recent paper published in the *Journal of Biological Chemistry*. In this study, dietary cholesterol intake was an important factor in the prevention of amyloid plaque buildup, which can contribute to the development of Alzheimer's disease.[97] Considering how saturated fat is actually one of the main components of brain cells and how significant cholesterol is in terms of brain health as demonstrated by the studies examined above, cutting them out of your diet may have deleterious effects on your overall health.

It is also important to remember that eating foods high in saturated fat does not equal skyrocketing saturated fat levels in the blood. In a 2014 study published by Ohio State University, for example, participants who remained on a diet high in saturated fat did not necessarily have higher levels of saturated fatty acids in their blood. Rather, it was an increased intake of *carbohydrates* that increased the level of saturated fat found in the blood, potentially increasing the risk of heart disease and diabetes.[98]

Of course, the fact that this study was financially supported by the meat and dairy industries does highlight a potential publication bias, yet the urgent need to change our overly simplified understanding of saturated fat and cholesterol is corroborated by several other papers.[99] According to one recent Finnish study that examined the dietary habits of children, the quality of carbohydrates consumed appears to be as important as saturated fat intake in terms of the fatty acid composition in our blood.[100] In another study, elderly subjects were assigned to one of two dietary groups: one group ate three eggs per day and the other ate the same amount in egg substitutes for a one-month period. There was a significant increase in both LDL and HDL cholesterol for those who ate eggs, but the ratio between the two was not affected significantly. In other words, if the LDL cholesterol went up, the HDL cholesterol did too, thereby counteracting the effect of higher LDL levels.[101] Indeed, in an eight- to fourteen-year follow-up study of around thirty-eight thousand men and eighty thousand women at Harvard University, there was no statistically significant difference in risk for heart attacks and strokes among people who ate eggs less than once a week compared with those who ate more than one egg per day.[102]

Along with organ meats, eggs contain high-quality protein and are the richest source of phospholipids in average diets, have all the essential amino acids in the closest thing to a perfect ratio, and are a great source of choline (a B-complex vitamin needed for transmission of electrical charges across synapses, thereby improving memory), while the egg's lecithin is a good "bad cholesterol" lowering agent.[103] Eggs, as long as they are treated the way God intended (that is, the laying hens are pasture-raised without the use of synthetic chemicals or hormones), are literally a superfood that can lower cholesterol!

### Too Many Researchers Spoil the Broth?

What do all these studies on fat and cholesterol ultimately tell us? Eating saturated fat–containing foods like eggs can potentially raise your cholesterol, but can do so in a way that maintains a healthy cholesterol balance in your body. Cholesterol acts as a nutrient in the body, as does saturated fat. Eating saturated fat, however, does not always raise your cholesterol levels. Even if saturated fats may raise your cholesterol levels, they can do so in a way that maintains a healthy balance of LDL and HDL cholesterol in the body. Carbohydrates can also increase the level of fatty acids in your blood.

As Dr. Fred A. Kummerow, a leading researcher on cholesterol, notes, "You do not need a source of cholesterol to develop heart disease."[104] Your cholesterol levels will even change according to the amount and types of protein you consume, and the amount of calories you consume in general—from *any* food source.[105] I think it is quite safe to say that we need to reexamine the overly simplified understanding that saturated fat will raise your cholesterol and potentially kill you.

169

## What Is the "Fat" of the Matter?

Ultimately, Keys's diet-heart hypothesis, much like Norman Borlaug's wheat-breeding experiments discussed in chapter 6, was a
notable, if imperfect, achievement for its time.[106] Yet it should be
the start of our expeditions into the world of nutrition, not the end
of them. It should be transformed by our growing understanding
of nutritional information; it should not constrain the way we
carry out nutritional science.

The diet-heart hypothesis is not infallible. It was built on a
foundation of animal experiments, the results of which cannot
be relied on as conclusive evidence in terms of human health, and
observational studies with correlations that are often interpreted,
dangerously, as cause and effect, which were supported by physicians with little or no training in biochemistry at the time.[107] In
fact, the lipid hypothesis discussed briefly above originated from
an experiment that fed animal fat to rabbits, which should also
strike our logical alarm bells, so to speak. God never created rabbits to eat meat or dairy or any other animal products; of course
they will have an adverse reaction to eating such foods.[108] Needless
to say, humans are not rabbits. We cannot merely copy and paste
the results of this experiment onto humans. Just as the absence
of harm does not equal the presence of safety (in terms of what
we consume), the presence of safety does not always equal the absence of harm in terms of real life, such as the differences between
species and types of saturated fat.[109] Research is a little bit more
complicated than that.[110]

We essentially have to remember that nutritional science is almost
"impossible to do,"[111] as we saw in part 1. By singling out lone enti-
ties like saturated fat, we forget the context of real-life food consumption.[112] Saturated fat in real, whole foods plays an important
part in a healthy, balanced diet, as the studies above indicate, not to
mention the other health benefits of these saturated fat–containing
foods.[113] On the other hand, even a small increase in saturated fat

intake may be the straw that broke the camel's back (or heart, in this particular context) if we have grown up on the MAD diet or eat a diet that is dominated by refined and processed foods, as one recent review indicates. In these cases, it could possibly be wise to decrease saturated fat intake while transitioning to an unprocessed, whole food diet, or it could do more harm than good.[114]

The key is not to focus solely on individual pieces of the puzzle like saturated fat or cholesterol. We need to look at the bigger picture: Are you eating *real food*? As a 2015 meta-analysis by the *BMJ* noted, official US and UK low-fat guidelines were not supported by strong randomized control trial evidence in the 1970s and the 1980s, and the subsequent vilification of saturated fat has obscured the complex interplay between the human diet and disease, including the role carbohydrates play in health.[115] Ultimately, fearing fat, just like fearing carbohydrates or gluten or sugar, is not the right way to approach a healthy diet.[116] Instead, we should fear the way our current industrial food system has transformed our foods into food-like products.

### Artificial Trans Fats: The Real Public Enemy

By avoiding the MAD diet, we actually avoid the one fat that we cannot tolerate as human beings: the artificial trans fatty acids found in foods such as margarine and processed vegetable oils like canola and soybean oil.[117] These trans fats are hydrogenated fats produced by the overheating and refining of oils, and are abundant in heavily refined and processed food-like products such as fried and industrially prepared pastries, pizza, pies, cookies, chips, crackers, cereals, breads, and drinks.[118] In fact, they are present in an estimated three thousand products in food establishments today, even products with the "0g Trans Fat" label. Government regulators allow the food industry to put minimal amounts of trans fats in their products, and thus "0g Trans Fat" can contain up to 0.5g of trans fats.[119] However, as many health authorities note, the only safe amount of trans fats in the diet is *no* trans fats.[120]

On the other hand, many of these same health authorities note that we need to avoid butter, since butter contains not only saturated fat but also trans fats. However, this is an oversimplification of the biochemistry of natural versus artificial trans fats. Unlike the naturally occurring trans fats in butter, these commercial fats have migrated double bonds, which have created fourteen artificial types of trans fats.[121] As a result, they do not provide any nutritional benefit and are stored in the body, inhibiting the creation of prostacyclin, which is necessary for blood flow and the prevention of cardiovascular disease.[122] In fact, trans fats increase the amount of oxidized LDL in the blood, which can lead to heart disease and can cause memory problems.[123] And these are just a few of the major health dangers associated with the consumption of *artificial* trans fats. Again, it is not the food per se; it is what we have done to the food. God created fat; we have changed the wired-for-love form of God's creation.

Research on the dangers of industrial trans fatty acids, in particular their link to heart disease, began appearing in the scientific literature in the 1950s, pioneered by the aforementioned biochemist Dr. Kummerow.[124] However, only recently has the FDA decided to take notable, if slow, measures against the use of trans fats in food products—predominantly due to the activist efforts of the remarkable Kummerow, who is a hundred years old and still doing research as I write this.[125] The FDA's hesitation was in many ways a result of the food industry, which needs trans fats to make its products taste good and store well.[126] Needless to say, it does us good to remember that official dietary recommendations are not always reliable, based on the latest scientific research, or bias-free—and should never just be taken at face value.[127]

The bottom line: avoid trans fats by avoiding fast foods and prepackaged foods, including margarine and shortening. Now let's apply this same type of research-based reasoning to a big problem in the MAD diet: sugar.

# 17

## Sugar: The Forbidden Fruit?

Sugar: we hate to love it and we love to hate it. Today, this substance seems to polarize the conversation as much as religion, politics, and sports, while it is found in abundance throughout the globe, in countless food establishments. Is it making us fat and sick? Is it killing us? Is it harmless? Is sugar in all forms bad for us? Is sugar the real bad guy?

Yes and no. MAD sugar, the refined and processed sugar so many of us consume today, disrupts the intricately balanced environments in our brain and body.[1] It is a powerful epigenetic factor—for the worse. Unfortunately, processed sugar affects the brain in many toxic ways, and the more we eat it, the worse these effects get.[2] Evidence suggests that processed sugar acts on the brain in ways similar to well-known addictive substances such as alcohol and drugs, where both the opioid (natural painkillers in the brain) and dopaminergic (dopamine pathway) systems are upset, which can cause neurophysiological and structural confusion.[3]

This addictive process is part of the reward systems in your brain. Endorphins are peptide hormones that bind to the opioid receptors in your brain and act as neurotransmitters. Endorphins reduce the sensation of pain and affect our emotions.[4] Exorphins, on the other hand, are compounds that we can eat that activate our opioid receptors, thereby giving us pleasure as we consume our food.[5] A growing body of research indicates that these exorphins can be found not only in wheat and gluten-containing products but also in meat, eggs, dairy, green leafy vegetables, chocolate, and green tea. In fact, they may be ubiquitous in our food supply.[6] They appear to account for the desire to eat more of these foods. God wants us to enjoy eating!

MAD sugars, however, highjack these natural reward systems, distorting the desire for *real*, whole food, and replacing it with cravings for processed and refined food-like products.[7] Dr. Stephan Guyenet, a neurobiologist and researcher, suggests that "the palatability of a food, regardless of its exorphin content, is a major determinant of the food's interaction with the opioid [reward] system."[8] By manipulating the palatability of industrial food-like products, such as calculating the bliss points discussed in part 1, food manufacturers go to enormous lengths to capitalize on the addictive properties of their wares.

### You Are Not Your Addiction

Nevertheless, sugar cravings and addictions are actually *learned* behaviors. According to recent research, the abnormal craving for sugar is *not* innate in children and adults; it is the result of the massive amounts of sugar being added to highly processed foods and drinks.[9] The increasingly sweet MAD diet is driving the desire *to learn* to crave more and more sugar.

Although it may not seem like it at first, this is good news! If a behavior or habit is learned, it can be unlearned. What we wire into the brain we can wire out of the brain, because the brain is neuroplastic, as we saw at the beginning of this section. It can change! We choose to follow temptation; God does not tempt us (James 1:13–15). Even though it may be difficult to resist these foods, the mind is stronger than the body and we can choose to overcome the craving and retrain our brains and bodies through our minds.

Yet how exactly do we learn to love sugar? Sugar eventually ends up in the pleasure centers in our brains, such as the orbital frontal cortex, where we consciously experience the pull of the "sugar rush."[10] If this pull is repeated enough times daily, over about sixty-three days, a memory craving sugar will have been implanted in our nonconscious mind (see page 97 for a reminder of how the sixty-three days works). For example: we eat a refined, processed donut at the office because that's what everyone does on Fridays. Over the next couple of days we think about the donut, recalling its taste. This process of imagining activates the same pathways in the brain as though we were actually eating a donut. By day four we find ourselves craving a donut. On day five we buy and eat two donuts. And so this cycle carries on repeatedly, for sixty-three days, after which we have willfully *learned* to crave donuts, entrenching this memory in our nonconscious mind. Next time we see a donut? We will definitely battle resisting it!

### The Love of MAD Sugar Is One of the Roots of Evil

Of course, there are sugars in *real* foods as well, such as honey and fruit. God created these foods in such a way as to give us pleasure when we eat them, just as eating them nourishes us and fills our body with good nutrients. In fact, we have sugar receptors all the way down the esophagus, which appear to be intricately linked to our appetites.[11] Our taste buds in particular are designed to help us recognize and pursue important nutrients: we have receptors for essential salts, for energy-rich sugars, for amino acids (the building blocks of proteins), and for energy-bearing molecules called nucleotides.[12] Not just our brains but also our bodies show how God wants us to enjoy the pleasures of *real* food.

We can essentially become addicted to anything, even kale! As my daughter Jessica often jokes, our family may have to go to kale rehab (we each eat about two large bunches a day). Yet "the 17 teaspoons of added sugar in a 20-ounce Coke is the same amount of sugar found in roughly 3 pounds of carrots, 7 ½ oranges, 230 stalks of asparagus, or 531 cups of spinach—with none of the nutrition of those whole foods."[13] We can eat a whole bag of oranges, which have natural fruit sugars in them, and technically consume a lot of sugar, yet these sugars are encased in their whole-food packages and are full of fiber and nutrients that sustain life. And, as anybody who has eaten a whole bag of oranges knows, this is a difficult task and the end result may not be so pleasant.

MAD sugars, on the other hand, are *empty* calories. When we eat these refined and processed sugars, we consume an excess of calories because sugars (both sucrose and fructose, such as can be found in the infamous high fructose corn syrup, or HFCS) block the signal in our brains that tells us we have had enough.[14] Highly processed sugars, just like any processed and refined food products, actually disturb our taste buds.[15] In 2001, scientists identified the actual protein molecule, T1R3, that detects sugar. When excessive amounts of sugar are eaten, this protein is disturbed, contributing to the development of a toxic sugar craving.[16]

Indeed, as we saw above, food corporations craft these food-like products in such a way as to get us to consume more and more of these empty sugars, without realizing that this will make us sick.[17] It can set up the conditions for type 2 diabetes, obesity, fatty liver disease, mental health issues, and tooth decay, to mention just a few of the health consequences of refined MAD sugars.[18] And this stuff is legally consumed by millions and given to our children as "treats."

God never intended for us to eat foods that will kill us. As Jesus himself said, "Which of you fathers, if your son asks for a fish, will give him a snake instead?" (Luke 11:11 NIV). God loves and cares for us, and for his entire creation. He came to heal us and set us free—body, spirit, and soul. He made us more than conquerors through him. But we have to choose to follow his promises. We have to choose to change the way we eat, as we have to choose to give every other part of our life to him.

### Hungry as a Horse . . . on High Fructose Corn Syrup

Before entering the bloodstream from the digestive tract, sugar is broken down into two simple sugars, glucose and fructose.[19] Each type of sugar performs different yet complementary functions. Glucose, which is produced mainly by the breakdown of complex carbohydrates, is the type of energy our body is designed to run on. Every living thing uses glucose for energy.[20] Fructose, on the other hand, activates the taste cells found on our pancreas, a reaction that slightly increases our body's secretion of insulin, which we need to move the glucose into our cells for energy.[21] This is a complementary relationship.

Glucose and fructose are metabolized differently in the body. Glucose has been found to reduce brain activity in regions that regulate appetite and reward, but fructose does not.[22] Fructose only weakly stimulates the secretion of insulin, a hormone that can increase satiety and reduce hunger. It also reduces the amount of the hormone glucagon, such as peptide-1 (GLP-1), which contributes to a feeling of satiety.[23] Researchers are concerned that fructose alone, as is found in processed HFCS, could significantly increase hunger and eating. Similarly, research indicates that glucose decreases cerebral blood flow in the hypothalamus, thalamus, insula, and the striatum, but fructose increases cerebral blood flow in these areas.[24] Glucose essentially reduces activity in the hypothalamus, an event that is associated with feelings of metabolic fullness and satiety, whereas fructose has the opposite effect: it can make you crave more food. Likewise, the brain's response to fructose on its own produces abnormal activation in the nucleus accumbens, which is part of the reward circuit. This activation increases the desire for food, just as fructose's effects on the hypothalamus increase the desire for food.[25]

In fact, one of the main functions of the hypothalamus is to keep a handle on how much long-term energy is stored as fat—the conversion of extra glucose into fat for a rainy day, so to speak. The hypothalamus does this by detecting levels of the fat-derived hormone leptin. It also carefully monitors the body's levels of blood glucose, which as we saw impact feelings of satiety. When we eat, the hypothalamus sends out signals that make us less hungry. When food is restricted, the hypothalamus sends signals that increase our desire to eat, potentially leading to weight gain, obesity, and lifestyle-related diseases.[26]

Processed sugars like HFCS put these carefully controlled wired-for-love signals into disarray. One recent study has shown how a glucose drink can cause blood flow and activity in the brain areas controlling appetite, emotion, and reward to decrease with a feeling of fullness. Drinking fructose, on the other hand, continued to stimulate the brain's appetite and reward areas, and the participants did not report feeling full. They even said they could have easily carried on eating and drinking.[27] Now imagine how a soda with HFCS can confuse the brain and lead to overeating. Talk about being as hungry as a horse!

### It's All about Connections

The brain's many structures and circuits work on the principle of connectivity, which means all the parts work together in an intricate and balanced way. As I have noted many times throughout this book, this connectivity can be upset by toxic thinking and toxic eating. In terms of connectivity between different brain regions, glucose increases activity between the hypothalamus and the thalamus and striatum by providing energy.[28] These regions are a part of the thinking pathway (known as the science of thought) that deals with our state of mind, connects existing thoughts moving from the nonconscious to the conscious mind, and determines cognitive fluency.[29]

Fructose, when it is balanced with glucose in real, whole foods, increases connectivity between the hypothalamus and thalamus, but not the striatum, which deactivates once a person is full.[30] This means fructose gives an extra boost to the dynamic and active regulation of what is coming into the conscious mind (what you are choosing to eat: say, for example, cake or kale?), the conscious evaluation of this with existing thoughts (*I love this cake, it is my comfort food, but I read how good kale is for me the other day, so I really should choose that . . .*), and the final choice made (*I am going to eat the kale!*).[31] Fructose is therefore more responsible for activating hunger by creating epigenetic conditions that increase the communication between the hypothalamus and thalamus, while glucose makes sure you stop eating when you are full by activating all three regions, including the striatum.

Yet when the fructose-glucose love affair, so to speak, is out of kilter, the connectivity between these regions is compromised. This feels like fogginess and lack of clarity and slowness in the mind. The fructose in the HFCS activates our hunger without increasing activity in the striatum, so we do not feel that full and continue to eat more and more of the food-like products. Similarly, the cortical brain control area, which is activated when we think critically and self-evaluate, is inhibited by fructose but activated by glucose.[32] When we eat *real* food and think good thoughts, this area is activated correctly and enables us to balance our reactions to everyday circumstances. A healthy, connected cortical brain control area allows us to be both excited and sharp, yet cautious and wise, truly following Jesus's commands: "Therefore be wise as serpents and harmless as doves" (Matt. 10:16). MAD sugars, on the other hand, significantly affect our critical thinking skills. In fact, since this brain control area includes sites important in determining how our senses respond to foods, the extent to which the public is bombarded with "eat more processed food" messages is alarming.[33] What are we doing to our poor brains?

## As Sweet as Honey

God designed glucose and fructose to be eaten together, the way they are found in fruits and honey, in small, controlled quantities and seasonally available—that is why they are so hard to obtain in nature. As Dr. Lustig, one of the leading experts on childhood obesity and sugar, notes, our ancestors could only access sugary foods as fruit or honey or another naturally occurring sweetener, and then only for a few months of the year.[34] Moreover, within vegetables and fruits, fructose is mixed with everything it needs to make it beneficial to our bodies and brains: fiber, vitamins, minerals, enzymes, and phytonutrients, for example. The correct amount of these sugars, in real, whole foods, activates the nucleus accumbens, hypothalamus, thalamus insula, and striatum in a biochemically balanced way. If, for example, you have just finished a power walk, the fructose will be turned into glycogen and stored in the liver until you need it, while the glucose will be used for energy.[35]

When sugar is eaten in fruit and honey, glucose increases production of insulin in a healthy, wired-for-love kind of way. The insulin enables sugar in the blood to be transported into the cells where it can be used for energy, increases the production of leptin, a hormone that helps regulate appetite and fat storage, and suppresses the production of ghrelin, a hormone made by the stomach that helps regulate food intake.[36] Because of this reaction, after eating glucose, feelings of hunger actually decrease, unlike the aforementioned effect of HFCS.

Yet today, refined MAD sugars, primarily in the form of HFCS, are widely available and added to virtually all processed foodstuffs and drinks. Even regular table salt now contains sugar! Lustig certainly hit the nail on the head, observing that "nature made sugar hard to get; man made it easy."[37] Although we should be proud of many modern advances, the production of refined sugars like HFCS should not be one of them. If the liver is already full of glycogen from all these processed sugars, any excess fructose will be stored as fat.[38] If this fat gets lodged in the liver it can cause nonalcoholic fatty liver disease, among other health issues.[39] Not every modern development should be embraced as "progress."

It is not that fructose in itself is bad. It is the reductionist, *lab-manufactured, biologically inappropriate amounts* of HFCS and other refined sugars that is the problem.[40] High fructose corn syrup in particular is a cheap sweetener (it is actually sweeter than regular sugar) and is used in most soft drinks, processed foods, condiments, and, sadly, many baby foods.[41] It makes sense economically for food corporations to use HFCS, yet it makes no sense biologically for us to consume HFCS, or any other highly refined and processed sugar. As we have already discussed, not only does it overload the liver but it also confuses the receptors on the pancreas's cells, as well as the taste buds, and neurophysiological turmoil ensues.

However, HFCS is not the only bad guy. Any processed and refined form of sugar is toxic. Raw, unfiltered, and unprocessed honey, for example, contains royal jelly, bee pollen, and propolis—three major sources of antioxidants, vitamins, and minerals.[42] These elements all work together in a balanced way so there will not be any negative metabolic effects when incorporating raw and unfiltered honey into the human diet. When heated and filtered, however, the honey loses vitamins A, C, D, E, and K, various B vitamins, calcium, potassium, magnesium, and live enzymes.[43] It becomes toxic to our health, just like HFCS.

We are not supposed to have a lot of fructose floating about in our heads. Molecularly speaking, fructose has the same number of calories but is sweeter than glucose.[44] Unlike glucose, however, fructose is almost entirely removed from the blood by the liver: very little of it actually gets into the brain if we eat a balanced diet of real, whole foods.[45] When we eat excessive amounts of fructose in the MAD diet, more fructose enters the brain than it should, and problems ensue since our brain is not designed to handle large amounts of this processed sugar.[46]

The moral of the story is that when we isolate fructose in a laboratory, we disrupt the delicate balance of God's created foods. This is just one more example of a theme that I have discussed throughout this book: it is not the food per se, but what humanity does to the food. We would do well to follow the advice in Proverbs 25:16: "Do you like honey? Don't eat too much, or it will make you sick!" (NLT).

## HFCS and AGEs: An Alphabet Soup You Won't Like

The manufacturing process for HFCS is different than that of table sugar. HFCS contains free and unbound fructose molecules that are more easily absorbed in the body.[47] These molecules do not have to go through an extra metabolic step like other sugars.[48] Fructose, as in HFCS, can cause up to seven times more cell damage than glucose because it binds to cellular proteins seven times *faster*—this is called glycation.[49] It even releases more free radicals than glucose, which can cause tissue damage and aging.[50]

Normally, sugar binds to a protein under the direction of an enzyme, forming glycoproteins that are essential to the proper functioning of our body.[51] These enzymes attach glucose to proteins at specific sites, on specific molecules, for specific purposes.[52] Sugar and protein are not, however, supposed to bind nonenzymatically. When they do so, say if you eat a MAD donut, the glycation of blood proteins takes place when the levels of glucose shoot up and stay high.[53] The product of this nonenzymatic binding is a glycated protein called an *advanced glycation end-product* (AGE).[54]

How do these AGEs come about? Hemoglobin is found in red blood cells, which carry oxygen throughout your body. When your blood sugar is too high, sugar builds up in your blood and combines with your hemoglobin: it has become glycated. Excess sugar molecules that cross the blood-brain barrier combine with proteins and fats.[55] This reaction causes the proteins to fold incorrectly, and then they become less functional and even toxic.[56] These dangerous new structures are AGEs.[57]

These AGEs affect how cells function, thereby causing damage to the body, which puts a strain on the immune system. AGEs cause inflammation, free radical damage and damage to blood vessels, and increased oxidation—all these can create major cognitive issues.[58] This type of degeneration usually takes place over time: it can start as minor biological disturbances or disabilities, and later continue on to become specific disorders, contributing to major brain degeneration and reduced mental functioning.[59]

Research shows that AGEs come from fats and proteins as well, not just glucose. Our body actually has a natural way of removing AGEs, since these glycated proteins form inside our cells as well—not just from our food. They are dealt with within the cell by being degraded and are flushed out by the kidneys.[60] Zinc, insulin, and glutathione, acting as antioxidants, also fight the AGEs that are produced within the cell.[61] As long as our kidneys and intestines are working properly, and our antioxidant systems are functioning, the majority of dietary AGEs will be eliminated very quickly—unless, of course, we are eating the MAD diet, which puts all our bodily functions at risk by creating a toxic epigenetic environment around our cells.

The fructose in HFCS directly affects the brain. It is believed to cause a sensation of pleasure and trigger a craving for more HFCS, without curbing the appetite. Essentially, it gives us a pleasurable boost without the "downside" of feeling full, so we think we can consume more of it, but in fact we are overconsuming empty sugar calories.[62] High levels of HFCS in the brain have been linked to brain damage and depression.[63] A number of scientists now believe HFCS to be more dangerous and insidious to our health than alcohol![64]

Although people may feel a temporary "high" when they eat MAD foods high in processed salt, sugar, and fat, doing so on a regular basis will eventually lead to a learned craving that is self-destructive. Their brains have been altered, and now they feel like they need the food-like product to function normally. Indeed, because these foods create disarray in the brain, we crave more and more of them to try to get order back.[65]

Yet through choosing to change, this can be reversed because of the incredible process of neuroplasticity. I really cannot say this enough: we are not victims of our biology. We can renew our mind and remodel the biology of our brain.[66] We are more than conquerors through Christ (Rom. 8:37). What incredible hope there is when we apply God's principles and his science correctly!

### This Is Your Reward Circuit on Sugar

Apart from regulating satiety, the hypothalamus, thalamus, insula, and striatum regions of the brain act as our "metabolic analysis team."[67] They "read and analyze" our metabolic state and, in doing so, help influence and balance motivation and reward.[68] Glucose stops us wanting to eat more, as we saw earlier, while fructose increases our desire to eat. In *real*, whole foods their respective functions complement each other. Too much fructose, out of the context of real, whole foods, confuses this "read and analyze" function, and we end up wanting more and more of the wrong foods to keep experiencing these reward highs.[69]

In a secular sense, scientists treat motivation and reward as though we are animals that can be trained. This approach is essentially defeatist and mechanistic. They see brain scans light up in the same regions as in a drug-user's brain, and label the sugar eater an addict. Indeed, as we have seen, several leading scientists and doctors believe that food addiction and even obesity are incurable diseases, and that they are just something individuals have to learn to cope with—usually with significant amounts of drugs involved.[70]

Yet our brains are designed to latch on to something: God![71] The more we align our thinking with God's Word, the more we will develop a healthy relationship with food, since we latch on to him first and foremost. Become addicted to God, and "all these things shall be added to you" (Matt. 6:33). In his perfect design, motivation and reward come from the fact that we can be aware of our thinking and eating, bring those thoughts captive to God, choose to override bad eating patterns, and build good eating habits into our minds. Why? Because we treasure our bodies, neighbors, and the whole of creation as gifts from God—gifts we must steward wisely. To eat food is a beautiful thing, because God created eating and he created food.

### The Shrinking Hippo[campus]

Dendrites are the branches on the top of neurons and look somewhat like branches on a tree. But do not let the simplicity of their shape fool you. Dendrites act like mini supercomputers and play a critical role in thinking and long-term thought formation.[72] When we put our body and brain into toxic stress by unhealthy eating and unhealthy thinking, the hippocampal neurons became shorter and the dendrites shrink in a phenomenon called *dendritic remodeling*, which means that their supercomputer functions become compromised.[73] This affects long-term memory. Furthermore, there are fewer synaptic connections and therefore less opportunity for optimal information flow. In turn, this affects information processing and short-term memory.

185

In fact, the hippocampus is involved in processing information, converting short-term to long-term memory and spatial memory, so any damage here means that information processing is slowed down in all these areas, negatively impacting cognition.[74] In the synapses themselves the vesicles, which are like little bags of excitatory neurotransmitters, begin to dry up if we do not take our thoughts captive to Christ and if we continue to eat the MAD diet.[75] Because neurons use excitatory neurotransmitters to tell each other to increase their level of activity, fewer of these vesicles means that fewer signals can be sent, slowing down information processing.[76] Toxic food habits can break down communication pathways and short-term processing, resulting in a compromised memory.

When the hippocampus functions like it should, which happens when we think and eat properly, a neurotrophin (proteins that allow survival, development, and function of neurons) called BDNF is found in large quantities in the hippocampus, hypothalamus, and cerebral cortex.[77] It is involved in neuroplasticity, neurogenesis, and the maintenance and growth of many types of neurons.[78] If there is not enough BDNF, then the thinking process and the formation of short and long-term memories will be negatively affected, the structure of our blood vessels will be damaged, our brain can become inflamed, and synaptic plasticity will be reduced.[79] And, according to a recent study, it takes only three months of eating the MAD diet (high in processed sugars, salt, and fat) to lower levels of BDNF.[80] Consuming food-like products instead of real, whole foods, actually affects spatial memory within seventy-two hours and other types of memory within twenty-eight to thirty days.[81] Imagine what a continual lifestyle of eating a MAD diet does!

## Those MAD Sugars

And the evil of decontextualized, processed, lab-manufactured HFCS continues. Fructose in excess and out of the context of real, whole foods reduces blood flow not only in the hippocampus but also in other regions in the brain. This loss of blood flow affects cognitive function.[82] If you consume HFCS on a regular basis, for instance, you compromise the anterior cingulate cortex's ability to shift between thoughts, and you get "stuck" in your thinking.[83] Inflexible thinking, in turn, disrupts your intellect and ability to think things through by considering all options for any given situation. Likewise, processed and refined sugars like HFCS also reduce blood flow to the fusiform, which is involved in visual processing and facial recognition, thereby upsetting the visual cortex.[84] When there is reduced blood flow to these areas, the ability to recognize faces and process visual cues is damaged. This can affect how you relate to others.[85] Simply put: eating HFCS can affect your relationships.

Yet God's mercies are renewed each morning (Lam. 3:22–23). Recent research has shown how a shrinking hippocampus and other damages caused by the MAD diet are reversible.[86] Change your thinking and your eating, and you can remodel your dendrites and increase blood flow! This is truly God's grace in action.

### In a MAD Rush of Insulin

Eating a diet high in processed and refined foods can also cause resistance to the anabolic hormone insulin, which in turn can contribute to the onset of chronic diseases and even early death. When the cells are saturated in excess insulin, such as when we eat a lot of MAD sugars, the receptors (doorways) on our cells that let in the insulin are desensitized. The insulin cannot deliver the sugars to the cells, so now there is a lot of excess sugar floating about in the bloodstream (*hyperglycemia*). The pancreas then secretes more insulin, since the tissues cannot "hear" what is going on correctly, so they feel they need more of this hormone to do the job. The body compensates for excess insulin in the blood by developing insulin resistance syndrome, the precursor to type 2 diabetes. This will eventually lead to a state called *hyperinsulinemia*—too much insulin in the blood. Similarly, other hormones also become affected by the high levels of insulin in the body, and the process of metabolism is thrown into chaos.[87]

Needless to say, both hyperglycemia and hyperinsulinemia are bad news. In fact, they are major epigenetic factors in the development of type 2 diabetes.[88] It is therefore not surprising that people who drink sugar-sweetened beverages have up to an 83 percent higher risk of developing type 2 diabetes.[89] Other health issues associated with insulin resistance and high blood glucose levels include blindness, obesity, heart disease, nerve damage, cancer, compromised fatty liver (which is a precursor to cirrhosis and liver failure), and the formation of amyloid beta plaques, the hallmark of Alzheimer's.[90] Some researchers now even refer to Alzheimer's as type 3 diabetes.[91]

And pure sugar is not the only culprit. There is consensus among nutrition scientists that simple, refined carbohydrates such as white bread, pasta, and processed cereals are not good fuel sources, since they release sugar too quickly into the bloodstream.[92] Their chemical composition once metabolized is not much different from that of pure sugar—they are often referred to as "sweet poison" because of their toxic effects in excess on the body.[93] These types of food continually force the body to compensate by making the pancreas produce excessive amounts of insulin, leading to hyperinsulinemia.[94]

Like everything in the body, insulin in and of itself is important, and not just for glucose metabolism. It can pass through the blood-brain barrier and trigger neurological processes that are important for learning and memory, if the environment in our body is healthy. However, consuming large amounts of MAD sugars on a regular basis blocks insulin's ability to regulate how our brain cells store and use sugar for the energy needed to fuel thoughts and emotions, thus having a negative impact on learning and memory.[95] Essentially, high blood sugar and insulin levels from eating incorrectly also upset the brain's neurotransmitters that regulate mood, thinking, and learning.[96] The synaptic function between neurons gets disrupted, which directly affects emotions, memory, and thinking: the brain's connectivity is thrown into disarray, and this affects short-term memory and thinking since the brain cells will have trouble signaling each other.[97]

Indeed, hyperinsulinemia impacts the insulin receptors in the brain, including the hypothalamus. The brain does not respond well to the increased blood insulin, which signals the brain, along with leptin, if we are eating too much and putting on weight. Since the brain can no longer suitably detect excess fat production in the body, our response will be to eat more, and therefore gain more weight—a vicious cycle.[98]

## MAD Stress

We turn now from insulin to cortisol. While commonly known as the "stress hormone," in a negative sense, cortisol is actually an essential steroid hormone derived from cholesterol.[99] It increases available energy by increasing blood glucose and releasing fatty acids from fat, which, in healthy doses, can do amazing things in our brain such as promoting attention, storing memory, and maintaining a balance between healthy and toxic stress.[100] However, when we eat MAD foods, or think toxic thoughts, our cortisol levels are elevated and become toxic, impairing attention and memory, causing changes in the hippocampus (thereby affecting the conversion of short-term memory to long-term memory), and shrinking nerve cells (which will eventually die).[101] Is it any wonder, then, that a diet high in fructose throughout adolescence can worsen learning, memory, and depressive- and anxiety-like behavior, and alter how the brain responds to stress?[102]

The amygdala in the brain has receptors for cortisol and insulin and is therefore also affected by excessive consumption of refined and processed sugars.[103] This structure is also part of the aforesaid thinking pathway, working with the hypothalamus to provide the emotional and perceptual information that puts memories in context.[104] When our amygdala is affected by MAD food-like products, we can become reactive and impulsive, since we no longer have strong emotional and perceptual clarity.[105] To put it simply, thinking and emotions are affected in a negative way by anything that is not *real*, whole food.

## The Soul, Stress, and Sugar

As I discussed earlier, the hypothalamus is a central player in how the mind (soul) controls the body's reaction to stress and foods. The hypothalamus is actually referred to as the "brain" of the endocrine system.[106] It integrates signals from the mind and body, sending them throughout our bodies so that we can react in an appropriate and functional manner, "so that the whole body is healthy and growing and full of love" (Eph. 4:16 NLT).

Stress, like *real* food, is not inherently bad—it depends on how we react to it.[107] Stage 1 of stress is only short term and makes us alert and ready for action.[108] It is an appropriate response to certain situations. During this stage, corticotropin-releasing factor (CRF) is secreted from the hypothalamus and stimulates the pituitary glands to produce adrenocorticotropic hormone (ACTH).[109] ACTH travels via the blood to the adrenal glands (above the kidneys) and stimulates them to produce the stress hormone cortisol.

On the other hand, if we react incorrectly to stress due to a "spirit of fear" (2 Tim. 1:7), our stress reaction is prolonged and becomes toxic. According to one study, increased stress can potentially increase the risk of mortality by 43 percent—but only for the individuals who *believed that stress was harmful for their health*. People who didn't view stress as harmful actually *decreased* their risk of dying. Over the eight years of the study, the researchers estimated that the 18,200 people who died, died from the belief that stress is bad for you—that is more than two thousand deaths a year.[110] This is a real eye-opener, because it shows that how we perceive stress determines its impact on our mental and physical health.

If you change your mind about stress, however, you can change your body's response to stress. Instead of viewing the stress response as negative, when faced with a stressful situation you can view it as your body being energized to help you meet the challenge—rethink the stress response as helpful! Imagine your pounding heart preparing you for action; if you are breathing faster, good! You are getting more oxygen to your brain.[111]

If we choose to react wrongly to a challenging situation, we will enter stage 2 of the stress reaction. During this stage, high levels of cortisol circulate in the blood for extended periods of time, in turn contributing to prolonged high blood sugar that can also lead to insulin resistance, prediabetes, and weight gain, since prolonged high levels of cortisol lead to the accumulation of fat instead of fat breakdown. In this toxic situation, fat tends to accumulate around the middle of the body and is a risk factor for heart disease.[112] In fact, prolonged, high levels of cortisol can in some extreme cases lead to Cushing's syndrome, with its characteristic fat accumulation around the middle and back of the human body, but not on the legs, which remain thin due to muscle wastage.[113] If we continue to release cortisol, we enter stage 3 of the stress reaction, which can lead to adrenal exhaustion and eventually death.[114]

So a maladaptive stress response that arises from our perceptions of stress and from excessive MAD sugar intake can interact to make us ill and gain weight. Likewise, both a bad stress response and elevated insulin levels from too much sugar intake feed back through the brain, especially the hypothalamus. These interactions are a profound example of the interconnected nature of the brain and body, and how both signals from our thinking (the 80 percent) and our environment, or in this case eating (the 20 percent), can influence our health both physically and mentally.

Yet there is good news! Since the mind (soul) controls the brain, including the hypothalamus, the *mind is the key* to breaking the maladaptive stress/sugar cycles. We can choose with our minds how we react to the circumstances of life, including stress and the foods we choose to eat. I will explain in greater detail how we can overcome the stress/sugar problem in part 3.

## Is Sugar Making You Fat?

The urgency of choosing good food and good thoughts is prevalent throughout the scientific literature. The science of thought and developing intellect has been a large part of my research. A growing body of research examining the link between sugar consumption and obesity, for example, has found a significant statistical association between these two factors: thinking and eating.[115] The link is especially strong in children, where each daily serving of sugar-sweetened beverages is associated with a 60 percent increased risk of weight gain and obesity, and thus the diet-related diseases.[116]

These findings should cause us to question current business practices. How ethical is it to use children to determine how sweet or salty something should be, calculating "bliss points" so that big companies can make more money? How ethical is it to market MAD foods to children and youth? Indeed, the mental and physical health effects of consuming MAD processed and refined foods as a child can persist into adulthood.[117] As investigative journalist Michael Moss notes in *Salt, Sugar, Fat: How the Food Giants Hooked Us*, the food corporations are "manipulating or exploiting the biology of the child."[118] How can we allow this to continue?

## Go MAD and Lose Your Mind?

With the increasing rates of not only obesity but also Alzheimer's in our world today, allowing food manufacturers to sell products that can affect both our physical and mental health poses a threat to us all. The number of people with Alzheimer's disease is projected to increase fourfold over the next forty years, reaching approximately fourteen million by 2050.[119] The MAD diet affects the gastrointestinal (GI) system in multiple ways, including damaged memory, as we already saw.[120] The exponentially increasing obesity rates within Western societies over the last thirty years have been a cause for alarm, yet primarily in terms of associated health problems like type 2 diabetes and cardiovascular disease.[121]

However, recent research is showing how Alzheimer's disease and dementia are an equal cause for concern in terms of the MAD diet. Considering how over one-third of Americans today are classified as obese, there is a strong possibility these people will suffer from cognitive decline.[122] More and more studies are highlighting the frightening association between the consumption of MAD foods, weight gain, and dementia.[123] This body of research underscores the fact that the MAD diet has dire effects on learning and memory processes (which, if you recall, are dependent on the hippocampus).

Excessive amounts of processed and refined foods actually accost the small intestine, which in response secretes elevated levels of amyloid beta protein.[124] This excess amyloid beta protein moves through the blood, damaging the blood-brain barrier. The blood-brain barrier is the brain's security system; it is a network of blood vessels lined with endothelial cells wedged tightly together, creating a nearly impermeable barrier between the brain and the bloodstream.[125] Every thought we have and action we take involves precise types of communication within and between the nerve cells in our brain. The blood-brain barrier is how the brain separates itself from the natural chemical fluctuations that occur in the environments around the cells, which will affect this communication and, therefore, affect our thinking. The only things that can pass through the blood-brain barrier are very small compounds and fat-soluble molecules. These, unfortunately, include antidepressants, antianxiety medications, alcohol, cocaine, and many hormones. Larger molecules like glucose or insulin must be carried across by proteins.[126]

A healthy blood-brain barrier allows essential nutrients to get in and blocks harmful substances. So what happens if it is damaged? Some molecules, like amyloid beta, are able to break down the blood-brain barrier. Amyloid beta in the blood from incorrect eating breaks down the tight junction proteins of the blood-brain barrier (it does this by reducing the gene expression of these protein junctions), gets into the brain, and damages the hippocampus.[127] Because the blood-brain barrier has been broken down, there is an increase in the accumulation of amyloid beta in the hippocampus, which contributes to the development of dementia and Alzheimer's disease (which are characterized by amyloid beta plaques that cause memory and processing problems).[128]

Unfortunately, the story does not end there. The damaged blood-brain barrier now leaves the hippocampus and the other structures of the brain vulnerable to circulating toxins, like heavy metals and inflammatory markers, with resultant increasing levels of cognitive damage.[129] The surrounding environment of the brain is no longer stable, and this can occur from both an unhealthy thought life and an unhealthy diet—MAD thinking and MAD eating! If a MAD diet becomes a lifestyle, the damage will continue; if unforgiveness, bitterness, toxic thinking, stress, and negative emotions become a lifestyle, the damage will continue. God wants us whole and healthy in spirit, soul, and body.

Of course, reading all these studies can be frightening and disheartening, which is why I am glad I can turn to God! He has given us an incredible mind, which can change our brains—we can reverse this cognitive damage![130] We are not victims of our biology, of the food corporations, of the government, of our grandparents' eating and thinking habits. We are more than conquerors in Christ. We can renew our minds. We can change our biology.

## Prescribe Produce, not Prozac

Although the ancient Greek physician Hippocrates famously said that "food should be our medicine, and medicine should be our food," only recently is the idea of food as medicine becoming a resurgent field of research. The fields of medicine and psychiatry are beginning to rediscover the many connections between food and mental illness after more than a half century of depending primarily on prescription drugs for relief.[131]

Steve Holt, summarizing Dr. Bonnie Kaplan's work in this area, hit the nail on the head when he said that "we may soon see psychiatrists prescribing produce rather than Prozac."[132] Kaplan's research, particularly in the field of learning disabilities, shows that eating correctly is "consistently and reliably" associated with better moods and mental health.[133] These findings are exciting, since they lay the foundation for the positive effect of a broad-spectrum micronutrient approach to learning disabilities, as opposed to traditional medications that have a number of unwanted and dangerous side effects including structural and chemical changes in the brain.[134] Similarly, other researchers have found lower rates of depression, anxiety, and bipolar disorder among those who ate a traditional, real-food diet of protein and vegetables, compared to people who followed a modern diet heavy with processed and fast foods—or even compared with a health-food diet of just tofu and salads![135]

We need to change the way we view nutrition science. "Magic-bullet" methodology, where we praise certain foods and demonize others, fits comfortably within the reductionist pharmaceutical paradigm and traditional scientific methodology, where drugs are typically single ingredient and independent variables are potentially manipulated one at a time.[136] What is needed is multi-nutrient *real* food studies showing the impact of *real* whole foods, in context, on mental and physical health, if this is at all possible within our current scientific framework. Nutritional science, on the other hand, is almost impossible to do, and we are far better off eating foods the way they have been historically grown, the way God designed (with biomimicry-inspired improvements), rather than eating the laboratory-manipulated ones we have today.

Now that we have discussed how proteins, fats, and sugars epigenetically affect our bodies and brains, we turn to a subject that has gotten a lot of attention recently: Should we or should we not eat gluten? We'll see that the concern over gluten sensitivity is valid but its solution is not what is commonly recommended.

# 18

## To Eat Gluten or Not to Eat Gluten: That Is the Question

The current wheat-gluten debate and the epidemic of gluten intolerance tends to say more about our modern "diet fad" psychology than what is truly happening in our environments, food supplies, physiology, and biology.[1] By making gluten the root of all dietary evils, we once again step into reductionist thinking, where one ingredient or chemical is blamed for most of the woes of mankind, and where the small subset of those genuinely afflicted is made to represent the larger population.

Research shows that one out of five people are self-diagnosing gluten intolerance, and about one-third of the American population claim to have gluten intolerance.[2] Yet there is no solid scientific research to back up this trend. Statistics show that a handful of people are truly gluten intolerant, such as individuals who are allergic to wheat or gluten, or people who have an autoimmune disorder called celiac disease.[3] And while celiac disease is a well-established entity, the evidence base for gluten as a trigger of symptoms in patients without celiac disease (so-called non-celiac gluten sensitivity or NCGS) is limited.[4] Indeed, the exact mechanisms by which gluten triggers the gastrointestinal symptoms have yet to be identified.[5] Scientists have not "proven" nor do they even really understand what is exactly behind gluten "intolerance," let alone that it is a real thing for most of the people who claim to have it.

Testimonials of how cutting out gluten "changed my life," especially from celebrity doctors, actors, and sports people, are in no short supply, popularizing the gluten-free fad even more. It is not uncommon these days to blame every neuropsychological, neurological, and learning disorder on gluten, even though the actual evidence for this is scant. You may certainly benefit from reducing your wheat and gluten intake, especially the MAD variety (eliminate the MAD kind completely!), but not necessarily because you have an allergy to gluten. No one can tolerate the MAD diet, whether it is highly processed, refined, and industrially manufactured meats or breads or vegetables. Eating *real*, whole foods, not food-like products, will pay dividends.

Our MAD food system has dramatically changed the grains we eat and the way we eat grains. As we saw in part 1, wheat and other grains have been bastardized through industrial methods that have damaged their ability to nourish us. Equally, people cannot tolerate the MAD diet in general, of which highly processed and refined gluten is a part. Yet gluten-free eating is financially driven by industry: if more people can be labeled as gluten intolerant, food corporations can make more money manufacturing these types of foods.

## MAD Science

In 2011, Dr. Peter Gibson, professor of gastroenterology at Monash University, led a study that remains one of the most-cited pieces of evidence for non-celiac gluten sensitivity (NCGS).[6] His research gave impetus to the gluten-free diet, which is predicted to increase gluten-free product sales to an estimated $15 billion by 2016. Gibson, however, has reevaluated his results and has become dissatisfied with them, in particular due to the other variables that were not controlled for in the study.[7]

Questioning the causal links between the consumption of gluten and his subjects' reactions, he repeated the trial.[8] Gibson attempted to remove all potential dietary triggers, including lactose (from milk products), certain preservatives like benzoate, propionate, sulfites, and nitrites, and fermentable, poorly absorbed short-chain carbohydrates (also known as FODMAPs), except gluten.[9] Based on his findings, Gibson came to the *opposite* conclusion of his original research: "In contrast to our first study . . . we could find absolutely *no specific response* to gluten."[10] Gluten itself was not necessarily the cause of the gastrointestinal symptoms under investigation. What is known as the *nocebo effect* was occurring among the participants: people suffered digestive issues when they consumed foods containing gluten because they *expected* to suffer from eating gluten.[11] Gluten intolerance among the participants was predominantly *psychological*.

The work of Gibson and his colleagues has highlighted another dietary issue we should be more concerned about, rather than isolating gluten and putting it in the naughty corner. According to Biesiekierski, who worked with Gibson on the research, "some of the largest dietary sources of FODMAPs (short-chain carbohydrates such as oligosaccharides and sugar alcohols)—specifically bread products—are removed when adopting a gluten-free diet, which could explain why the millions of people worldwide who swear by gluten-free diets feel better after going gluten-free."[12] In a number of individuals, these FODMAPs are poorly absorbed in the small intestine and could potentially be responsible for the impetus behind the gluten-free movement.

Ultimately, however, we should not make FODMAPs the new villain just yet. Nutritional science, as we have seen throughout this book, is a complicated and messy business. Indeed, both Biesiekierski and Gibson conclude that much more research is needed on NCGS, research that is as well controlled as possible and is reproducible. This scientific rigor is especially necessary in light of the fact that non-celiac gluten sensitivity seems "predominantly driven by consumers and commercial interests, not quality scientific research."[13] When money is involved, research that is already complicated gets even more complicated by competing interests.

Yet I have noticed a positive trend in the area of nutritional science. Many researchers, like the aforementioned Gibson and Biesiekierski, cite the need for more research, especially for research that moves beyond the realm of animal studies. Moreover, food needs to be looked at in the context of whole, *real* food, and in the context of the whole human being. We cannot approach nutrition from a reductionist standpoint, where we pinpoint individual "bad foods" based on complicated correlations with a strong sense of causation. Lastly, scientists and other sources of scientific information ought to think carefully before making sweeping statements that claim that going gluten free is something *everyone* should do because gluten is the cause of most neurological diseases in the brain.[14]

These questions do not have easy answers. I cannot write a book telling you what types of *real* food you as a unique human being should and should not eat, although I can tell you, as I have throughout this book, how eating MAD food-like products instead of *real* food is always a bad idea. Throughout this book I have tried to find as many of the scientists who question current nutritional practices as I could. You can read their research, books, blogs, and other materials, and then think this through for yourself. In the end, you have to make your own dietary choices, including whether you should go gluten free or not. Remember, the Holy Spirit "will guide you into all the truth" (John 16:13 NIV).

## MAD Wheat

Gluten has played an incredibly important role in human history.[15] In the Bible alone, gluten-containing grains such as wheat are often referred to throughout both Old and New Testaments. Wheat, which is perhaps the most well-known source of gluten today, is an ancient grain and incredibly nutritious when grown and prepared in the way God designed it to be grown and prepared, according to the way his creation works (biomimicry). It is a good source of B vitamins, potassium, vitamin E, calcium, magnesium, iron, and zinc, to name just a few of the health benefits. And it certainly is delicious too!

Grains of wheat, or *wheat berries*, have three layers. The bran layer is the hard outer shell where the fiber is contained. The endosperm is the largest part of the grain and is made up of mostly starch. The germ is the embryo of the grain, loaded with nutrients and fatty acids and capable of sprouting a new wheat plant. *Whole grain* refers to wheat that has all three of these layers intact—the high nutrient value of wheat is only present when all three of these layers are intact. By grinding grains between large stones (a traditional way of grinding wheat), the flour that is produced contains everything that is in the grain, including the germ, fiber, starch, and a wide variety of vitamins and minerals.[16] Without refrigeration or artificial preservatives, fresh stone-ground flour spoils quickly, since the natural wheat-germ oil becomes rancid at about the same rate that milk becomes sour; refrigeration of whole grain breads and flours is necessary.

Today's wheat, however, is far removed from its ancestors. Modern industrial farming methods have reduced the number of wheat varieties from thirty thousand to roughly a few handfuls.[17] In particular, most of us today consume a high-yield, hybrid dwarf wheat variety that originated in the 1960s (through the research efforts of Norman Borlaug, whom I discussed in part 1). This type of wheat has fewer nutrients and is less digestible than its predecessors, like spelt and einkorn. Yet since it is a high-yield variety, food producers have by and large adopted it.[18]

Even worse, the way this dwarf wheat is processed further destroys its capacity to nourish us. The high spoilage rate of traditionally prepared wheat makes earning large profits off the mass transportation and distribution of thousands of loaves of bread very difficult. The modern food industry's answer to these "problems" has been to apply faster, hotter, and more refined techniques of processing.[19]

The result? Finely ground flours that do not spoil in bread products and that can last for months on grocery store shelves—served with a side of *real* health problems. Refined wheat flour has a larger surface area than coarsely ground wheat grains because the protective, hard-to-digest, and fibrous outer coat that temporarily fends off enzymes from digesting the starch inside too quickly has been stripped away.[20] God designed our bodies to use indigestible fiber to carry along partly digested food, shielding it from immediate digestion, which can cause gastrointestinal distress and other health issues like high blood sugar levels and an increased amount of toxins in our bodies. Indeed, according to Walter Willett, head of Harvard's Nutritional Department, "constipation is the number one gastrointestinal complaint in the United States, costing more than two million physician visits a year, and costs of $1 billion a year on over-the-counter laxatives. By keeping the stool soft and bulky, *the fiber in intact whole grains* helps prevent this troubling problem."[21] The fiber in whole wheat can save you a lot of stomach pain and social discomfort, to say the least.

Likewise, the refining process used to prepare modern wheat increases the gluten content of flour by removing the germ and keeping the endosperm.[22] Many of us today now consume gluten out of context of whole, real wheat, which, as I have discussed in many places throughout this book, is a health accident waiting to happen. Is it any wonder many of us feel we cannot tolerate gluten?

As the wheat grains are first exposed to high temperatures, moreover, the proteins are denatured, and under the high-speed rollers, important nutrients are nearly eliminated. The wheat grains lose up to 77 percent of their thiamine (B1), 80 percent of their riboflavin (B2), 81 percent of their niacin, 72 percent of their pyridoxine (B6), 50 percent of their pantothenic acid, 86 percent of their vitamin E, 60 percent of their calcium, 71 percent of their phosphorus, 84 percent of their magnesium, 77 percent of their potassium, 78 percent of their sodium, 40 percent of their chromium, 86 percent of their manganese, 76 percent of their iron, 89 percent of their cobalt, 78 percent of their zinc, 68 percent of their copper, and 16 percent of their selenium.[23] The wheat grains subsequently go through various stages of milling as they are refined even further.[24] The wheat that most of us eat today is so far removed from the wheat our ancestors ate that it is any wonder we still call it wheat.

And of course I cannot forget to mention all the added chemicals! Conventional wheat seeds are treated with a fungicide before they are even planted in the ground; the crops are sprayed with pesticides and hormones in the field; after harvest the wheat is stored in bins that have been sprayed with various chemicals to kill insects; and, finally, the wheat is given a final spray of pesticide to kill any "superbugs" (or bugs that have developed a resistance to the previous chemicals) that may have made it through the previous treatments.

Unfortunately, that is not the end of the chemical processing of wheat. As Dr. Chirag R. Patel notes in *Brain Foods: Eat Your Way to a Better Brain and Live the Life You and Your Brain Deserve*, "chlorine oxide is used to age, bleach, and oxidize the flour."[25] Chlorine oxide can react with the natural proteins in wheat flour, thereby producing alloxan, a compound that may in turn contribute to the onset of diabetes. Similarly, the potentially dangerous chemicals nitrogen oxide, benzoyl peroxide, and nitrosyl can contaminate the wheat flour as it is being milled.[26] And, as if all these artificial substances are not alarming enough, hormones are added to influence wheat characteristics.[27] What effects can all these substances have on our bodies? MAD wheat is a BAD idea, particularly since the consumption of processed grains can be addictive in a negative sense and has been shown to raise bad cholesterol levels, may interfere with the body's use of essential fatty acids, and can upset insulin levels, to name just several of the potential health issues.[28]

## Celiac: A MAD Problem?

Celiac disease is an autoimmune disorder triggered by gluten that affects a significant portion of the world population—an estimated 1 in every 100 people.[29] Celiac disease appears to have its roots in a preexisting infection or dysbiosis (microbial imbalance on or inside the body).[30] The immune system has to recognize that the gluten protein fragment is problematic, so there has to be a "memory" of the problematic protein before it is recognized. In order for a T cell of the immune system to properly recognize the gluten protein, this little protein fragment must first be deamidated. Deamidation involves the removal of nitrogen from certain amino acids to produce their acidic counterparts by an enzyme called *tissue transglutaminase*. For example, the nitrogen is removed in glutamine by transglutaminase to produce glutamate, a necessary compound for cellular metabolism. Our cells only release transglutaminase when they are attempting to recover from tissue damage. So, first the tissue damage occurred in some way—perhaps due to a poor diet consisting of MAD foods—then tissue transglutaminase was released in response to this damage to remove nitrogen from the relevant amino acids (deamidation happened) and a "memory" of this was formed in the immune system, in case of similar damage in the future.[31]

What does all this complex scientific information have to do with the price of bread, literally and figuratively? As the nutritional biochemist Chris Masterjohn notes, "What has the food industry decided to do to the wheat gluten it adds to processed junk food in the last several decades? Deamidate it! Sometimes by chemical treatment, and sometimes by treating it with . . . [*drumroll please*] tissue transglutaminase!"[32] The MAD diet adds the very enzyme that is activated when there is tissue damage in the body into processed and refined foods like your average loaf of white bread. Essentially, the substances being added to the bread are the very substances your body produces in response to tissue damage. The epigenetic triggers that signal damage are potentially being activated with every mouthful of this bread, possibly leading to a rising incidence of celiac disease.

Unfortunately, little research is being carried out in this area of gluten intolerance, which should deeply concern us.[33] What other questions are not being asked as people buy these types of MAD foods on a daily basis? How can governmental bodies like the FDA deem a food safe, when we know so little about the process in terms of the *whole* human body?

We should fear the way our current, industrial food system has transformed our *real* foods into food-like products. In answer to the question posed as the header of this chapter, "To eat gluten or not to eat gluten: that is the question," here is my proposed answer: your diet should be MAD free, not gluten free!

# 19

## Sleep In, Then Move It

We close part 2 with two practices that go hand in hand with healthy eating. God commands us to focus on the health of our triune being, as we saw at the beginning of part 2, and this includes healthy sleeping patterns and regular physical activity. Sleep is needed to regenerate and protect the proper biological function of both our bodies and minds and to consolidate memory.[1] We cannot think good food thoughts without sleep, and we can't digest the food we eat well without sleep. Likewise, exercise is equally important. Not only does it make our blood circulate more efficiently through our bodies, bringing the chemicals of life to the cells and removing the debris of metabolism, but regular exercise also benefits the mind.

**Sleep Less, Eat More**

A lack of sleep has actually been associated with junk food cravings, confused food desires, and weight gain. In one study, people who were deprived of just one night's sleep spent more money on MAD food-like products loaded with empty calories and bought more grams of food, in a mock supermarket, the following day. The researchers also found higher levels of a hormone that increases hunger, ghrelin, in the blood of the participants who lost one night's sleep.[2] Thus a lack of sleep can potentially make you hungrier, increasing your risk of unhealthy weight gain. Other studies have supported this finding, with a significant correlation between sleep deprivation and obesity.[3]

Indeed, scientists widely acknowledge that sleep deprivation impairs self-control and higher levels of self-reflection, self-control, and decision making.[4] For instance, evidence from fMRI scans shows how a lack of sleep impacts higher-order thinking by specifically reducing activity in the frontal lobe region of the brain, an area that is important for controlling thinking and making complex choices.[5] In fact, when you worship, pray, and meditate, this area fires up.[6] And just as worship feeds our spirits, so food feeds our brains and bodies. The more we focus on God and the more we sleep, the more we will be inclined to follow a healthy diet, have healthy thinking, and have bodies and brains that work as they ought to work.

We need to be still and know that God is God (Ps. 46:10). Indeed, social jet lag—a syndrome related to the mismatch between the body's internal clock and the harsh realities of our daily schedules—is also believed to be a contributing factor to today's obesity epidemic by upsetting our sleeping patterns.[7] Although our brains like the speedy rush of modern-day life, as we saw earlier, we need to learn to do busy well, which means sleeping well, not just for our digestion but for our mental and physical health in general.

There is also mounting evidence that sleep issues disturb neuroendocrine control of appetite, leading to overeating, which can decrease insulin and/or increase insulin resistance, both pathways to type 2 diabetes.[8] Our brains change after chronic sleep deprivation, which in turn influences how much we eat and how well our metabolism functions to digest and use the food we eat—it affects the whole body.[9]

Ultimately, the combination of hunger and poor decision making can create the "perfect storm" when it comes to our daily food choices.[10] Keeping a regular sleep pattern is therefore really important for good thinking habits and good food choices.

## Get off Your Bottom

We all know we need to move. We are designed to move, for the sake of both the brain and body. Exercise potentially improves all areas of cognitive function, including thinking, learning, and memory, especially with age. In children, exercise is incredibly important for memory development. Yet the older you get, the more you need to move on a daily basis, even if it is in short bursts or power walking up those stairs instead of going in the elevator.[11] Add worship, prayer, and constant internal dialogue with the Holy Spirit, and you have the winning formula: you get better and wiser with age![12]

Our overall ability to think and understand through intellectualizing and shifting through our thoughts is improved with exercise, regardless of our age. Physical activity increases blood flow to the anterior cingulate cortex (deep inside the middle of the brain), which is activated when we shift between thoughts in a flexible manner.[13] Not only are we better able to form memories when we move but we also improve communication between these memories, facilitating deep understanding. Adding to these benefits, certain hormones, which are increased during exercise, help improve memory and thinking. These hormones are growth factors called brain-derived neurotrophic factor (BDNF), vascular endothelial growth factor (VEGF), and insulin-like growth factor 1 (IGF-1).[14] In fact, people who exercised often improved their memory performance and showed greater increase in brain blood flow to the hippocampus, the key brain region that deals with converting short- to long-term memory and is particularly affected by Alzheimer's disease.[15] In short, your brain loves exercise!

A growing body of research indicates that it is aerobic exercise such as power walking and cardio, not just physical activity in general, which specifically leads to improved and flexible cognition.[16] Unhealthy lifestyle habits, such as the MAD diet with little or no exercise, will actually speed up the process of senescence (cell death), and, in turn, the release of damaging substances from dying cells. These substances unfortunately increase the toxic load in the body and brain and are responsible for early aging.[17] Exercise, on the other hand, can help prevent or delay cell death.[18]

Physical activity essentially changes our DNA for the better. The epigenetic pattern of genes that affect fat storage in the body actually changes with exercise—the more we move, the better our bodies get at using and storing fat. Remember, from chapter 15, how the methyl groups on genes can be influenced in various ways, through exercise, diet, and lifestyle, in a process known as DNA methylation? Researchers have found that when we exercise, epigenetic changes occur in 7,000 of the 20,000 to 25,000 genes, with positive changes in genes linked to type 2 diabetes and obesity![19] Other studies have shown that when we exercise, our body almost immediately experiences genetic activation that increases the production of fat-busting proteins.[20] So thinking well, eating well, *and* physical exercise are therefore necessary to maintain a healthy body weight and lifestyle.

Although exercise fads come and go, the main thing to remember is to stay off your bottom as much as possible![21] Find out what works well for your body type, and maintain a disciplined exercise schedule. The mind dominates over everything, as I have mentioned throughout this book. So when you exercise, *put your mind behind it.*

## So How Exactly Do I Change?

You are more than your biology. You have the mind of Christ and are a conqueror in him. You can renew your mind. You can change your life, including your eating patterns, so that you are a good steward of not only your own body but the rest of creation too.

Yet with all the information presented in the past two sections, what does this change look like in real, everyday life? Where do you even begin? Part 3 is filled with practical tips, both physical and mental, to help you start your journey to health—spirit, soul, and body. I've also provided twenty-one of my family's favorite recipes to get you back into the kitchen and reignite your love affair with real, whole foods. Bon appétit!

# BEAT IT!

# 20

# Twelve Tips to Beat It

What do I eat? Where do I buy my food? Do I ever "cheat"? What are the foods I avoid? What foods do I eat a lot of? How do I cook my food? It seems as if not a day goes by that I do not have someone asking me about food.

My answer is simple. It is not so much about eating or avoiding specific foods for your mental and physical health; it is all about *thinking* right and eating *real* food. It is a completely "renewed" lifestyle, and it starts in your head (Rom. 12:2).

As we saw in part 2, the brain controls the body but the mind controls the brain. And for the mind to function optimally, it needs to be controlled by your choices, which in turn need to be led by the Holy Spirit. Eating right begins with following the wisdom of God's Word. In this chapter, I shall summarize the fundamental principles outlined in parts 1 and 2 into practical, *mind*-driven lifestyle tips that will help you beat the MAD food system we are all confronted with today.

213

I have also included a selection of my favorite recipes, twenty-one in total, to get you started on your journey. Since it takes twenty-one days to begin reforming neural pathways in the brain, these recipes serve as a habit "kick-starter." They do not need to be followed to the letter—if you want to change them, find alternatives, or create your own, go for it! Indeed, a true love of food comes from experimenting in the kitchen—whether the experiment fails or succeeds. If you can only do one recipe a day, that is perfectly fine. The key is to *renew* the way you think about food and thereby *renew* your food choices.

I am not offering an overnight, quick-fix, magic-bullet, or reductionist solution. I am not going to tell you it will be easy and that everything will start going right in your life. Although the mind can change (remember our neuroplasticity), true change requires hard work and consistent perseverance. I can, however, guarantee that if you choose to make this long-term commitment to changing your food lifestyle, you will be amazed at the results.

I am not going to give you a fish. I am going to *teach* you to fish, so you can think good thoughts and eat *real* food, just as God intended, thereby reaping long-term benefits for you, your family, future generations, and our beautiful planet.

### Tip 1: Develop a *Real* Food Mindset

Our brains and bodies function well when we eat *real* food, since it is full of the essential nutrients needed to maintain everyday biological processes. *Real* food helps us think well.

Memorize the criteria for *real* food:

1. It is largely whole and unprocessed, and all "processing," such as roasting, baking, or preserving, should be done in a kitchen.
2. It is free of synthetic chemicals, both when grown and when prepared.

3. It is predominantly local, fresh, and varies according to the seasons.

4. It is grown in an ecologically diverse environment, which maintains the health of the ecosystem and thus the nutritional content of the foods.

5. It is as wild and sustainable as possible, both in terms of produce and meat.

6. It is processed in a way that treats both the people and animals involved humanely and respects the way animals are meant to eat (grass-fed beef, for instance).

7. It contains just one or a few recognizable ingredients.

8. It does not require a complicated label or make eye-catching health claims.

9. It can rot (with the exception of honey and other natural foods that do not expire in a short amount of time).

10. It is fairly traded. Food production takes a lot of work, and we should respect the individuals who grow our food as much as we would like them to respect us as customers.

Find as many products as possible in your pantry that fulfill these criteria, and compare them with the products in your pantry that cannot be classified as *real* food. Avoid purchasing these products in the future.

Find as many products as possible that fulfill these criteria when you go to the store, farmers' market, or any other establishment that sells food. If they do not fulfill the criteria, avoid purchasing them. Think about what you are buying and make deliberate, health-based food choices rather than following your cravings.

Prepare a delicious meal, using *real* food! Before saying grace, think of the way it was grown, raised, and prepared; how it got to your plate; and how eating this food allows you to be a good steward of God's creation. Pray with a *real* food mindset.

## Tip 2: You Are, and You Become, What You Think

Your mind controls your brain and your brain controls your body. If you want a healthy body, you need a healthy mind. *You are, and you become, what you think.*

### 1. Reexamine Rather Than React

The first, and loudest, unprocessed signal/information coming in through your five senses will dominate your mind if you permit it to, such as a flashing fast-food sign or the smell of popcorn at the movies. It is the signal that has had the most sensory information and the strongest emotions attached to it. It will dominate other signals.

This loudest signal may be an internal existing memory or an external sensory input or both, yet allowing it to dominate your conscious thinking and choosing can be dangerous for your mental and physical health. For example, if your first reaction to a soda commercial is a feeling of contentment and desire for the good life, practice reexamining your *motive* for reaching for that soda.

As you think about, shop for, and plan your meals, become aware of what signals and information are coming into your mind. Become aware of what memories are popping up from your nonconscious mind in response to this information. You may, for instance, have an existing memory such as *Real food costs too much and takes too much time*. Remind yourself of the true cost of cheap food and the true cost of convenience, discussed in part 1.

### 2. Take Those Thoughts into Captivity

If you randomly allow any thought into your mind, and do not bring those thoughts into captivity, damage can ensue on a mental and physical level. If you are not selectively paying attention to what you are thinking about when it comes to food and eating, then you will become reactive and driven by whatever thoughts (and their dynamic emotional energy) come into your mind. Don't allow the fast-food thought to stay in your mind, for example, because then you will want to eat fast food.

The apostle Paul wrote that we have to bring all thoughts into captivity to Christ Jesus (2 Cor. 10:5). *All means all.* Never let any thought go unchecked through your mind. This goes for everything, including *what* and *how* you eat.

Bring those thoughts into captivity: when you are about to make a food-related choice, ask the Holy Spirit what you need to buy, grow, or eat. Ask yourself whether the food choice you are about to make fulfills the criteria of *real* food. Discipline your mind.

### 3. Take the Time to Process Sensory Information

Deep critical thinking, which I have researched for years, involves asking, answering, and discussing incoming sensory information and existing internal thoughts as they move into the conscious mind. This means we consider all the options from as detached and informed a position as possible. This is what it means to *think objectively*, or in quantum physics terms, get into *superposition.* Superposition involves stopping, standing back, observing our own thoughts and the information coming in through the five senses, setting up a dialogue with the Holy Spirit, considering all the options, and then choosing which thoughts we want to implant in our nonconscious mind. This is discussed in depth in chapter 10.

There are a number of options we can choose, just as there are a number of dishes we can choose to eat! These options are called probabilities. The large group of options or probabilities we can choose from is called *Schrödinger's probability wave.*[1] This is a quantum physics principle named after Austrian scientist Erwin Schrödinger.[2] It is a way of mathematically describing all the probable choices we could make, when in superposition, about all the information we come across and every issue we face, including what we put on our plates—even the information offered in this book.[3] We should think carefully and deliberately about all the information we encounter and ask a lot of questions! Just because a professional dietician or "expert" calls something a fact does not mean it *is* a fact.

Likewise, when you are about to make a food-related decision, ask yourself why you are eating and why you want to eat a particular food. Are you really hungry? Are you just craving a snack or something sweet? Are you bored? Happy? Sad? Why? How will you feel later if you indulge now? Do not act reactively.

### 4. Choose Life

Choice is single-handedly the most powerful and creative part of the human mind. As soon as we choose, we collapse a probability into an actuality.[4] Schrödinger's probability wave therefore goes hand in hand with the *observer effect*, another quantum physics law, which states that it is the observer outside of the system (you and me, for example) who collapses probabilities into actualities. This simply means that it is through our choices that things happen. Nothing happens until *we choose*. This is the powerful, sound mind God has given us (2 Tim. 1:7). We set the observer effect in motion each time we think and make a food choice.

We have to understand that *choice is real* and will have *real consequences*, which is why Deuteronomy 30:19 is so powerful: "I call heaven and earth as witnesses today against you, that I have set before you life and death, blessing and cursing; *therefore choose life*, that both you and your descendants *may live*" (emphasis added). It is imperative that we become informed, so that we do not become a "my people are destroyed for lack of knowledge" statistic (Hosea 4:6).

Ask yourself if your food choices will be based on health and life or on sickness and death. Choose life.

## Tip 3: My Brain Didn't Make Me Do It

Remember that the brain and mind are separate, and the mind controls the brain. We have to take personal responsibility for the way we think, speak, and act. We need to stop being victims of our biology, of what happens to us, and start being victors.

A neurocentric view of thought is, *My brain is in control and made me do it*, or *My brain scan shows I have an overactive amygdala, so it is hard for me to control my emotions and that is why I cannot control my eating.* Once you start down this path, you will ultimately have to question your belief in free will, since a predominant focus on the brain takes the control away from the individual and places the blame squarely on the brain.

I do not deny that very real changes will happen in the brain when we lead a toxic eating and thinking lifestyle, nor do I deny the fact that some individuals do have damaged brains through no fault of their own. Yet for the most part our minds (our thoughts and choices) come first and cause problems in the brain and body, which in turn feed back into the mind, making us feel awful if our mind is toxic. The only way weight will come off, and stay off, is through our minds: when we plant healthy food "trees" in our heads, we will eat healthy food in reality. To help with this I recommend my twenty-one-day brain detox.[5]

Do not blame your biology: your mind controls your brain. Regardless of your circumstances, you can change the way you think about and eat food. This does not mean you can eat every single type of food and not get a reaction. It does, however, mean that you can stop eating the MAD diet, and you can choose to follow a *real* food way of eating. Take responsibility for your food choices—past, present, and future.

Food addiction is *not* a disease. *Our brains are wired to latch on to something, and that something is God.* Any toxic addiction, whether it be food, drugs, or even a person, is the result of misplaced choice. Yet, as a growing body of research shows, the majority of people can quit addictions. Individuals who stay addicts usually subscribe to the biomedical model of "once an addict, always an addict." Yet God came to set us free, not lock us in (Luke 4:18). Do not make food your idol, nor any other created thing. It will always disappoint you, but God never will.

Never forget that you are more than a toxic addiction. Even thinking *I can't give up soda* is a toxic addiction resulting from choice. The toxic choices you may have made in the past do not define you. Your identity is in Christ alone (Gen. 1:27; 1 Cor. 6:17; 12:27; Gal. 3:27–28; Col. 2:9–10).

The more you align your thinking with God, the more you will find eating correctly to be both possible and sustainable. We experience true reward when we do things God's way, for his glory, including eating correctly. Faith is the substance (what we choose to wire into our brains) and the evidence (the physical thought that is built as a result of our thinking and choosing) of all that we are hoping for, which leads to physical changes in our brains and bodies (Heb. 11:1). Have faith in your ability to change your eating habits.

### Tip 4: Change Habits over Sixty-Three Days

As I discussed in chapter 10, it takes around twenty-one days to rewire neural pathways and begin building a new way of thinking about food and forty-two days (another two sets of twenty-one days, for a total of sixty-three days) to establish a new habit.

The talk between the conscious and nonconscious mind requires discipline and practice, but if you put the above tips into action for just seven minutes a day, within three weeks you will have removed a toxic food habit and built a new way of thinking about and eating food—through your choices and perseverance!

Here is an example: for dinner tonight, prepare a pasture-raised chicken from the local farmstead, farmers' market, grocery store, or your community-supported agriculture (CSA) box instead of choosing that convenient take-out chicken sandwich from the fast-food establishment down the road. (One of our favorite soup recipes with chicken can be found in the recipe section, if you want a delicious suggestion.) Think about why you are preparing dinner, what care went into your food before it hit your plate, the care you used to prepare it, and how thankful to God you are to have this food and the nourishment it will provide. Think about why you are preparing this meal and the positive eating habits you are establishing. Think about how your brain and body are benefitting. You are changing your epigenetics and your genetics by your choices! Think about how wonderful God is, who has given us such magnificent food, and the pleasure of eating well and enjoying good health. Perhaps discuss these thoughts with your loved ones at the dinner table and definitely enjoy your meal! This is real grace.

You will have to do this thinking at least once a day for a minimum of seven minutes over sixty-three days, when you are shopping, eating, or doing anything food-related, to establish a new habit. Remember, you are rewiring commercials, advertisements, billboards, tastes, and other sensory information that you would on average have seen sixteen times a day, or 5,900 times per year. It is going to take a further two cycles of twenty-one days (forty-two more days, for a total of sixty-three days) to make these new food choices a lifestyle habit. Practice these kinds of choices daily for sixty-three days. You are literally creating a new eating lifestyle, based on life, through the principle of renewing your mind (Rom. 12:2).

True change will take time and commitment. You have to *choose* to change. Constantly thinking about something or listening to something creates genetic change, and learning takes place. This happens—whether you like it or not—when we are constantly exposed to MAD food or *real* food. New thoughts become entrenched and implanted in your nonconscious mind. Be aware of what thoughts you are planting in your mind. Do they lead to life or death?

## Tip 5: Evaluate Your Emotions and Attitude

Remember, the mind and the gut are intensely interconnected. The GI tract is very sensitive to our emotions and works closely with the hypothalamus in the brain, which responds to our emotions *and* the feeling of satiety. Yet emotional awareness in terms of your food choices goes beyond the gut-brain connection: a healthy emotional thought life is necessary to make every food-related decision, including what to buy. Emotions, choices, and actions cannot be separated, since they are part of the perfect circle of thinking in your mind, which in turn impacts your entire body. Your thoughts, with their associated emotions, determine what you choose to eat: you are what you eat *and what you think.*

Beware of how you are feeling when you make a food choice; become a strict observer of your emotions. Do not eat when you are upset, jealous, bitter, angry, or experiencing any other negative emotions. These will affect your digestion. Do not eat just because you are happy or excited. This, too, is an emotional form of eating. Make sure that you are hungry as well, as ridiculous as this may sound.

Eat in a *deliberative* and intentional, not *reactive*, way. Do not grab the ice-cream tub when you are stressed or upset, for example (even if it is organic, local, and grass-fed!). Calm down, and perhaps enjoy a bowl later with your loved one.

Deliberative, intentional eating requires that you deeply think about your food choices and the linked emotions when shopping for, preparing, and eating food. Make sure these decisions are based on positive emotions: love, gratitude, hope, happiness, contentment, satisfaction, excitement, peace, and similar emotions are the perfect condiments to any meal.

If you are stressed, view the situation as a challenge to overcome, not a threat to overwhelm. Stress is designed to work for you and not against you—including in your digestion. How you view a situation will determine this. Do not let toxic stress get the better of you—you can control how you react by your choices.

222

Fear of food is also a negative emotion. Fearing fat, just like fearing carbohydrates or gluten or salt or sugar, is not the right way to approach a healthy diet. Instead, we should fear the way our current industrial food system has transformed our foods into MAD food-like products. It does us good to remember that official dietary recommendations are not always reliable, based on the latest scientific research, or bias-free, and should never just be taken at face value.

Being obsessed about healthy eating and panicking about what you eat will also affect your ability to digest food—no matter how healthy it is! If you bake a chocolate cake (with *real* whole foods, of course), enjoy it! As Oscar Wilde notes, "Everything in moderation, including moderation."[6] We were created to enjoy our food, which is a gift from God.

Get "dressed" mentally for dinner. Before eating, listen to your favorite song, watch your favorite movie, or read your favorite book. Talk to a loved one. Pay it forward with a random act of kindness. Put on your favorite song and dance like no one is watching. Read the Bible and think of how much you have to be grateful for. Whatever you love, whatever makes you happy, do it; this will get a whole host of positive chemicals running about your body and prepare you for a great meal.

## Tip 6: There Is No One Diet

As we saw in part 1, there is no one particular way of eating that works for everyone. God created fat, carbohydrates, and proteins, as well as all the other important nutritional building blocks that make up the food we eat—all perfectly and intricately balanced within the *real* foods we eat. Stick to *real* foods, and avoid the MAD diet and diet fads. Learn to listen to what your body needs.

To help identify what your body uniquely needs, plan to do a fast. (See chapter 12 for more on fasting.) Start with intermittent fasting (skipping a meal), giving up a specific type of food or drink for ten or more days, or something like the Daniel Fast.[7] If you have been eating the MAD diet, your brain and body will be confused by all the food-like products you have been consuming. Fasting helps clear the confusion in your brain and body. When you add a type of food back to your diet after several days, you can see how your body responds to it. (Obviously, if you have allergies, first consult with a medical professional.)

The different types of fasting are excellent lifestyle choices for our brain, body, and mental health, and, of course, have many spiritual benefits. As we discipline our *mind* and choose to reduce our *bodily* food intake as we focus on God, our *spirit* develops. Jesus wants us to be integrated spirit, soul, and body (1 Thess. 5:23).

Any diet that promises *instant* results should come under our intellectual radar. Real, permanent change always takes *time and effort*. Do not expect immediate results. Do expect difficult days. But always remember that you are more than a conqueror through Christ, with whom all things are possible.

### Tip 7: Buying Food

When purchasing any food item, make sure it is *real* food insofar as possible, not a food-like product. Try to shop outside of the supermarket: visit local CSAs, farmers' markets, and farmstead stores, or start growing or raising your own food.

Get to know the people who produce your food: ask them questions and learn the story behind your food. Generally avoid food producers who are evasive about how the food is grown, raised, or made, or do not allow visitors (such as on a farm). Ask your local and seasonal food producers what they have a lot of, and buy it. This helps prevent food waste and supports local businesses.

Buy local, organically produced foods: they support your community and ecosystem and they reduce fossil fuel use, as well as ensuring that you get food that is as fresh, synthetic chemical–free, and nutritious as possible, especially in terms of fresh produce.

Buy whole foods, such as wheat grains and whole produce, which can be "processed" in your kitchen. You will also find that buying whole foods and processing them at home can be a cheap way to make your diet healthy. Potato chips, for instance, can cost $8 per pound, where an heirloom potato variety at a farmers' market costs less than half that.[8]

If you eat out, support establishments that serve local, farm-to-table, and organically produced foods as much as possible. If you visit a grocery store, be aware of the structured environment and how the layout is designed to grab your attention and get you to buy and eat more processed MAD foods. Healthier products are often put close to the bottom of the shelves, while the healthiest foods are on the perimeter, such as fresh produce. The center aisles are usually filled with processed and refined MAD foods. And remember, avoid impulse buys at the counter!

Buy wild foods: these are generally more nutritious and make a meal both exciting and impressive. This tip applies to all food types. If you buy animal products, they should ideally be pasture-raised or grass-fed (aim for 100 percent grass-fed, not just grass-finished), organically raised, free of added hormones or antibiotics, and always humanely raised. It is a good idea to buy these meats in bulk and freeze them for future use. Often several individuals buy shares in a whole animal from a local farm.

Try to avoid purchasing too much muscle meat: go for bone broths, organ meats, and other parts of the animal that are more nutrient dense.

Buy a diverse range of foods. If you try to shop as seasonally as possible, you often eat a more varied diet. Farmers' markets are particularly good places to begin. Japanese turnip and kohlrabi with your heirloom purple potatoes, anyone?

Buying bulk in season, and freezing or preserving the foods, can save time and money. For example, buy berries or tomatoes in the summer when they are widely available and less expensive, and freeze or puree them for the winter months.

Try to buy whole nuts, seeds, and grains and process them at home. For example, make your own wheat flour for your own homemade bread, or make your own almond milk. There are countless recipes online for free. If you buy bread, make sure it is fresh, whole grain, with optimally a few simple and well-known ingredients—it should start going stale after a day. Buy fats that are unrefined, unfiltered, extra-virgin (when possible), and cold-processed.

Remember, "If it ain't decomposing in your kitchen, it ain't decomposing in your tummy." Avoid all food that does not rot (with certain exceptions, such as honey). Avoid MAD foods, foods with added nutrients, and/or foods that make health claims. Think of an apple: Does it have any health claims plastered on its skin?

### Tip 8: Respect the Environment

The apostle Paul declares, "Whether you eat or drink or whatever you do, do it all for the glory of God" (1 Cor. 10:31 NIV). As stewards of God's creation, we glorify him when we steward the earth's resources well and we eat food that nourishes us and glorifies the creation of our own bodies.

Before you purchase any food, think deeply about how that food was produced. If you purchase it, ask yourself whether you are stewarding God's creation well. Each day, make an effort to think about how the food in your basket or on your plate got there. Perhaps say a prayer for the people who produced it, and thank God for the opportunity to glorify his creation with your food.

Volunteer at a local farm, farmers' market, farmstead store, or CSA, or start a garden and begin raising chickens. By coming face-to-face with your food, you will develop a deeper appreciation for God's creation and the gift of life.

Think of ways you can reduce food waste. Compost leftover foods or regrow vegetables from food scraps, for example. Start raising chickens and feed them kitchen scraps as a supplement to their diet. See *Folks, This Ain't Normal: A Farmer's Advice for Happier Hens, Healthier People, and a Better World* by Joel Salatin and *Waste: Uncovering the Global Food Scandal* by Tristram Stuart for more suggestions.

Think of ways you can vote not only with your fork but with your political vote as well. Get involved in grassroots movements that promote local, sustainable, agroecological farming methods. Get in touch with your local and state representatives to fight for a better food system. Send letters to the government officials handling dietary guidelines. There are many, many ways you can make a more sustainable food system a reality for not only you but every person on the planet, while stewarding God's creation well and bringing "heaven to earth."

Be a "hipster" and start an agroecological garden, or even a farm—even if you have just one chicken and a zucchini shrub in the beginning. As is often said, "Little by little, one travels far."

### Tip 9: How to Cook

Often, diet books are so concerned about what you eat that they do not explain how you should prepare these meals to preserve the most nutrients possible. Cooking is not just about nutrient preservation, however; it also entails the bioavailability of nutrients, or how readily these nutrients can be absorbed. The following points are cooking tips we use as a family.

1. Some vegetables are better eaten raw, such as lettuce greens, while other vegetables are better eaten cooked, such as carrots and tomatoes. For a full list of fruit and vegetable preparation, see *Eating on the Wild Side* by Jo Robinson.

2. Eat your produce with a type of fat, in order to absorb the fat-soluble nutrients.

3. There are several main factors in terms of nutrient loss and cooking: heat, duration of cooking time, amount of water, amount of fat in the food, direct or indirect sources of heat used, and type of fuel used.[9] Be aware of this as you cook any food. For instance, overcooking at high temperatures activates the Maillard reaction, when glucose and protein molecules bind at high temperatures. This is toxic because it forms AGEs (advanced glycation end products).[10] In turn, this changes the structure of a protein, potentially making it a problem for the body to digest, assimilate, and metabolize, with negative health effects such as the possible development of cancer.[11] Most processed foods in the MAD are heated to very high temperatures and for long lengths of time—one more reason to stay clear of them![12]

4. Ideally, cook vegetables in a soup, *sous-vide* in silicone bags (a water bath method), stew in a slow cooker, poach, or steam them.[13] Occasionally roast or sauté—although avoid high temperatures with long cooking times. We usually roast vegetables for a maximum of twenty to thirty minutes, or sauté them for just a minute in a small amount of fat (coconut oil, olive oil, lard, grass-fed butter, or ghee) after steaming on medium-low heat. We do not boil our fruit or vegetables, as the nutrients can leech out into the water.[14]

5. For meat, steaming, a *sous-vide* method, and cooking in soups, stews, and broths on low heat are healthier options. Avoid direct and open sources of heat as much as possible.[15] Open-flame grills can be carcinogenic, especially if you like your meat well done, which can produce potentially carcinogenic levels of heterocyclic amines (HCAs) and polycyclic aromatic hydrocarbons (PAHs), for instance.[16] To get a crispy exterior, you can quickly sauté or grill the meat, constantly

turning it over the source, after you have used one of the methods above. We have the occasional roast chicken, ham, beef, turkey, or lamb, which will braise in an acidic liquid such as lemon juice or wine (see below), and bake in parchment paper or in a covered roasting dish.

6. Acids, such as vinegar and lemon juice, also reduce the risk of unwanted cooking side effects, so use them when cooking all types of food.[17] They are also great for flavor!

7. In terms of nuts, beans, seeds, and grains, soaking and sprouting may be better options than regular whole grains, both in terms of digestibility and nutrient content and nutrient bioavailability.[18] We as a family personally do not experience any additional benefit from soaking or sprouting our quinoa. My daughters, however, do feel that sprouted nuts and beans are more digestible. You may feel otherwise. They can be expensive, so sprout them at home to save money (there are many online resources showing how to do this).

8. Avoid artificial additives, seasonings, and preservatives when cooking. Sodium in salt is a necessary nutrient, and a deficiency in sodium can harm your health as much as an excess of sodium can, yet it should form part of a balanced *real* food diet. You will find that local, fresh, organically produced, and seasonal foods do not need salt to replace flavor (unlike the MAD foods). Rather, salt such as Himalayan pink salt and black lava salt, in moderate amounts, enhances rather than replaces the beautiful flavors of these *real* foods.

9. Use a separate cutting board for meat than you use for produce and grains.

10. Do not wash your meat—this can spread germs around the kitchen. But always wash your hands, before and after handling meat! We generally take meat out of the package with a fork and try to handle the raw meat with our bare hands as little as possible.

11. Thoroughly wash all your produce items. Salad spinners and fruit and vegetable sprays are indispensable in the kitchen.

12. Use pots, pans, and dishes that are free of heavy metals, PFOA, and PTFE, as these chemicals can have adverse health effects.[19] We use stainless steel and ceramic cookware, or nonstick cookware that is free of heavy metals, PFOA, and PTFE.

13. As Michael Pollan notes, "Treat treats as treats."[20] For the most part, if we crave something sweet we will eat some fruit. On occasion, we love a good dessert, prepared with delicious *real* food. For a recipe suggestion, try our apple pie recipe—you won't regret it!

14. Of course, it goes without saying that you should eat lots of vegetables and fruits.

### Tip 10: How to Eat

Our fast-paced modern lifestyles have produced the mindset of *I am too busy to sit down to a home-cooked meal*. If you value your health and your relationships, begin changing this mindset. A home-cooked family meal has more benefits than just bodily health!

Modern technology has made it easier in many respects for us to work *all the time*. Do not fall into the trap of living under an unnecessary sense of urgency, which can put you in chronic toxic stress and make you ill—and give you terrible indigestion. Remember the gut-brain connection!

Eat less from a box and eat less in front of a box: avoid TV, reading, or listening to the radio while eating. These forms of entertainment make you pay less attention to how you are eating and how much you are eating.

The joy of preparing a meal and sharing it with people is incredibly powerful and therapeutic. Do not view cooking as a task; see it as a fun adventure and an opportunity to spend time with those you love, family and friends, as much as is possible in your lifestyle.

Eat slowly. If we eat too fast we will eat more, since it takes up to twenty minutes for our body and brain to signal satiation and for us to realize we are no longer hungry.[21] Make sure that most of your meals last more than twenty minutes. And remember, the first two bites of any food are the most flavorful, so take time to enjoy them!

*Hara hachi bu!* Take this Okinawan saying to heart: stop eating when you are 80 percent full.[22] Eighty percent is not a strict calculation per se—it just means that if you feel quite full, you have eaten too much. It is based on calorie restriction and, paired with fasting, can help maintain a healthy lifestyle. The Okinawans live in one of the seven identified "blue zones"—areas that have the highest life expectancy—and thus their advice is worth taking to heart. The key is *eating less*, which will be different for everyone. We have somewhat adapted this saying in our house: only seconds for salad, or you will make a *hara hachi* "boo boo."

Avoid snacking, as your body will not have had time to digest your previous meals and you may end up eating too much.[23] Generally, eat when you are hungry, which requires that you learn to listen to your body's demands. Limiting your food intake to three meals a day is a good start. If you overeat, you will carry on eating—the more you eat the less able you are to judge how much you have eaten.

Let your mind, not your eyes, be your guide—it is not a good idea to decide visually how much to eat, since you will have a tendency to finish what is on the plate rather than stopping when full.[24] Put less food on your plate or use a smaller plate.

Be aware of habits you may have developed over time, such as eating when you are sad or excited (but not hungry), or coming home and going straight to the fridge or pantry out of habit (even if you are not hungry).

Prepare and eat meals together as a family and/or with friends as much as possible. Not only will this help your health but it has added benefits for your children: research shows that family time over meals is associated with lower drug and alcohol abuse, less depression and suicide risk, and even better grades in school.[25] Moreover, good company is associated with positive emotions, which aid digestion and promote mental wellbeing.

Do not eat in your car and on the run. Make your eating habits as *deliberate* as your thinking habits. Also, your posture is important to digestion, whether you are at the table or going about your daily tasks.[26] Pay attention to the way you sit and stand.

Whoever cooks should not clean, if possible—divide the tasks and the work will be finished in a shorter amount of time. You can even draw lots; it certainly makes mealtime fun.

## Tip 11: Sleep, Schedules, and Digestion

The brain and the gut are connected in many things, including sleep and schedules. Healthy sleeping patterns contribute to healthy eating patterns.

Do not go to sleep worrying about your circumstances; this can upset your sleep cycle, digestion, and weight. Hand all your issues over to God—even if unsolved—and fall asleep quoting a Scripture or thinking of all the good things that have happened to you or anything that makes you happy and feel at peace. Write your cares down before you sleep and read the promises in God's Word. A good Scripture to memorize is 1 Peter 5:7: "Give all your worries and cares to God, for he cares about you" (NLT). Give him your fears.

Everyone has their own sleep cycle, a cycle that is as unique as everything else about them. You have to sleep—that is a no-brainer—but there is no agreement among scientists on exactly how much sleep you need or when you should sleep. You will do damage to your health if you worry about your sleep, wondering what will happen and then panicking that you are not getting exactly eight hours of sleep and are not going to digest your food properly and will get sick and fat and have brain damage. These fears will cause more brain damage and worsen your sleep pattern, so just relax, read the Bible, and pray if you cannot sleep. Even start a discussion with the Holy Spirit about whatever you want to talk about.

Give your eating habits over to God each night before you sleep. Ask him to guide your food decisions. Pray over your brain and your body before you go to sleep.

Ask the Holy Spirit to help you with your schedule. You are designed to "do busy well," but only if this "busy" is led by God. Not doing busy well will affect your sleeping patterns and your food choices, including how much you eat, since a lack of sleep is associated with a greater intake of food the next day. Healthy, peaceful sleeping patterns and balanced schedules mean you will eat well, and this will help maintain good health.

**Tip 12: Exercise**

Eat less, move more: we have all heard this saying at some point in our lives. Not only does exercise make our blood circulate more efficiently through our bodies, bringing the chemicals of life to the cells and removing the debris of metabolism, but it can also improve all areas of cognitive function, including thinking, learning, and memory, especially with age. The older you get the more you need to move, even if it is for short bursts or just walking up those stairs instead of going in the elevator.

Research indicates that aerobic exercise in particular (such as cardio and walking) creates improved and flexible cognition and maintains good bodily health. When you exercise, your cognition becomes more flexible, your metabolism increases, and great hormones flow! Remember, however, that exercise can never make up for unhealthy food choices. Both regular physical activity and a healthy *real* food diet are necessary for a healthy lifestyle.

Unhealthy lifestyle habits, such as the MAD "TV" diet with little or no exercise, will speed up the process of senescence, or cell death.

As you are running, power walking, spinning, doing high-intensity training, lifting weights, or whatever you choose to do, these exercises are changing your DNA, hormones, brain, and your entire body for the better. And to enhance your exercise routine, you can add a cup of organic, freshly roasted, fair-trade and whole bean coffee. Coffee can change your genetic expression in the same way exercise does—but obviously does not replace exercise.[27]

Your mind makes exercise much more effective. After all, exercise is a choice you make with your mind, so when you exercise, put your mind behind it! Be as deliberative about your exercise habits as you are about your eating habits.

# 21

# A Twenty-One Recipe Kick Start

## —— Avocado-Cilantro Hummus ——

| | |
|---|---|
| 1 med | ripe avocado, peeled and pitted |
| 1 cup | chickpeas (garbanzo beans), drained and rinsed |
| ¼ cup | fresh cilantro (coriander), chopped |
| 2 Tbs | freshly squeezed lemon juice |
| 1 tsp | freshly squeezed lime juice |
| pinch | lemon zest |
| ½ tsp | cumin |
| | salt and fresh ground pepper to taste |
| 1 | clove fresh garlic, minced |
| 1 | chili pepper, finely chopped and seeded (optional) |
| 3 Tbs | tahini (homemade is always the most flavorful) |
| 1 tsp | nutritional yeast (optional) |
| dash | cayenne pepper |

Blend all ingredients together in a food processor or strong blender until creamy. Add a little water if needed. Serve with fresh, seasonal raw vegetables such as carrots, bell peppers, celery, and cucumber; homemade pita bread (whole grain or grain free); or homemade crackers. Serve as an appetizer or as lunch or dinner—whatever suits your fancy!

If you want a more interesting taste variation, make your own tahini: toast raw sesame seeds on low in the oven, grind them into a smooth paste, then add them to the other ingredients. Or, if you cannot handle chickpeas, use 1 cup steamed cauliflower or 1 cup diced zucchini instead. Generally, it is a good idea to experiment with vegetables that are in season.

Tired of the flavor? Replace the cilantro with fresh chopped parsley, mint, basil, chives, or oregano—you may have to adjust quantities depending on your preference. Mint works especially well with preserved lemons in a hummus. Can't handle the heat? Leave out the chili pepper and replace the cayenne with a dash of mild paprika (smoked or regular).

Want a sweeter version? Use 1 large roasted red beet instead of chickpeas and avocado. This version works particularly well with mint or basil instead of cilantro. To roast beet, preheat oven to 400°F (204°C), scrub the beet's exterior, put it in a parchment bag, and bake it for 30 minutes or until soft. Peel beet and add to the food processor with other ingredients. Raw fennel (or anise) is particularly tasty with this variation.

Another tummy-friendly version: replace avocado and chickpeas with two cups zucchini, chopped, and slowly pour in ¼ cup of olive oil in a steady, thin stream on low speed (to emulsify) after you have blended all the other ingredients into a creamy paste.

Generally, a mortar and pestle is a brilliant investment for grinding all herbs instead of just chopping them: it brings out their flavor perfectly.

## ———— Avocado Dandelion Salad ————

|       |                              |
|-------|------------------------------|
| 4     | carrots, julienned           |
| 2 cups| dandelion greens, chopped    |
| 1 lg  | ripe avocado, peeled and pitted |
| 1 Tbs | fresh squeezed lemon juice   |

1   clove garlic, minced
    salt and black pepper to taste
dash   cayenne pepper
½ tsp   paprika
1 Tbs   nutritional yeast (optional)

1. Julienne the carrots with a peeler (we usually leave the skins on) and mix with chopped dandelion greens.
2. Blend the avocado, lemon juice, garlic, salt and black pepper, cayenne, paprika, and nutritional yeast, and massage into the salad. Leave to set for 5 minutes, then serve.

## —— Simple Arugula and Kale Salad ——

1 cup   baby arugula
2 cups   kale of choice
½ cup   cherry tomatoes, halved
1   lemon, juiced
    salt and pepper to taste
1 Tbs   olive oil
1 tsp   Dijon mustard (optional)

1. Toss arugula, kale, and tomatoes with lemon juice, salt, black pepper, and olive oil.
2. Massage in Dijon mustard, if using (this softens the kale and makes it more digestible). Let stand for 5–10 minutes, then serve.

## — Mint and Red Pepper Quinoa Salad —

1 cup   fair-trade quinoa
2 cups   water or homemade broth
2   red peppers (capsicum), diced
2 Tbs   olive oil, divided
    salt and black pepper to taste
½   clove garlic, finely minced
1   lemon, halved

1 lg   cucumber, diced
1½ Tbs   mint, freshly chopped
3 cups   salad greens
2 tsp   balsamic vinegar
(or other vinegar of choice)

1. Rinse quinoa thoroughly in a small strainer. Place quinoa and water (or homemade broth) in a 1½ quart saucepan and bring to a boil. Reduce heat to simmer. Cover and cook until liquid is absorbed, about 10–15 minutes.
2. Place cooked quinoa into a salad bowl with peppers, 1 tablespoon of olive oil, salt and freshly ground black pepper (be generous with the black pepper!), minced garlic, and the juice of half a lemon. Allow this mixture to cool.
3. Once the quinoa has cooled to room temperature, add in the cucumber, mint, salad greens, remaining olive oil, balsamic vinegar, and the juice of the other lemon half, plus more salt and pepper if needed. Toss and let set for 5–10 minutes before serving.

## Simply Steamed Carrots

10   rainbow carrots, whole, with tops chopped off (leave the skin on, just make sure you wash them well)
1 Tbs   ghee (or olive oil to make it vegan)
salt and pepper to taste
½   clove garlic, minced

1. Steam carrots whole for about 8 minutes or until tender, depending on their size.
2. Chop carrots and mix with ghee or olive oil, salt, pepper, and garlic.

If you want to spruce up the dish, sprinkle with cumin or two sprigs of thyme.

If you cannot find rainbow carrots, use regular orange carrots (and grow your own for the future!).

# —— Cinnamon and Cumin —— Butternut Mash

| | |
|---:|:---|
| 1 | whole butternut squash, peeled, seeded, and cubed (rinse and reserve seeds) |
| 1 tsp | balsamic vinegar |
| 2 dashes | cinnamon |
| 1 dash | cumin |
| 1 Tbs | ghee (or olive oil to make it vegan), plus a little extra for the seeds |
| ½ | clove garlic, minced |
| | salt and pepper to taste |

1. Preheat the oven to 325°F (163°C). Toss reserved seeds in balsamic vinegar and a bit of fat of choice and roast on parchment paper for around 15 minutes. Toss the seeds again and roast for another 10 minutes. Set aside to cool.
2. While the seeds are roasting, steam squash for about 12 minutes until it pierces easily with a fork.
3. Combine all ingredients (except the seeds) and mash.
4. Before serving, sprinkle with roasted seeds.

# —— Balsamic Brussels Sprouts —— with Roasted Chestnuts

| | |
|---:|:---|
| 2 cups | Brussels sprouts |
| 1 | clove garlic, minced |
| 1 Tbs | ghee (or oil of choice) |
| 1 Tbs | balsamic vinegar |
| | salt and pepper to taste |
| 2 strips | bacon of choice (such as pork, turkey, or beef), chopped and sautéed, or 4 slices of prosciutto (optional) |
| ½ cup | roasted chestnuts, chopped |

1. Lightly steam Brussels sprouts (we usually steam them for around 6–7 minutes).
2. Mix in all other ingredients except chestnuts. Let stand for 15 minutes.
3. Add chestnuts, let it stand for another 5 minutes, and serve.

## —— Sweet Potato Ricotta Lasagna ——

|  |  |
|---|---|
| 1 | onion (yellow or red), diced |
| 2 | cloves fresh garlic, minced |
| 1 cup | basil, freshly chopped |
| 1 cup | oregano, freshly chopped |
| 3 sprigs | rosemary, freshly chopped |
| ¼ cup | thyme, freshly chopped |
| ¼ cup | marjoram, freshly chopped |
| 1 Tbs | parsley, freshly chopped |
|  | salt and pepper to taste |
| 2 lbs | ground meat of choice (try to find a "primal" version that is mixed with organ meats) |
| 3 cups | tomatoes, diced |
| 3 cups | tomato puree |
| 1 cup | tomato paste |
| ¼ cup | red wine (sulfite-free is a good option) |
| 3 lg | sweet potatoes, peeled and sliced into lasagna-style pasta sheets, about half a finger's thickness |
| 2 Tbs | oil or fat of choice |
| 1½ cups | whole milk mozzarella cheese, shredded and divided |
| 1½ cups | ricotta cheese |
| ½ cup | heavy whipping cream |
| 1 lg | egg |
| ¼ cup | Parmesan cheese, freshly shredded |

1. On medium-low heat, sauté onions, garlic, herbs, salt, and pepper in fat until onions are translucent.
2. Add meat on low heat and cook (stirring vigorously to avoid clumping) until lightly browned.

3. Add all tomatoes and wine, and simmer for about two and a half hours (one hour with the lid on, one and a half hours with the lid off) to create the Bolognese sauce.
4. Meanwhile, preheat oven to 425°F (220°C). Drizzle sweet potato slices with oil or fat (very, very little or they will be too soggy!) and bake on parchment paper until soft (about 20 minutes).
5. Combine 1 cup mozzarella, ricotta, heavy whipping cream, and egg in a saucepan, and cook on medium-low heat until mozzarella is melted.
6. Layer the lasagna in a 9x13 pan as follows: one-third of the sweet potato "pasta," one-third of the Bolognese sauce, then half of the ricotta sauce. Repeat. For the third layer, use remaining sweet potato and Bolognese, then top with remaining ½ cup mozzarella and Parmesan, which will enable the top to bake to a light golden layer. Optional: top with any leftover fresh basil or oregano before placing in the oven.
7. Preheat oven to 350°F (180°C). Bake the lasagna for 20 minutes, or until the top is a golden color.

In place of the sweet potato, you can use whole-grain or gluten-free lasagna pasta sheets, or even sliced eggplant, zucchini, or another vegetable for variation or for a less sweet taste. Experiment with what is in season. You can use this Bolognese sauce on any kind of pasta as well, including zucchini pasta.

For a vegan Bolognese sauce, shred carrots, onions, cauliflower, zucchini (or whatever vegetables are in season) in a food processor to yield about 6 cups. Quickly sauté on medium-low heat. Add tomatoes and wine and simmer for 45 minutes. For a thicker sauce, add 1 cup of drained and rinsed chickpeas that have been made into a paste in the food processor, and simmer up to an hour. Replace the ricotta sauce with a vegan bechamel sauce—there are many great recipes online and in books. Our personal favorite is Diana Sanfilippo's sauce in *Mediterranean Paleo Cooking*.

There are many great recipes online and in books for making and preserving your own tomato sauces. If you have to buy store bought, aim for organic sauces in glass jars, BPA-free cans, or boxes that can be reused or recycled. We use so much tomato sauce that inevitably we run out and have to buy it from the store during the colder months when tomatoes are not in season.

If you cannot tolerate tomatoes, find a tomato-free marinara sauce online and use the same quantities. Our favorite with this recipe is Jenni Hulet's marinara sauce, which you can find on her blog, *The Urban Poser.*

## — Beet and Pink Peppercorn Salmon —

| | |
|---|---|
| 1 sm | red beet |
| 4 | salmon fillets |
| 1 | whole lemon |
| 2 | garlic cloves, thinly sliced at an angle |
| 2 tsp | olive oil (or fat of choice) |
| | salt and pepper, to taste |
| 2 tsp | pink peppercorns |
| 2 tsp | dried hibiscus leaves |
| 1 tsp | chickpea miso |
| 2 | lemons, juiced |
| 2 | shallots, minced |
| 1 | clove garlic, minced |

1. Roast the beet. Preheat oven to 400°F (204°C), scrub the beet's exterior, put it in a parchment bag, and bake for 30 minutes or until soft. Let cool, then peel and dice.
2. Preheat oven to 320°F (160°C). Grease your baking dish or line it with parchment paper. Place salmon fillets side by side in the pan.

   Cut the whole lemon in four quarters, take out the seeds, and squeeze the juice over the fish, then drizzle olive oil over and sprinkle the sliced garlic and a dash of salt and pepper evenly on each fillet. Cover fillets in more parchment paper and bake for 20–30 minutes. Alternatively, you can place fillets in a parchment bag with the lemon quarters and bake them, or steam the salmon. If steaming, drizzle with oil, lemon, salt and pepper, and garlic. Lemon-infused water also works particularly well when steaming. A sous vide (with reusable silicone bags) works well too.
3. While salmon is cooking, put remaining ingredients (roasted beet, pink peppercorns, hibiscus flowers, chickpea miso, juice of two lemons, minced shallot, minced garlic, and a dash of salt) into a food processor or strong blender and blend until creamy.

4. Drizzle the beet sauce over the salmon and serve with a side dish of choice. Fennel (anise) works well with this dish.

If you are a vegan or vegetarian, or just do not want fish, this beet and pink peppercorn sauce pairs well with lightly steamed fennel and quinoa or another whole grain of choice (we usually toss the quinoa in a bit of olive oil, salt, and pepper in this recipe).

Can't handle chickpeas? Try substituting the miso with 1 teaspoon of tahini and a dash of coconut aminos (a "soy" sauce made from coconut rather than soy).

## Chicken Vegetable Soup

| | |
|---|---|
| 1 | yellow onion, diced |
| 2 | leeks, chopped |
| 3 lg | zucchini, diced |
| 1 cup | celery, diced |
| 1 cup | carrots, diced |
| 1 cup | broccoli florets |
| 1 | turnip, diced |
| 3 | cloves garlic, freshly minced |
| 10 cups | homemade broth (for more flavor) or water |
| 1 Tbs | coconut vinegar or apple cider vinegar |
| 2 heaping tsp | black pepper |
| 1 dash | cayenne pepper |
| 1 tsp | celery seed |
| 2 Tbs | parsley, freshly chopped |
| 1 Tbs | oregano, freshly chopped |
| 1 Tbs | thyme, freshly chopped |
| 1 Tbs | basil, freshly chopped |
| 1 Tbs | sage, freshly chopped |
| | ground coriander, to taste |
| | salt, to taste |
| 1 | whole chicken |

1. Add the vegetables to a large pot over medium-low heat (or slow cooker on low) with the water or broth.
2. Add the vinegar, pepper, herbs, and salt to taste, and stir in.
3. Carefully add the whole chicken, and leave on low heat for 6 hours.
4. Remove chicken, let cool slightly, then clean meat from the bones and return the meat to pot (you can save the chicken carcass to make stock for future recipes).
5. Serve as-is or blend for a more creamy consistency.

For a vegan/vegetarian version, leave out the chicken, use water or vegetable stock instead of chicken broth, and add an extra 3 cups of vegetables of choice. Cook for about 1 hour on simmer/low.

This soup can be changed based on what is in season. We usually use whatever vegetables are growing or we have in our CSA box.

# ——— Mustard and Mushroom ——— Chicken Sauté

|  |  |
|---:|---|
| 4 | chicken breasts |
| 2 | garlic cloves, minced |
| 1 | shallot, chopped |
| 1 Tbs | ghee, or fat of choice |
| 2 cups | fresh mushrooms of choice, chopped |
|  | salt and pepper to taste |
| 2 | fresh sprigs of thyme |
| 3 Tbs | Dijon mustard |
| 1 | lemon, juiced |

1. Steam chicken until cooked through, then chop into small pieces.
2. Sauté garlic and shallots in fat of choice on medium-low heat until shallots are translucent.
3. Add mushrooms and sauté until water has evaporated.
4. Add cooked chicken, thyme, dijon mustard, and lemon juice, sauté for around 2–3 minutes, and serve with a side of choice.

For a vegan/vegetarian version, add mustard and thyme to the mushrooms, sauté for half a minute, and substitute 1 cup of quinoa or whole grain of choice (cooked with water or vegetable broth) for the chicken.

## —— Simple and Sweet Potato Waffles ——

| | |
|---|---|
| 2 cups | sweet potato, peeled and shredded |
| 1 | egg |
| dash | cinnamon |
| 1 tiny pinch | salt |
| ½ tsp | coconut oil or fat of choice |

1. Mix shredded sweet potato with the egg, cinnamon, and salt.
2. Melt the fat on the waffle griddle and cook the sweet potato mixture. (We use a ceramic waffle iron.) Cook until golden.
3. Top with your favorite fruits; spices such as cinnamon; proteins to make the waffles savory; fats such as nut butters, coconut cream, or grass-fed organic cream or butter. Be adventurous!

To make the waffles savory, omit cinnamon and add another spice, such as cumin, if you want!

## ——— No-Cook Avocado Oatmeal ———

| | |
|---|---|
| ¼ cup | oat groats or steel-cut oats, soaked overnight in water |
| ½ | ripe avocado |
| 3 Tbs | homemade almond milk or milk of choice |
| 1 | date, pitted (add an extra date if you prefer it sweeter) |
| 2 dashes | cinnamon |

Blend all the ingredients on high until smooth. Add more milk if necessary.

## Egg Cupcakes

|      |      |
|-----:|:-----|
| 12 | cherry tomatoes, diced |
|  | a bit of ghee or fat of choice |
| 6 | eggs |
| 2 Tbs | red onion, finely chopped |
| 6 | sprigs of fresh chives, chopped |
|  | salt and pepper to taste |
| 6 strips | cooked bacon of choice (optional) |

1. Preheat oven to 350°F (180°C).
2. Grease a six-count cupcake pan with fat, or line cups with parchment paper.
3. Sauté the tomatoes over medium-low heat with a bit of ghee or other fat for around 1–2 minutes.
4. Whisk together egg, onion, chives, salt, and pepper, and add the tomatoes.
5. Put one slice of bacon around the edge of each cupcake (so it will wrap around the egg mixture).
6. Pour egg mixture into the cupcake pan, dividing evenly, and bake for around 15–20 minutes.

Shredded cheese is a great addition on top, if you can tolerate dairy.

## Seed Bread

|      |      |
|-----:|:-----|
| ½ cup | raw, shelled pumpkin seeds |
| 1½ cups | raw hemp seeds |
| ½ cup | ground flax seeds |
| 1 cup | raw sunflower seeds |
| 2 Tbs | chia seeds |
| 1 tsp | salt |
| small dash | stevia powder |
| 3 Tbs | psyllium husk powder |
| 1½ cups | water |
| 3 Tbs | melted coconut oil or ghee |

1. Mix seeds, salt, stevia, and psyllium in a bowl.
2. Whisk water with melted coconut oil (or ghee). Add to seed mixture. After mixing well, let set for 2½ hours.
3. Preheat oven to 350°F (180°C). Pour mixture into a bread loaf pan that has been lined with parchment paper. Bake for 20 minutes. Rotate the pan and bake for another 50 minutes to an hour.

If you don't like stevia, replace with 1 tsp coconut nectar, whisked into the water and coconut oil.

For a crispier toast, switch the oven off, slice the baked bread, and leave in the oven for 10–15 minutes.

## —— Orange, Plum, and Apricot Jam ——

| | |
|---:|:---|
| 3 | dates, pitted |
| ½ cup | dried plums |
| ½ cup | dried apricots |
| ½ tsp | lemon juice |
| ½ lg | orange, juiced |
| 1 Tbs | chia seeds |

1. Soak dates, apricots, and plums in boiling water to cover for twenty-five minutes, and then drain.
2. Blend all the ingredients on high until smooth (using either a food processor or high-speed blender). Add a little more water or orange juice if necessary.

## ——— Pineapple Almond Shake ———

| | |
|---:|:---|
| 1 cup | whole raw almonds |
| 1 whole | pineapple, peeled, cored, and diced |
| 3–4 Tbs | freshly squeezed orange juice (or more if needed) |

1. In a food processor, grind the almonds into a flour.
2. Add pineapple and orange juice. Blend until smooth and serve.

## ——— Green "Ice Cream" Smoothie ———

| | |
|---|---|
| 2 cups | baby kale |
| 2 cups | spinach |
| 1 cup | raw coconut water |
| 1 scoop | vanilla protein powder (we use Vega Vanilla Smoothie) |
| ½ | frozen banana |
| 1 Tbs | chia seeds |
| 2 Tbs | homemade almond milk, or milk of choice |

Blend all the ingredients until smooth and creamy.

## ——— Coconut Mango Sorbet ———

| | |
|---|---|
| 1 cup | chopped, peeled, frozen mango |
| ¾ cup | coconut milk |
| 1 tsp | coconut sugar or maple sugar |
| dash | vanilla |

Blend all ingredients together and serve.

## ——— Apple Pie ———

For the crust:

| | |
|---|---|
| ½ cup | coconut flour |
| ¼ cup | tapioca flour |
| ¼ tsp | salt |
| 2 Tbs | ghee or coconut oil |
| 1 Tbs | coconut nectar |
| 2 | eggs |
| ½ lg | apple, peeled, cored, diced, and blended into applesauce in a food processor (reserve peels) |

For the filling:

| | |
|---|---|
| 1 Tbs | ghee or coconut oil |
| 4 lg | apples, peeled, cored, and sliced (reserve peels) |

248

|           |                  |
|----------:|------------------|
| dash      | cloves           |
| ½ tsp     | nutmeg           |
| 1 heaping tsp | cinnamon     |
| 3 Tbs     | coconut nectar   |
| 2 tsp     | coconut flour    |
| 1 tsp     | vanilla          |

For the topping:

|           |                     |
|----------:|---------------------|
|           | reserved apple peels |
| ½ tsp     | ghee or coconut oil |
| 1 tsp     | lemon zest          |
| 3 tsp     | coconut sugar       |
| 1 tsp     | cinnamon            |

For crust:
1. Preheat oven to 400°F (204°C).
2. Mix the flours and salt together.
3. Whisk oil, coconut nectar, eggs, and applesauce together.
4. Carefully add the flour mixture, stirring with a wooden spoon (but do not overmix, as the dough can get crumbly). Keep a tablespoon or two of water nearby in case you need to moisten the dough.
5. Line your pie pan with parchment and pat in the dough. Evenly poke it with a fork and bake for around 8 minutes, or until golden.

For filling:
1. Preheat oven to 350°F (180°C).
2. Melt the ghee or coconut oil in a saucepan over medium-low heat. Add the apples, spices, and coconut nectar. Mix well, and leave on the heat for 5 minutes.
3. Mix in coconut flour and leave on the heat for another 5 minutes.
4. Add vanilla, take off the heat, and let the mixture cool for 10 minutes. Once cool, pour into the pie crust and bake for around 8 minutes, until top has crisped slightly.

For topping:
1. Preheat oven to 400°F (204°C).
2. Toss the apple peels in the ghee or coconut oil, lemon zest, sugar, and cinnamon.

3. Bake on a cookie sheet for around 12 minutes or until golden and crispy.
4. When cool, crumble over the baked apple pie.

We generally bake the apple peels directly after the crust, while we are making the filling.

You can make extra pie crust dough if you want to do a more traditional lattice topping, but bake for an extra 8 minutes or so in the final stage.

# ——— Dark Chocolate Bundt Cake ———

For the cake:

| | |
|---|---|
| 1½ cups | whole wheat flour or other whole-grain baking flour of choice (or 1 cup buckwheat flour mixed with ½ cup tapioca flour to make it gluten free) |
| 1 cup | coconut sugar or maple sugar (use an extra ¼ cup if you prefer it sweeter) |
| ½ cup | cacao |
| 4 tsp | aluminum-free baking powder, divided |
| ¼ tsp | salt |
| 5 | eggs, separated |
| ½ cup | coconut oil |
| 1 tsp | vanilla |
| ¾ cup | warm water |

For the icing:

| | |
|---|---|
| 2 | ripe avocados, peeled and pitted |
| 2 Tbs | coconut nectar or maple syrup (add an extra tablespoon if you want it sweeter) |
| ½ tsp | vanilla |
| ¼ cup | cacao |

For the cake:

1. Preheat oven to 350°F (180°C). Grease a bundt pan with oil of choice or line with parchment paper.
2. Blend the flour, sugar, cacao, 3 tsp baking powder, and salt.
3. Beat the egg yolks with the coconut oil, vanilla, and water.

4. Beat the egg whites and remaining teaspoon of baking powder until peaks form. Add to egg yolk mixture and mix well.
5. Add the liquids to the dry mixture and mix well.
6. Pour batter into prepared bundt pan and bake for 25–30 minutes, or until a knife inserted in the cake comes out clean. Allow the cake to cool to room temperature before icing.

For the icing:
Blend avocados with coconut nectar (or maple syrup), vanilla, and cacao. Spread over cooled cake.

For the icing, we also use recipes from Jenni Hulet's incredible book, *My Paleo Patisserie: An Artisanal Approach to Grain Free Baking*. There are also a lot of great recipes online using unrefined sugars. Experiment!

# Conclusion

"Let food be thy medicine." We have been meditating on Hippocrates's famous quote; it certainly is a simple yet profound way to think about food. However, I would say that it is also only one side of the coin. We need to "let eating *and thinking* be thy medicine." We will never change our eating habits unless we change the way we think about food.

True, positive lifestyle changes, which can be both exasperating and exhausting, are worth the effort. Science and Scripture are in sync (and so they should be, since God gave us science to better understand ourselves and the world we live in) when it comes to the benefits of lifestyle change. "Think and eat yourself smart, healthy, and happy" is a lifestyle change that draws on a formula of knowledge, attitude, and skills. I provided the knowledge of our food systems in part 1. Attitude was handled in part 2. And the skills to change are provided in part 3.

Knowledge, attitude, and skills—hence your lifestyle—are driven and controlled by your *thinking*. If your thinking is not right, nothing else in your life will go right, including your eating habits. Thinking governs eating, and the two activities are inseparable. This is why I have placed such emphasis throughout this book on the mindset behind the meal being the 80 percent, and the meal behind the mindset being the 20 percent.

If we want to see a healthier world, we need to look in the mirror and see a healthier person, mentally and physically. It starts with us: we have to begin thinking and eating ourselves smart, happy, and healthy . . . and plant healthy trees not only in our gardens but wherever we go, in the footsteps of our Lord and Savior.

> *In the middle of its street, and on either side of the river,*
> *was the tree of life, which bore twelve fruits,*
> *each tree yielding its fruit every month.*
> *The leaves of the tree were for*
> *the healing of the nations. (Rev. 22:2)*

# Notes

**Prologue**

1. World Health Organization. "Obesity and Overweight: Fact Sheet." January 2015. http://www.who.int/mediacentre/factsheets/fs311/en/; World Food Program. "Hunger Statistics." 2014. http://www.wfp.org/hunger/stats; Patel, Raj. *Stuffed and Starved: The Hidden Battle for the World Food System*. Brooklyn, NY: Melville House, 2014. 9–29; Gustafson, Ellen. *We the Eaters: If We Change Dinner, We Can Change the World*. New York: Rodale, 2014. v–xx.

2. Dolnick, Sam. "The Obesity–Hunger Paradox." *New York Times*. March 14, 2010; Bogart, W. A. *Regulating Obesity?: Government, Society, and Questions of Health*. Oxford University Press, 2013. 168; Bauer, Jean W. *Rural Families and Work Context and Problems*. New York: Springer, 2011. 80; Gustafson, *We the Eaters*, 1–30.

3. Wright, N. T. *Surprised by Scripture: Engaging Contemporary Issues*. San Francisco: HarperOne, 2014. 83–106.

**Chapter 1: *Real* Food and the MAD Way of Eating**

1. Schlosser, Eric. *Fast Food Nation: The Dark Side of the All-American Meal*. Boston: Mariner Books/Houghton Mifflin Harcourt, 2012. Kindle Edition, 4, 282.

2. Gustafson, *We the Eaters*, 191; Graham, Tyler, and Drew Ramsey. *The Happiness Diet: A Nutritional Prescription for a Sharp Brain, Balanced Mood, and Lean, Energized Body*. Emmaus: Rodale, 2012. Kindle Edition, 15–33.

3. Price, Weston A. *Nutrition and Physical Degeneration: A Comparison of Primitive and Modern Diets and Their Effects*. Redlands, CA: Price Pottenger Nutrition Foundation, 1945; Minger, Denise. *Death by Food Pyramid*. Malibu,

CA: Primal Blueprint Publishing, 2013. Kindle Edition, 215–44; Ungar, Peter S., and Mark Franklyn Teaford. *Human Diet: Its Origin and Evolution.* Westport, CT: Bergin & Garvey, 2002. 78; Fitzgerald, Matt. *Diet Cults: The Surprising Fallacy at the Core of Nutrition Fads and a Guide to Healthy Eating for the Rest of Us.* 2014. Kindle Edition, 3, 83; Nabhan, Gary Paul. *Why Some Like It Hot: Food, Genes, and Cultural Diversity.* Washington, DC: Island Press, 2004.

4. Laudan, Rachel. *The Food of Paradise: Exploring Hawaii's Culinary Heritage.* Honolulu: University of Hawai'i Press, 1996; Fitzgerald, *Diet Cults,* 150.

5. Rosenbaum, MW, et al. *Okinawa: A Naturally Calorie Restricted Population.* In: Everitt A. V., ed. *Calorie Restriction, Aging and Longevity.* New York: Springer Science, 2010. 43–53; Willcox, DC, et al. "The Okinawan Diet: Health Implications of a Low-Calorie, Nutrient-Dense, Antioxidant-Rich Dietary Pattern Low in Glycemic Load." *Journal of the American College of Nutrition* 28 (2009): 500S–516S.

6. Matalas, Antonia-Leda. *The Mediterranean Diet: Constituents and Health Promotion.* Boca Raton, FL: CRC Press, 2001. 205–25; Fitzgerald, *Diet Cults,* 34.

7. Mandel, Abigail L., and Paul A. S. Breslin. "High Endogenous Salivary Amylase Activity Is Associated with Improved Glycemic Homeostasis Following Starch Ingestion in Adults," *Journal of Nutrition* 142, no. 5 (2012): 853–8; Minger, *Death by Food Pyramid,* 206.

8. Pollan, Michael. *The Omnivore's Dilemma: A Natural History of Four Meals.* New York: Penguin, 2007. Kindle Edition, 3–17; Pollan, Michael. *In Defense of Food: An Eater's Manifesto.* New York: Penguin, 2008. Kindle Edition, 1–27.

9. Pollan, *In Defense of Food,* 1–27.

10. Ibid.; Patel, *Stuffed and Starved,* 9–19; Graham and Ramsey, *The Happiness Diet,* 15–33; Cheney, Ian, et al. *King Corn.* New York: Docurama Films, 2008; Kenner, Robert, et al. *Food, Inc.* Los Angeles: Magnolia Home Entertainment, 2009; Nestle, Marion, and Mike Peters. *Eat Drink Vote: An Illustrated Guide to Food Politics.* New York: Rodale, 2013. 2–6; Gustafson, *We the Eaters;* Hesterman, Oran B. *Fair Food: Growing a Healthy, Sustainable Food System for All.* New York: Public Affairs, 2011. Kindle Edition, 4–50; Barber, Dan. *The Third Plate: Field Notes on the Future of Food.* New York: Penguin, 2014. Kindle Edition, 2–26; Nestle, Marion. *What to Eat.* New York: North Point Press, 2006. Kindle Edition.

11. Pollan, *The Omnivore's Dilemma,* 84.

12. Robinson, Jo. *Eating on the Wild Side: The Missing Link to Optimum Health.* New York: Little, Brown, 2013. Kindle Edition; Rule, Cheryl Sternman, and Paulette Phlipot. *Ripe: A Fresh, Colorful Approach to Fruits and Vegetables.* New York: Running Press, 2011; Barber, *The Third Plate,* 88–89.

13. Daley, Cynthia A., et al. "A Review of Fatty Acid Profiles and Antioxidant Content in Grass-Fed and Grain-Fed Beef." *Nutrition Journal* 9, no. 1 (2010): 10.

14. Barber, *The Third Plate;* Waters, Alice, et al. *The Art of Simple Food: Notes, Lessons, and Recipes from a Delicious Revolution.* New York: Clarkson Potter, 2007.

15. Ronald, Pamela C., and Raoul W. Adamchak. *Tomorrow's Table: Organic Farming, Genetics, and the Future of Food.* New York: Oxford University Press, 2008. Kindle Edition, 17.

16. Pollan, *The Omnivore's Dilemma*; Pollan, *In Defense of Food*; Patel, *Stuffed and Starved*; Graham and Ramsey, *The Happiness Diet*, 15–33; Cheney et al., *King Corn*; Nestle and Peters, *Eat Drink Vote*, 2–6; Gustafson, *We the Eaters*; Hesterman, *Fair Food*, 4–50; Barber, *The Third Plate*; Pollan, *In Defense of Food*, 2–26.

17. Ibid.; Kristiansen, Paul, Acram Taji, and John Reganold. *Organic Agriculture: A Global Perspective*. Collingwood, VIC (Australia): CSIRO Publishing, 2006; Lockeretz, William. *Organic Farming: An International History*. Wallingford, UK: CABI, 2007; Hansen, Ann Larkin. *The Organic Farming Manual: A Comprehensive Guide to Starting and Running a Certified Organic Farm*. North Adams, MA: Storey Pub, 2010; Allen, Will and Charles Wilson. *The Good Food Revolution: Growing Healthy Food, People, and Communities*. New York: Gotham Books, 2012. Kindle Edition; Pollan, *In Defense of Food*; Lichtfouse, Eric. *Sociology, Organic Farming, Climate Change and Soil Science*. Dordrecht: Springer, 2010. 275–302.

18. Ronald and Adamchak, *Tomorrow's Table*; Pollan, *In Defense of Food*; Salatin, Joel. *Folks, This Ain't Normal: A Farmer's Advice for Happier Hens, Healthier People, and a Better World*. New York: Center Street, 2011. Kindle Edition; Kristiansen, Paul, Acram Taji, and John P. Reganold. *Organic Agriculture: A Global Perspective*, 279.

19. Brown, Ed, et al. *Unacceptable Levels*. Macroscopic Media, 2013. DVD.

20. Fernandez-Cornejo, Jorge, et al. "Pesticide Use in US Agriculture: 21 Selected Crops, 1960–2008." No. 178462. United States Department of Agriculture, Economic Research Service, 2014.

21. Brown et al., *Unacceptable Levels*; Vandenberg, Laura N., et al. "Hormones and Endocrine-Disrupting Chemicals: Low-Dose Effects and Nonmonotonic Dose Responses." *Endocrine Reviews* 33, no. 3 (2012): 378–455.

22. Environment America. "Wasting Our Waterways: Toxic Industrial Pollution and Restoring the Promise of the Clean Water Act." June 2014. http://envir onmentamericacenter.org/sites/environment/files/reports/US_wastingwaterway s_scrn%20061814_0.pdf; Halden, Rolf U. and Kellogg J. Schwab. *Environmental Impact of Industrial Farm Animal Production*. Pew Commission on Industrial Farm Animal Production, 2008.

23. Interviewed in Brown et al., *Unacceptable Levels*.

24. Vandenberg et al., 378–455.

25. Martić-Kehl, Marianne I., Roger Schibli, and P. August Schubiger. "Can Animal Data Predict Human Outcome? Problems and Pitfalls of Translational Animal Research." *European Journal of Nuclear Medicine and Molecular Imaging* (2012): 1–5; Van Norman, Gail A. *Clinical Ethics in Anesthesiology: A Case-Based Textbook*. Cambridge: Cambridge University Press, 2010. 174–79.

26. Popper, Karl. *The Logic of Scientific Discovery*. London: Routledge, 2005. 318; Gigerenzer, Gerd. *Reckoning with Risk: Learning to Live with Uncertainty*. London: Penguin, 2003; Edwards, Adrian. "Communicating Risks Means That Patients Too Have to Learn to Live with Uncertainty." *BMJ: British Medical Journal* 327, no. 7417 (2003): 691; Satel, Sally L., and Scott O. Lilienfeld. *Brainwashed: The Seductive Appeal of Mindless Neuroscience*. New York: Basic Books, 2013.

Kindle Edition; Fukuoka, Masanobu. *The One-Straw Revolution: An Introduction to Natural Farming.* New York: New York Review Books, 2010. Kindle Edition, 29; Salatin, *Folks, This Ain't Normal*, 235–36.

27. United States Department of Agriculture. "National Organic Program." 2014. http://www.ams.usda.gov/AMSv1.0/nop.

28. Pollan, *The Omnivore's Dilemma*; Pollan, *In Defense of Food*, 134–83.

29. Ibid., 140.

30. Ibid., 134–83.

31. Ibid.

32. Ibid.; Pollan, Michael. *Food Rules: An Eater's Manual.* New York: Penguin Books, 2009. Kindle Edition, 34–36; Hesterman, *Fair Food*, 3–44; Ackerman-Leist, Philip. *Rebuilding the Foodshed: How to Create Local, Sustainable, and Secure Food Systems.* Santa Rosa: Post Carbon Institute, 2013. Kindle Edition; Chase, Lisa, and Vernon P. Grubinger. *Food, Farms, and Community: Exploring Food Systems.* 2014. Kindle Edition; Barber, *The Third Plate*; Nabhan, Gary Paul. *Coming Home to Eat: The Pleasures and Politics of Local Foods.* New York: Norton, 2009. Kindle Edition, 17–28; The Prince of Wales HRH. *The Prince's Speech: On the Future of Food.* New York: Rodale, 2012.

33. Pollan, *The Omnivore's Dilemma*, 134–83.

34. Robinson, *Eating on the Wild Side*; Pollan, *In Defense of Food*, 30, 101–36; Pollan, *Food Rules*.

35. Robinson, *Eating on the Wild Side*, 160–62; Nath, A., et al. "Changes in Post-Harvest Phytochemical Qualities of Broccoli Florets during Ambient and Refrigerated." *Food Chemistry* 127 (2011): 1510–14; Cantwell, Marita, and Trevor Suslow. "Broccoli: Recommendations for Maintaining Postharvest Quality." *Perishables Handling* 92 (1997); Vallejo, Fernando, Francisco Tomás-Baberán, and Cristina García-Viguera. "Health-Promoting Compounds in Broccoli as Influenced by Refrigerated Transport and Retail Sale Period." *Journal of Agricultural and Food Chemistry* 51 (2003): 3029–34.

36. Robinson, *Eating on the Wild Side*, 323–24; Conesa, A., J. M. Brotons, F. J. Manera, and I. Porras. "The Degreening of Lemon and Grapefruit in Ethylene Atmosphere: A Cost Analysis." *Scientia Horticulturae* 179 (2014): 140–45; Yuncheng, et al. "Effect of Commercial Processing on Pesticide Residues in Orange Products." *European Food Research and Technology* 234 (2012): 449–56; Stewart, William S. "Storage of Citrus Fruits: Studies Indicate Use of 2,4-D and 2,4,5-T Sprays on Trees Prolong Storage Life of Citrus Fruits." *California Agriculture* 3 (1949): 7–14.

37. Pollan, *Food Rules*, 30; Pollan, *In Defense of Food*, 101–36; Nestle, *What to Eat*, 28–70; Robinson, *Eating on the Wild Side*.

38. Pollan, *Food Rules*, 30; Pollan, *In Defense of Food*, 101–36; Nestle, *What to Eat*, 28–70.

39. Hesterman, *Fair Food*, 7–8; Pollan, *In Defense of Food*, 1–27; Pollan, *The Omnivore's Dilemma*, 1–183.

40. Pollan, *Food Rules*, 30.

41. Ibid.; Pollan, *In Defense of Food*, 1–14, 101–36; Pitt, John I. *Fungi and Food Spoilage.* Boston: Springer, 2013. 469–507; Nestle, *What to Eat*, 247–400;

Deville, Nancy. *Death by Supermarket: The Fattening, Dumbing Down, and Poisoning of America*. Austin: Greenleaf Book Group Press, 2011. Kindle Edition; Moss, Michael. *Salt, Sugar, Fat: How the Food Giants Hooked Us*. New York: Random House, 2013. Kindle Edition; Gustafson, *We the Eaters*; Graham and Ramsey, *The Happiness Diet*.

42. Barber, *The Third Plate*, 341–42; Gustafson, *We the Eaters*, 79–102; Masterjohn, Chris. "Wheat Belly—The Toll of Hubris on Human Health." *The Daily Lipid*. October 12, 2011. http://blog.cholesterol-and-health.com/2011/10/wheat-belly-toll-of-hubris-on-human.html.

43. Gustafson, *We the Eaters*, 184, 196.

44. Ibid.; FDA, "Frequently Asked Questions on Azodicarbonamide (ADA)." 2014. http://www.fda.gov/Food/IngredientsPackagingLabeling/FoodAdditivesIngredients/ucm387497.htm.

45. CDC, "International Chemical Safety Cards (ICSC): AZODICARBON-AMIDE." 2014. http://www.cdc.gov/niosh/ipcsneng/neng0380.html; World Health Organization, "Concise International Chemical Assessment Document 16: Azodicarbonamide." 1999. http://www.who.int/ipcs/publications/cicad/en/cicad16.pdf; Gustafson, *We the Eaters*, 184, 196.

46. Smith, Jim, and Lily Hong-Shum. *Food Additives Data Book*. 2nd ed. Chichester, West Sussex: Wiley-Blackwell, 2011. 548; Office Journal of the European Union, "Commission Directive 2004/1/EC of 6 January 2004 amending Directive 2002/72/EC as Regards the Suspension of the Use of Azodicarbonamide as Blowing Agent." 2004. http://eur-lex.europa.eu/LexUriServ/LexUriServ.do?uri=OJ:L:2004:007:0045:0046:EN:PDF.

47. Lofstock, John. "Boosting Impulse Sales at the Checkout Counter." *Convenience Store Decisions*. January 11, 2006. http://www.cstoredecisions.com/2006/02/01/boosting-impulse-sales-at-the-checkout-counter/; Patel, *Stuffed and Starved*; Nestle, *What to Eat*.

48. Klein, Ezra. "Big Food: Michael Pollan Thinks Wall Street Has Way Too Much Influence Over What We Eat." *Vox*. April 23, 2014. http://www.vox.com/2014/4/23/5627992/big-food-michael-pollan-thinks-wall-street-has-way-too-much-influence.

49. Martinez, Steve. *Local Food Systems: Concepts, Impacts, and Issues*. Washington, DC: US Dept. of Agriculture, Economic Research Service, 2010.

50. Pollan, *Food Rules*, 34.

51. Warner, Keith. *Agroecology in Action: Extending Alternative Agriculture through Social Networks*. Cambridge, MA: MIT, 2007.

52. Gustafson, *We the Eaters*, 153.

53. Ackerman-Leist, *Rebuilding the Foodshed*, 26.

54. Tate, Carolyn. *Conscious Marketing: How to Create an Awesome Business with a New Approach to Marketing*. Hoboken: Wiley, 2015. 34–36.

## Chapter 2: The Trouble with Mass Production

1. Gustafson, *We the Eaters*, 123, 170; Pollan, *In Defense of Food*; Pollan, *The Omnivore's Dilemma*, 14–183; Shiva, Vandana. *The Vandana Shiva Reader*.

Lexington: The University Press of Kentucky, 2015. Kindle Edition; Taylor, Chris-topher, et al. *Food Fight: A Story of Culinary Revolt.* United States: C. Taylor, 2008; Faillace, Linda, et al. *Farmageddon.* Concord, MA: Kristin Marie Produc-tions, 2011; Cheney et al., *King Corn*; Berry, Wendell. *Bringing It to the Table: On Farming and Food.* Berkeley: Counterpoint, 2009. Kindle Edition; Fukuoka, *The One-Straw Revolution*; Salatin, *Folks, This Ain't Normal.*

2. Gustafson, *We the Eaters*, 166–67.

3. Ibid., 123, 170; Pollan, *In Defense of Food*; Pollan, *The Omnivore's Dilemma*, 14–183; Shiva, *The Vandana Shiva Reader*; Taylor et al., *Food Fight*; Faillace et al., *Farmageddon*; Cheney et al., *King Corn*; Berry, *Bringing It to the Table*; Fukuoka, *The One-Straw Revolution*; Salatin, *Folks, This Ain't Normal.*

4. Taylor et al., *Food Fight.*

5. Gustafson, *We the Eaters*, 103–70; Pollan, *In Defense of Food*; Pollan, *The Omnivore's Dilemma*, 14–183; Shiva, *The Vandana Shiva Reader*; Taylor et al., *Food Fight*; Faillace et al., *Farmageddon*; Cheney et al., *King Corn*; Berry, *Bringing It to the Table*; Fukuoka, *The One-Straw Revolution*; Salatin, *Folks, This Ain't Normal.*

6. Gustafson, *We the Eaters*, 103–26; Salatin, *Folks, This Ain't Normal*, 98; Kelly, John. *The Graves Are Walking: The Great Famine and the Saga of the Irish People.* New York: Henry Holt and Co., 2012.

7. Gustafson, *We the Eaters*, 103–26; Ricklefs, Robert E., and Rick Relyea. *Ecology: the Economy of Nature.* New York: W.H. Freeman, 2014. 550; Pollan, *In Defense of Food*; Pollan, *The Omnivore's Dilemma*, 14–183; Shiva, *The Vandana Shiva Reader*; Taylor et al., *Food Fight*; Faillace et al., *Farmageddon*; Cheney et al., *King Corn*; Berry, *Bringing It to the Table*; Fukuoka, *The One-Straw Revolution*; Salatin, *Folks, This Ain't Normal.*

8. Ibid.

9. Ibid.

10. Ibid.

11. Runge, C. F. and B. Senauer. "How Biofuels Could Starve the Poor." *Foreign Affairs.* May/June 2007. https://www.foreignaffairs.com/articles/2007-05-01/how-biofuels-could-starve-poor; Nestle and Peters, *Eat Drink Vote*, 31; Taylor et al., *Food Fight*; Gustafson, *We the Eaters*, 79–102; Pollan, *The Omnivore's Dilemma*, 14–183; Cheney et al., *King Corn.*

12. Ibid.

13. Gustafson, *We the Eaters*, 17.

14. Salatin, *Folks, This Ain't Normal*; Hesterman, *Fair Food*, 2–44; Nestle and Peters, *Eat Drink Vote*, 128–35; Taylor et al., *Food Fight*; Gustafson, *We the Eaters*, 31–78; Pollan, *In Defense of Food*; Pollan, *The Omnivore's Dilemma*, 14–183; Faillace et al., *Farmageddon*; Cheney et al., *King Corn*; Berry, *Bringing It to the Table*; Nestle, Marion. *Food Politics: How the Food Industry Influences Nutrition and Health.* Berkeley: University of California Press, 2002; Schlosser, *Fast Food Nation*; Imhoff, Dan. *The CAFO Reader: The Tragedy of Industrial Animal Factories.* Healdsburg, CA: Watershed Media, 2010. Kindle Edition; Kenner et al.,

*Food, Inc.*; Barber, *The Third Plate*; Graham and Ramsey, *The Happiness Diet*; Nestle, *What to Eat*, 67–305.

15. Ibid.

16. National Commission on Industrial Farm Animal Production. "Pew Commission on Industrial Animal Farm Production." 2009. http://www.ncifap.or g/_images/pcifapfin.pdf.

17. Salatin, *Folks, This Ain't Normal*; Hesterman, *Fair Food*, 2–44; Nestle and Peters, *Eat Drink Vote*, 128–35; Taylor et al., *Food Fight*; Gustafson, *We the Eaters*, 31–78; Pollan, *In Defense of Food*; Pollan, *The Omnivore's Dilemma*, 14–183; Faillace et al., *Farmageddon*; Cheney et al., *King Corn*; Berry, *Bringing It to the Table*; Nestle, *Food Politics*; Schlosser, *Fast Food Nation*; Imhoff, *CAFO Reader*; Kenner et al., *Food, Inc.*; Barber, *The Third Plate*; Graham and Ramsey, *The Happiness Diet*; Nestle, Marion. *What to Eat*. New York: North Point Press, 2006. Kindle Edition, 67–305.

18. Ibid.

19. Ibid.; American Cancer Society. "Recombinant bovine growth hormone." 2014. http://www.cancer.org/cancer/cancercauses/othercarcinogens/athome/reco mbinant-bovine-growth-hormone.

20. Ibid.

21. Ibid.; Barber, *The Third Plate*, 155–56.

22. Guay, K., et al. "Behavior and Handling of Physically and Immunologically Castrated Market Pigs on Farm and Going to Market." *Journal of Animal Science* 91 (2013): 5410–17; Sutherland, M. A., et al. "The Physiological and Behavioral Response of Pigs Castrated With and Without Anesthesia or Analgesia." *Journal of Animal Science* 90 (2012): 2211–21; McGlone, John J., and J. M. Hellman. "Local and General Anesthetic Effects on Behavior and Performance of Two- and Seven-Week-Old Castrated and Uncastrated Piglets." *Journal of Animal Science* 66 (1988): 3049–58; McGlone, John J. White. "Behavior of Immunologically Castrated Boars Compared to Surgically Castrated Pigs." Unpublished paper.

23. Salatin, *Folks, This Ain't Normal*; Hesterman, *Fair Food*, 2–44; Nestle and Peters, *Eat Drink Vote*, 128–35; Taylor et al., *Food Fight*; Gustafson, *We the Eaters*, 31–78; Pollan, *In Defense of Food*; Pollan, *The Omnivore's Dilemma*, 14–183; Faillace et al., *Farmageddon*; Cheney et al., *King Corn*; Berry, *Bringing It to the Table*; Nestle, *Food Politics*; Schlosser, *Fast Food Nation*; Imhoff, *CAFO Reader*; Kenner et al., *Food, Inc.*; Barber, *The Third Plate*; Graham and Ramsey, *The Happiness Diet*; Nestle, *What to Eat*, 67–305.

24. Ibid.; Hartcher, K. M., et al. "The Effects of Environmental Enrichment and Beak-Trimming during the Rearing Period on Subsequent Feather Damage Due to Feather-Pecking in Laying Hens." *Poultry Science* 94, no. 5 (2015): 852–59; Carruthers, C. T., et al. "On-Farm Survey of Beak Characteristics in White Leghorns as a Result of Hot Blade Trimming or Infrared Beak Treatment." *The Journal of Applied Poultry Research* 21, no. 3 (2012): 645–50.

25. Schlosser, *Fast Food Nation*.

26. Barnett, Erin, et al. *Food Chains*. New York: Screen Media Films, 2015.

27. Barnett et al., *Food Chains*; Schlosser, *Fast Food Nation*; Estabrook, Barry. *Tomatoland: How Modern Industrial Agriculture Destroyed Our Most Alluring Fruit*. Kansas City: Andrews McMeel, 2012. Kindle Edition; Bales, Kevin, and Ron Soodalter. *The Slave Next Door: Human Trafficking and Slavery in America Today*. Berkeley: University of California Press, 2009. Kindle Edition; Bales, Kevin. *Disposable People: New Slavery in the Global Economy*. Berkeley: University of California Press, 1999. Kindle Edition; Kenner et al., *Food, Inc.*; Human Rights Watch. "Blood, Sweat and Fear: Workers' Rights in U.S. Meat and Poultry Plants." 2004. http://www.hrw.org/sites/default/files/reports/usa0105.pdf; Worrall, Michael S. "Meatpacking Safety: Is OSHA Enforcement Adequate." *Drake Journal of Agricultural Law* 9 (2004): 300–321; Davidson, Julia O'Connell. "Troubling Freedom: Migration, Debt, and Modern Slavery." *Migration Studies* 1, no. 2 (2013): 176–95; Murphy, Laura. *Survivors of Slavery: Modern-Day Slave Narratives*. Columbia University Press, 2013; Ngwe, Job Elom, and O. Oko Elechi. "Human Trafficking: The Modern Day Slavery of the 21st Century." *African Journal of Criminology and Justice Studies* 6, nos. 1, 2 (2012).

28. Ibid.

29. Ibid.; Food and Agriculture Organization of the United Nations. "Livestock's Long Shadow: Environmental Issues and Options." 2006. ftp://ftp.fao.org/docrep/fao/010/a0701e/a0701e00.pdf; Sabaté, Joan, and Sam Soret. "Sustainability of Plant-Based Diets: Back to the Future." *The American Journal of Clinical Nutrition* 100, no. 1 Supplement (2014): 476S–82S; Ripple, William J., et al. "Ruminants, Climate Change and Climate Policy." *Nature Climate Change* 4, no. 1 (2014): 2–5; Dlamini, A. M., and M. A. Dube. "Contribution of Animal Agriculture to Greenhouse Gases Production in Swaziland." *American Journal of Climate Change* 3, no. 3 (2014): 253; Hedenus, Fredrik, Stefan Wirsenius, and Daniel J. A. Johansson. "The Importance of Reduced Meat and Dairy Consumption for Meeting Stringent Climate Change Targets." *Climatic Change* 124, nos. 1, 2 (2014): 79–91.

30. Ibid.

31. Ibid.; Bridges, Jeff, and Tom Colicchio. *A Place at the Table*. United States: Magnolia Home Entertainment, 2013; Stuart, Tristram. *Waste: Uncovering the Global Food Scandal*. New York: W.W. Norton & Co, 2009. Kindle Edition.

## Chapter 3: The MAD Diseases

1. Gustafson, *We the Eaters*, 190; Salatin, *Folks, This Ain't Normal*; Hesterman, *Fair Food*, 2–44; Nestle and Peters, *Eat Drink Vote*; Taylor et al., *Food Fight*; Pollan, *In Defense of Food*; Pollan, *The Omnivore's Dilemma*; Faillace et al., *Farmageddon*; Cheney et al., *King Corn*; Berry, *Bringing It to the Table*; Nestle, *Food Politics*; Schlosser, *Fast Food Nation*; Imhoff, *CAFO Reader*; Kenner et al., *Food, Inc.*; Barber, *The Third Plate*; Graham and Ramsey, *The Happiness Diet*; Nestle, *What to Eat*; Stuart, *Waste*; Moss, *Salt, Sugar, Fat*; Cordain, Loren S., et al. "Origins and Evolution of the Western Diet: Health Implications for the 21st Century." *The American Journal of Clinical Nutrition* 81, no. 2 (2005): 341–54;

Danaei, Goodarz, et al. "The Global Cardiovascular Risk Transition Associations of Four Metabolic Risk Factors with National Income, Urbanization, and Western Diet in 1980 and 2008." *Circulation* 127, no. 14 (2013): 1493–1502; Carrera-Bastos, Pedro, et al. "The Western Diet and Lifestyle and Diseases of Civilization." *Journal of Research Reports in Clinical Cardiology* 2 (2011): 15–35; Kanoski, Scott E., and Terry L. Davidson. "Western Diet Consumption and Cognitive Impairment: Links to Hippocampal Dysfunction and Obesity." *Physiology & Behavior* 103, no. 1 (2011): 59–68; Manzel, Arndt, et al. "Role of 'Western Diet' in Inflammatory Autoimmune Diseases." *Current Allergy and Asthma Reports* 14, no. 1 (2014): 1–8.

2. Ibid.

3. Ibid.

4. Ibid.

5. Walton, Alice G. "How Much Sugar Are Americans Eating?" [Infographic]. *Forbes*. September 30, 2012. http://www.forbes.com/sites/alicegwalton/2012/08/30/how-much-sugar-are-americans-eating-infographic/.

6. Statistic Brain Research Institute. "Fast Food Statistics." March 12, 2015. http://www.statisticbrain.com/fast-food-statistics/.

7. Gustafson, *We the Eaters*, 166.

8. Nestle, Marion. *Food Politics 101: The School Nutrition Association vs. Fruits & Vegetables*. Food Politics, 2015. http://www.foodpolitics.com/2015/02/food-politics-101-the-school-nutrition-association-vs-fruits-vegetables/; Huehnergarth, Nancy. "Big Food Dominates the School Nutrition Association's Latest Conference." *The Huffington Post*. March 29, 2015. http://www.huffingtonpost.com/nancy-huehnergarth/the-school-nutrition-asso_b_6546984.html?utm_hp_ref=tw; School Nutrition Association. "2015 Position Paper: Reauthorization of the Healthy, Hunger-Free Kids Act." 2015. https://schoolnutrition.org/uploadedFiles/Legislation_and_Policy/SNA_Policy_Resources/2015PositionPaperPrintable.pdf.

9. United Nations News Center. "UN Expert Warns of Global Public Health Disaster Caused by Unhealthy Foods." March 6, 2012. http://www.un.org/apps/news/story.asp?NewsID=41470#.VT8oPbqJnww.

10. Gustafson, *We the Eaters*; United Nations News Center, "UN Expert Warns"; Margulies, Phillip. *America's Role in the World*. New York: Facts On File, 2009. 300; Pan, An, Vasanti Malik, and Frank B. Hu. "Exporting Diabetes to Asia: The Impact of Western-Style Fast Food." *Circulation* 126, no. 2 (2012): 163–65; Thow, Anne-Marie, and Wendy Snowdon. "The Effect of Trade and Trade Policy on Diet and Health in the Pacific Islands." *Trade, Food, Diet and Health: Perspectives and Policy Options* 147 (2010); Goran, Michael I., Stanley J. Ulijaszek, and Emily E. Ventura. "High Fructose Corn Syrup and Diabetes Prevalence: A Global Perspective." *Global Public Health* 8, no. 1 (2013): 55–64; Moss, *Salt, Sugar, Fat*; Cordain et al., "Origins and Evolution of the Western Diet," 341–54; Danaei et al., "Global Cardiovascular Risk," 1493–1502; Carrera-Bastos et al., "Western Diet and Lifestyle"; Kanoski and Davidson, "Western Diet Consumption"; Manzel et al., "Role of 'Western Diet' in Inflammatory Autoimmune Diseases"; Patel, *Stuffed and Starved*; Salatin, *Folks, This Ain't Normal*; Hesterman, *Fair Food*, 2–44; Nestle and Peters, *Eat Drink Vote*; Taylor et al., *Food Fight*; Pollan, *In Defense*

*of Food*; Pollan, *The Omnivore's Dilemma*; Faillace et al., *Farmageddon*; Cheney et al., *King Corn*; Berry, *Bringing It to the Table*; Nestle, *Food Politics*; Schlosser, *Fast Food Nation*; Kenner et al., *Food, Inc.*; Barber, *The Third Plate*; Graham and Ramsey, *The Happiness Diet*; Nestle, *What to Eat*.

11. Gustafson, *We the Eaters*; Patel, *Stuffed and Starved*.

12. Ibid.; Koseff, Alexei. "AM Alert: Chef Jamie Oliver Launches Clean Water Initiative." *Capitol Alert: The Sacramento Bee*. January 6, 2015.

13. World Health Organization. "Obesity and Overweight Factsheet." 2015. http://www.who.int/mediacentre/factsheets/fs311/en/.

14. Ng, Marie, et al. "Global, Regional, and National Prevalence of Overweight and Obesity in Children and Adults During 1980–2013: A Systematic Analysis for the Global Burden of Disease Study 2013." *The Lancet* 384, no. 9945 (2014): 766–81.

15. Ibid.

16. Wang, Y. C., et al. "Health and Economic Burden of the Projected Obesity Trends in the USA and the UK." *The Lancet* 378 (2011): 815–25.

17. Ng et al., "Global, Regional, and National Prevalence"; Dor, Avi, et al. "A Heavy Burden: The Individual Costs of Being Overweight and Obese in the United States." Washington, DC: Health Policy and Management Faculty Publications. 2010. http://www.stopobesityalliance.org/wp-content/themes/stopobesityalliance/pdfs/Heavy_Burden_Report.pdf.

18. Gustafson, *We the Eaters*; United Nations News Center, "UN Expert Warns"; Margulies, *America's Role*, 300; Pan et al., "Exporting Diabetes to Asia"; Thow and Snowdon, "The Effect of Trade and Trade Policy"; Goran et al., "High Fructose Corn Syrup and Diabetes"; Moss, *Salt, Sugar, Fat*; Cordain et al., "Origins and Evolution of the Western Diet"; Danaei et al., "Global Cardiovascular Risk"; Carrera-Bastos et al., "Western Diet and Lifestyle"; Kanoski and Davidson, "Western Diet Consumption"; Manzel et al., "Role of 'Western Diet' in Inflammatory Autoimmune Diseases"; Patel, *Stuffed and Starved*; Salatin, *Folks, This Ain't Normal*; Hesterman, *Fair Food*, 2–44; Nestle and Peters, *Eat Drink Vote*; Taylor et al., *Food Fight*; Pollan, *In Defense of Food*; Pollan, *The Omnivore's Dilemma*; Faillace et al., *Farmageddon*; Berry, *Bringing It to the Table*; Nestle, *Food Politics*; Schlosser, *Fast Food Nation*; Kenner et al., *Food, Inc.*; Barber, *The Third Plate*; Graham and Ramsey, *The Happiness Diet*; Nestle, *What to Eat*.

19. Gustafson, *We the Eaters*, 80, 143, 183–85; Patel, *Stuffed and Starved*; Kenner et al., *Food, Inc.*; Nestle and Peters, *Eat Drink Vote*; Salatin, *Folks, This Ain't Normal*.

20. Ibid.

21. Ibid.

22. Salatin, *Folks, This Ain't Normal*, 44.

## Chapter 4: The Mad Truth about the MAD

1. Bridges and Colicchio, *A Place at the Table*.

2. Ibid.

3. Hesterman, *Fair Food*.

4. Taylor et al., *Food Fight*.

5. Bridges and Colicchio, *A Place at the Table*; Salatin, *Folks, This Ain't Normal*; Hesterman, *Fair Food*; Nestle and Peters, *Eat Drink Vote*; Taylor et al., *Food Fight*; Gustafson, *We the Eaters*; Pollan, *In Defense of Food*; Pollan, *The Omnivore's Dilemma*; Faillace et al., *Farmageddon*; Cheney et al., *King Corn*; Berry, *Bringing It to the Table*; Nestle, *Food Politics*; Schlosser, *Fast Food Nation*; Imhoff, *CAFO Reader*; Kenner et al., *Food, Inc.*; Barber, *The Third Plate*; Graham and Ramsey, *The Happiness Diet*; Nestle, *What to Eat*; Stuart, *Waste*.

6. Ibid.

7. Ibid.; Shiva, *The Vandana Shiva Reader*; Patel, *Stuffed and Starved*.

8. Ibid.

9. Gustafson, *We the Eaters*.

10. Ritz, Stephen. "A Teacher Growing Green in South Bronx." TED. February 2012. http://www.ted.com/talks/stephen_ritz_a_teacher_growing_green_in_the_south_bronx?language=en.

11. Finley, Ron. "A Guerilla Gardener in South Central LA." TED. February 2 013. http://www.ted.com/talks/ron_finley_a_guerilla_gardener_in_south_central_la?language=en.

12. Paul Quinn College. "We Over Me Farm." http://www.weovermefarm.com/#!about-us.

13. Café Momentum. "About." http://cafemomentum.org/?page_id=520.

14. Garden Harvests Farm. "About Us." http://gardenharvests.com/Get_To_Know_Us.html.

15. United Nations. "Universal Declaration of Human Rights." 1948. http://www.un.org/Overview/rights.html.

16. Gustafson, *We the Eaters*; Bridges and Colicchio, *A Place at the Table*; Salatin, *Folks, This Ain't Normal*; Hesterman, *Fair Food*; Nestle and Peters, *Eat Drink Vote*; Taylor et al., *Food Fight*; Pollan, *In Defense of Food*; Pollan, *The Omnivore's Dilemma*; Faillace et al., *Farmageddon*; Cheney et al., *King Corn*; Berry, *Bringing It to the Table*; Nestle, *Food Politics*; Schlosser, *Fast Food Nation*; Imhoff, *CAFO Reader*; Kenner et al., *Food, Inc.*; Barber, *The Third Plate*; Graham and Ramsey, *The Happiness Diet*; Nestle, *What to Eat*; Stuart, *Waste*.

17. Ibid.

18. Centers for Disease Control and Prevention. "Caloric Intake From Fast Food Among Adults: United States, 2007–2010." February 2013. http://www.cdc.gov/nchs/data/databriefs/db114.htm.

19. Gustafson, *We the Eaters*, 190; Salatin, *Folks, This Ain't Normal*; Hesterman, *Fair Food*; Nestle and Peters, *Eat Drink Vote*; Taylor et al., *Food Fight*; Pollan, *In Defense of Food*; Pollan, *The Omnivore's Dilemma*; Faillace et al., *Farmageddon*; Cheney et al., *King Corn*; Berry, *Bringing It to the Table*; Nestle, *Food Politics*; Schlosser, *Fast Food Nation*; Imhoff, *CAFO Reader*; Kenner et al., *Food, Inc.*; Barber, *The Third Plate*; Graham and Ramsey, *The Happiness Diet*; Nestle, *What to Eat*; Stuart, *Waste*.

20. Gustafson, *We the Eaters*, 80, 143, 183–85; Patel, *Stuffed and Starved*; Kenner et al., *Food, Inc.*; Nestle and Peters, *Eat Drink Vote*; Salatin, *Folks, This Ain't Normal*.

21. Ibid.

22. Ibid.

## Chapter 5: Marketing to Children and Other Scandals

1. Moss, *Salt, Sugar, Fat*.

2. Grow, H. Mollie, and Marlene B. Schwartz. "Food Marketing to Youth: Serious Business." *JAMA* 312, no. 18 (2014): 1918–19; Kraak, V. I., and M. Story. "Influence of Food Companies' Brand Mascots and Entertainment Companies' Cartoon Media Characters on Children's Diet and Health: A Systematic Review and Research Needs." *Obesity Reviews* (2015); Kelly, Bridget, et al. "New Media but Same Old Tricks: Food Marketing to Children in the Digital Age." *Current Obesity Reports* (2015): 1–9; Bernhardt, Amy M., et al. "Children's Recall of Fast Food Television Advertising—Testing the Adequacy of Food Marketing Regulation." *PloS One* 10, no. 3 (2015): e0119300; Vandevijvere, Stefanie, and Boydoyd Swinburn. "Food References and Marketing in Popular Magazines for Children and Adolescents in New Zealand: A Content Analysis." *Obesity Research & Clinical Practice* 8 (2014): 109; Moss, *Salt, Sugar, Fat*; Nestle, *Food Politics*; Nestle and Peters, *Eat Drink Vote*; Schlosser, *Fast Food Nation*; Taylor et al., *Food Fight*; Pollan, *In Defense of Food*; Jordan, Amy B. *Media and the Well-Being of Children and Adolescents*. New York: Oxford University Press, 2014. 57–69; Couric, Katie, et al. *Fed Up*. Santa Monica, CA: Atlas Films. Starz Media, 2014; Gustafson, *We the Eaters*; Salatin, *Folks, This Ain't Normal*.

3. The Rudd Center For Food Policy & Obesity. "Food Marketing." 2015. http://www.uconnruddcenter.org/food-marketing; Harris, J. L., A. Heard, and M. B. Schwartz. *Older but Still Vulnerable: All Children Need Protection from Unhealthy Food Marketing*. New Haven, CT: Yale Rudd Center for Food Policy & Obesity, 2014.

4. Grow and Schwartz, "Food Marketing to Youth"; Kraak and Story, "Influence of Food Companies' Brand Mascots"; Kelly et al., "New Media but Same Old Tricks"; Bernhardt et al., "Children's Recall"; Vandevijvere and Swinburn, "Food References and Marketing"; Moss, *Salt, Sugar, Fat*; Nestle, *Food Politics*; Nestle and Peters, *Eat Drink Vote*; Schlosser, *Fast Food Nation*; Taylor et al., *Food Fight*; Pollan, *In Defense of Food*; Jordan, "Media"; Couric et al., *Fed Up*; Gustafson, *We the Eaters*; Salatin, *Folks, This Ain't Normal*.

5. Centers for Disease Control and Prevention. "Childhood Obesity Facts." 2015. http://www.cdc.gov/healthyyouth/obesity/facts.htm; World Health Organization. "Childhood Overweight and Obesity." http://www.who.int/dietphysical activity/childhood/en/.

6. Grow and Schwartz, "Food Marketing to Youth"; Kraak and Story, "Influence of Food Companies' Brand Mascots"; Kelly et al., "New Media but Same Old Tricks"; Bernhardt et al., "Children's Recall"; Vandevijvere and Swinburn, "Food References and Marketing"; Moss, *Salt, Sugar, Fat*; Nestle, *Food Politics*; Nestle and Peters, *Eat Drink Vote*; Schlosser, *Fast Food Nation*; Taylor et al., *Food Fight*; Pollan, *In Defense of Food*; Jordan, "Media"; Couric et al., *Fed Up*; Gustafson, *We the Eaters*; Salatin, *Folks, This Ain't Normal*.

7. Ibid.

8. Ibid.

9. Gustafson, *We the Eaters*, 55–78.

10. Ibid.; Salatin, *Folks, This Ain't Normal*; Pollan, *In Defense of Food*.

11. Nestle, *Food Politics*; Pollan, *In Defense of Food*, 18–82; Nestle and Peters, *Eat Drink Vote*; Taylor et al., *Food Fight*; Gustafson, *We the Eaters*.

12. Pollan, 18–82.

13. Nestle, *Food Politics*; Pollan, *In Defense of Food*, 18–82; Nestle and Peters, *Eat Drink Vote*; Taylor et al., *Food Fight*; Gustafson, *We the Eaters*.

14. Pollan, *In Defense of Food*, 64–67.

15. Nestle, *Food Politics*; Pollan, *In Defense of Food*, 18–82; Nestle and Peters, *Eat Drink Vote*; Taylor et al., *Food Fight*; Gustafson, *We the Eaters*.

16. Ibid.; Choi, Candace. "Coke as a Sensible Snack? Coca-Cola Works with Dietitians who Suggest Cola as Snack." *The Star Tribune*. March 6, 2015. http ://www.startribune.com/296404461.html.

17. Pollan, *The Omnivore's Dilemma*.

18. Pollan, *In Defense of Food*, 1.

19. Nestle, *Food Politics*; Pollan, *In Defense of Food*, 18–82; Nestle and Peters, *Eat Drink Vote*; Taylor et al., *Food Fight*; Gustafson, *We the Eaters*; Patel, *Stuffed and Starved*, 9–29; Graham and Ramsey, *The Happiness Diet*, 15–33; Cheney et al., *King Corn*; Kenner, et al., *Food, Inc.*; Nestle and Peters, *Eat Drink Vote*, 2–6; Hesterman, *Fair Food*, 4–50; Barber, *The Third Plate*, 2–26; Allen, Will, and Charles Wilson. *The Good Food Revolution: Growing Healthy Food, People, and Communities*. New York: Gotham Books, 2013. Kindle Edition.

20. Nestle, *Food Politics*; Pollan, *In Defense of Food*; Offit, Paul A. *Do You Believe in Magic?: The Sense and Nonsense of Alternative Medicine*. New York: Harper, 2013. Kindle Edition, 44–108.

21. Kroll, David. "Cease-and-Desist Orders Hit Walmart, Walgreens and Others for Herbal Supplement Sales." *Forbes*. February 3, 2015. http://www.forbes .com/sites/davidkroll/2015/02/03/cease-and-desist-orders-hit-walmart-walgreens -and-others-for-herbal-supplement-sales/.

22. Nestle, *Food Politics*; Pollan, *In Defense of Food*; Offit, *Do You Believe in Magic?* 44–108; Goldacre, Ben. *Bad Pharma: How Drug Companies Mislead Doctors and Harm Patients*. London: Fourth Estate, 2013. Kindle Edition; Goldacre, Ben. *Bad Science*. London: Fourth Estate, 2009. Kindle Edition; Gøtzsche, Peter C., Richard Smith, and Drummond Rennie. *Deadly Medicines and Organised Crime: How Big Pharma Has Corrupted Healthcare*. London: Radcliffe Publishing, 2013. Kindle Edition.

23. Goldacre, *Bad Science*, 44–108.

24. Ibid.

25. Offit, *Do You Believe in Magic?* 61–62; Dawsey, Sonja P., et al. "A Prospective Study of Vitamin and Mineral Supplement Use and the Risk of Upper Gastrointestinal Cancers." *PLoS One* 9, no. 2 (2014): e88774.

26. Goldacre, *Bad Science*; Offit, *Do You Believe in Magic?* 44–108.

27. Offit, *Do You Believe in Magic?* 44–108.

28. World Health Organization. "Physical Activity." 2015. http://www.who.int/topics/physical_activity/en/. See also Ekelund, Ulf, et al. "Physical Activity and All-Cause Mortality across Levels of Overall and Abdominal Adiposity in European Men and Women: the European Prospective Investigation into Cancer and Nutrition Study (EPIC)." 2015: 123456. http://ajcn.nutrition.org/content/early/2015/01/14/ajcn.114.100065.abstract.

29. Ibid.

30. Abramowitz, Michael. "Bush Urges Stepped-Up Campaign Against Childhood Obesity." *The Washington Post*. February 2, 2007. http://www.washingtonpost.com/wp-dyn/content/article/2007/02/01/AR2007020101701.html; Pate, Elias, et al. *Killer at Large*. New York: Disinformation Co., 2009.

## Chapter 6: Who Rules the Economic Roost?

1. Barnett et al., *Food Chains*; Moss, *Salt, Sugar, Fat*; Cordain et al., "Origins and Evolution of the Western Diet"; Gustafson, *We the Eaters*; Patel, *Stuffed and Starved*; Salatin, *Folks, This Ain't Normal*; Hesterman, *Fair Food*; Nestle and Peters, *Eat Drink Vote*; Taylor et al., *Food Fight*; Pollan, *In Defense of Food*; Pollan, *The Omnivore's Dilemma*; Faillace et al., *Farmageddon*; Cheney et al., *King Corn*; Berry, *Bringing It to the Table*; Nestle, *Food Politics*; Schlosser, *Fast Food Nation*; Kenner et al., *Food, Inc.*; Barber, *The Third Plate*; Graham and Ramsey, *The Happiness Diet*; Nestle, *What to Eat*.

2. Allen and Wilson, *Good Food Revolution*, 261; United States Department of Agriculture, "Economic Research Service, Food Cost Review, 1984." *Agricultural Economic Report*, no. 537 (July 1985): table 13. http://naldc.nal.usda.gov/download/CAT87214690/PDF (accessed November 28, 2012); United States Department of Agriculture. "Economic Research, Food Dollar Series." 2015. http://www.ers.usda.gov/data-products/food-dollar-series/food-dollar-application.aspx.

3. Barnett et al., *Food Chains*; Pringle, Peter. *A Place at the Table: The Crisis of 49 Million Hungry Americans and How to Solve It*. New York: PublicAffairs, 2013. Kindle Edition; Moss, *Salt, Sugar, Fat*; Cordain et al., "Origins and Evolution of the Western Diet"; Gustafson, *We the Eaters*; Patel, *Stuffed and Starved*; Salatin, *Folks, This Ain't Normal*; Hesterman, *Fair Food*; Nestle and Peters, *Eat Drink Vote*; Taylor et al., *Food Fight*; Pollan, *In Defense of Food*; Pollan, *The Omnivore's Dilemma*; Faillace et al., *Farmageddon*; Cheney et al., *King Corn*; Berry, *Bringing It to the Table*; Nestle, *Food Politics*; Schlosser, *Fast Food Nation*; Kenner et al., *Food, Inc.*; Barber, *The Third Plate*; Graham and Ramsey, *The Happiness Diet*; Nestle, *What to Eat*; Allen, *Good Food Revolution*.

4. Ibid.

5. Ibid.

6. Allen, *Good Food Revolution*; Pringle, *A Place at the Table*, 45–58; Moore, Latetia and Ana V. Diez Roux. "Associations of Neighborhood Characteristics with the Location and Type of Food Stores." *American Journal of Public Health* 96 (2006): 325–31; Satia, Jessie A. "Diet-Related Disparities: Understanding the Problem and Accelerating Solutions." *Journal of the American Dietetic Association*

109, no. 4 (2009): 610–15; Kochanek, Kenneth D., et al. "Deaths: Final Data for 2009." *National Vital Statistics Reports* 60, no. 3 (December 29, 2011): 65, table B.

7. Pringle, *A Place at the Table*; Moss, *Salt, Sugar, Fat*; Cordain et al., "Origins and Evolution of the Western Diet"; Gustafson, *We the Eaters*; Patel, *Stuffed and Starved*; Salatin, *Folks, This Ain't Normal*; Hesterman, *Fair Food*; Nestle and Peters, *Eat Drink Vote*; Taylor et al., *Food Fight*; Pollan, *In Defense of Food*; Pollan, *The Omnivore's Dilemma*; Faillace et al., *Farmageddon*; Cheney et al., *King Corn*; Berry, *Bringing It to the Table*; Nestle, *Food Politics*; Schlosser, *Fast Food Nation*; Kenner et al., *Food, Inc.*; Barber, *The Third Plate*; Graham and Ramsey, *The Happiness Diet*; Nestle, *What to Eat*; Allen, *Good Food Revolution*.

8. Ibid.; Brownell, Kelly D., and Kenneth E. Warner. "The Perils of Ignoring History: Big Tobacco Played Dirty and Millions Died. How Similar Is Big Food?" *Milbank Quarterly* 87, no. 1 (2009): 259–94; Meghani, Zahra, and Jennifer Kuzma. "The 'Revolving Door' Between Regulatory Agencies and Industry: A Problem that Requires Reconceptualizing Objectivity." *Journal of Agricultural and Environmental Ethics* 24, no. 6 (2011): 575–99; Vidal, Jordi Blanes, Mirko Draca, and Christian Fons-Rosen. "Revolving Door Lobbyists." *The American Economic Review* 102, no. 7 (2012): 3731–48; Mindell, Jennifer S., et al. "All In This Together: The Corporate Capture of Public Health." *BMJ* 345 (2012): e8082.

9. Nestle, *Food Politics*; Sarasohn, J. "Ex-USDA Chief Glickman Joins Akin Gump." *The Washington Post*. February 8, 2001: A21.

10. Ibid.

11. Nestle, *Food Politics*; WHO. *Diet, Nutrition, and the Prevention of Chronic Disease*. WHO Technical Report Series 916. Geneva, 2003. http://whqlibdoc.who.int/trs/who_trs_916.pdf ; WHO. "Global Strategy on Diet, Physical Activity, and Health." May 2004. www.who.int/dietphysicalactivity/strategy/eb11344/strategy_english_web.pdf; Waxman, A. "The WHO Global Strategy on Diet, Physical Activity and Health: The Controversy on Sugar." *Development* 47 (2004): 75–82; Zarocostas, J. "WHO Waters Down Draft Strategy on Diet and Health." *The Lancet* 363 (2004): 1373.

12. Nestle, Marion. "Sugar Politics: The BMJ's Series 'Spinning a Web of Influence.'" February 13, 2015. http://www.foodpolitics.com/2015/02/sugar-politics-the-bmjs-series-spinning-a-web-of-influence/. Gornall, Jonathan. "Sugar's Web of Influence 2: Biasing the Science." *BMJ* 350 (2015): h215; Bes-Rastrollo, M., et al. "Financial Conflicts of Interest and Reporting Bias Regarding the Association Between Sugar-Sweetened Beverages and Weight Gain: A Systematic Review of Systematic Reviews." *PLoS Med* 10 (2013): e1001578; Lesser, L. I., et al. "Relationship Between Funding Source and Conclusion Among Nutrition-Related Scientific Articles." *PLoS Med* 4 (2007):e5.

13. Bes-Rastrollo et al., "Financial Conflicts."

14. Nestle, "Sugar Politics"; Gornall, "Sugar's Web"; Bes-Rastrollo et al., "Financial Conflicts."

15. Berry, Wendell. "17 Rules For A Sustainable Local Community." The Hummingbird Project. April 6, 2013. http://www.hummingbirdproject.org/regions/wendell-berry-17-rules/; Berry, *Bringing It to the Table*; Gustafson, *We the Eaters*; Patel,

*Stuffed and Starved*; Salatin, *Folks, This Ain't Normal*; Hesterman, *Fair Food*; Nestle and Peters, *Eat Drink Vote*; Taylor et al., *Food Fight*; Pollan, *In Defense of Food*; Pollan, *The Omnivore's Dilemma*; Faillace et al., *Farmageddon*; Cheney et al., *King Corn*; Nestle, *Food Politics*; Schlosser, *Fast Food Nation*; Kenner et al., *Food, Inc.*; Barber, *The Third Plate*; Allen, *The Good Food Revolution*.

16. Gustafson, *We the Eaters*, 4.

17. Berry, "17 Rules"; Berry, *Bringing It to the Table*; Gustafson, *We the Eaters*; Patel, *Stuffed and Starved*; Salatin, *Folks, This Ain't Normal*; Hesterman, *Fair Food*; Nestle and Peters, *Eat Drink Vote*; Taylor et al., *Food Fight*; Pollan, *In Defense of Food*; Pollan, *The Omnivore's Dilemma*; Faillace et al., *Farmageddon*; Cheney et al., *King Corn*; Nestle, *Food Politics*; Schlosser, *Fast Food Nation*; Kenner et al., *Food, Inc.*; Barber, *The Third Plate*; Allen, *The Good Food Revolution*.

18. Ibid.; Rabotyagov, Sergey, et al. "Least-Cost Control of Agricultural Nutrient Contributions to the Gulf of Mexico Hypoxic Zone." *Ecological Applications* 20, no. 6 (2010): 1542–55; Mitsch, William J., et al. "Reducing Nitrogen Loading to the Gulf of Mexico from the Mississippi River Basin: Strategies to Counter a Persistent Ecological Problem Ecotechnology—The Use of Natural Ecosystems to Solve Environmental problems—Should Be a Part of Efforts to Shrink the Zone of Hypoxia in the Gulf of Mexico." *BioScience* 51, no. 5 (2001): 373–88.

19. Ibid.

20. Stuart, *Waste*; Feed Back. "Global Waste Scandal." 2014. http://feedbackglobal.org/food-waste-scandal/; Gustafson, *We the Eaters*; Gustavsson, Jenny, et al. "Global Food Losses and Food Waste. Food and Agriculture Organization of the United Nations." *Rom* (2011); Cordell, Dana, Jan-Olof Drangert, and Stuart White. "The Story of Phosphorus: Global Food Security and Food for Thought." *Global Environmental Change* 19, no. 2 (2009): 292–305; de Lange, Willem, and Anton Nahman. "Costs of Food Waste in South Africa: Incorporating Inedible Food Waste." *Waste Management* 40 (2015): 167–72; Thi, Ngoc Bao Dung, Gopalakrishnan Kumar, and Chiu-Yue Lin. "An Overview of Food Waste Management in Developing Countries: Current Status and Future Perspective." *Journal of Environmental Management* 157 (2015): 220–29.

21. Ibid.; Garrone, Paola, Marco Melacini, and Alessandro Perego. "Opening the Black Box of Food Waste Reduction." *Food Policy* 46 (2014): 129–39.

22. Ibid.

23. Gustafson, *We the Eaters*.

24. Ibid., 88–91.

25. Ibid.

26. Stuart, *Waste*; Feed Back, "Global Waste Scandal"; Berry, "17 Rules"; Berry, *Bringing It to the Table*; Gustafson, *We the Eaters*; Patel, *Stuffed and Starved*; Salatin, *Folks, This Ain't Normal*; Hesterman, *Fair Food*; Nestle and Peters, *Eat Drink Vote*; Taylor et al., *Food Fight*; Pollan, *In Defense of Food*; Pollan, *The Omnivore's Dilemma*; Faillace et al., *Farmageddon*; Nestle, *Food Politics*; Schlosser, *Fast Food Nation*; Kenner et al., *Food, Inc.*; Barber, *The Third Plate*; Allen, *The Good Food Revolution*.

27. Gustafson, *We the Eaters*; Patel, *Stuffed and Starved*.

**Chapter 7: The Genetic Elephant in the Room**

1. Shiva, *The Vandana Shiva Reader*; Druker, Steven M., and Jane Goodall. *Altered Genes, Twisted Truth: How the Venture to Genetically Engineer Our Food Has Subverted Science, Corrupted Government, and Systematically Deceived the Public.* Salt Lake City: Clear River Press, 2015. Kindle Edition; Krimsky, Sheldon, and Jeremy Gruber. *The GMO Deception: What You Need to Know About the Food, Corporations, and Government Agencies Putting Our Families and Our Environment at Risk.* New York: Skyhorse Publishing, 2014. Kindle Edition; Salatin, *Folks, This Ain't Normal*, 225–39; Gustafson, *We the Eaters*; Patel, *Stuffed and Starved*; Berry, *Bringing It to the Table*; Newton, David E. *GMO Food: A Reference Handbook.* Santa Barbara: ABC-CLIO, 2014.

2. Furley, David J. *The Greek Cosmologists.* Cambridge: Cambridge University Press, 1987. 115–35.

3. Shiva, *The Vandana Shiva Reader*; Druker and Goodall, *Altered Genes*; Krimsky and Gruber, *The GMO Deception*; Salatin, *Folks, This Ain't Normal*, 225–39; Gustafson, *We the Eaters*; Patel, *Stuffed and Starved*; Berry, *Bringing It to the Table*.

4. Whitman, Elizabeth. "GMO Apples and Potatoes Approved by FDA; Labeling Not Required." *International Business Times.* March 20, 2015. http://www.ibtimes.com/gmo-apples-potatoes-approved-fda-labeling-not-required-1854280; Shiva, *The Vandana Shiva Reader*; Druker and Goodall, *Altered Genes*; Krimsky and Gruber, *The GMO Deception*; Salatin, *Folks, This Ain't Normal*, 225–39; Gustafson, *We the Eaters*; Patel, *Stuffed and Starved*; Berry, *Bringing It to the Table*.

5. Newton, *GMO Food*; Druker and Goodall, *Altered Genes*; Krimsky and Gruber, *The GMO Deception*.

6. Fernandez-Cornejo, Jorge, et al. "Genetically Engineered Crops in the United States." *USDA-ERS Economic Research Report* 162 (2014); Nabradi, Andras, and Jozsef Popp. "Economics of GM Crop Cultivation." *Crop Biotech Update* (2011): 7–19; Newton, *GMO Food*; Druker and Goodall, *Altered Genes*; Krimsky and Gruber, *The GMO Deception*.

7. Fernandez-Cornejo et al., "Genetically Engineered Crops."

8. International Service for the Acquisition of Agri-biotech Applications (ISAAA). "Pocket K No. 16: Global Status of Commercialized Biotech/GM Crops in 2014." 2015. http://www.isaaa.org/inbrief/default.asp; James, C. "Global Status of Commercialized Biotech/GM Crops: 2014." ISAAA Brief No. 49. Ithaca, NY: ISAAA, 2014.

9. Krimsky and Gruber, *The GMO Deception*; Druker and Goodall, *Altered Genes*; Salatin, *Folks, This Ain't Normal*, 225–39; Shiva, *The Vandana Shiva Reader*.

10. Diels, Johan, Mario Cunha, et al. "Association of Financial or Professional Conflict of Interest to Research Outcomes on Health Risks or Nutritional Assessment Studies of Genetically Modified Products." *Food Policy* 36, no. 2 (2011): 197–203.

11. Leaf, Caroline. *The Switch on Your Brain 5-Step Learning Process.* Dallas: Switch on Your Brain USA LP, 2009.

12. McGrath, Alister E. *Surprised by Meaning: Science, Faith, and How We Make Sense of Things*. Louisville: Westminster John Knox Press, 2011. Kindle Edition, 43–44; McGrath, Alister E. *Dawkins' God: Genes, Memes, and the Meaning of Life*. Malden, MA: Blackwell, 2005. Kindle Edition; Polkinghorne, J. C. *Science and Religion in Quest of Truth*. New Haven: Yale University Press, 2011. Kindle Edition.

13. Krimsky and Gruber, *The GMO Deception*; Druker and Goodall, *Altered Genes*; Salatin, *Folks, This Ain't Normal*, 225–39; Shiva, *The Vandana Shiva Reader*; Gustafson, *We the Eaters*; Patel, *Stuffed and Starved*; Berry, *Bringing It to the Table*.

14. Diels et al., "Association of Financial or Professional Conflict of Interest."

15. Ibid.; Fernandez-Cornejo et al., "Genetically Engineered Crops"; Nabradi and Popp, "Economics of GM Crop Cultivation," 7–19; Krimsky and Gruber, *The GMO Deception*; Druker and Goodall, *Altered Genes*; Salatin, *Folks, This Ain't Normal*, 225–39; Shiva, *The Vandana Shiva Reader*; Gustafson, *We the Eaters*; Patel, *Stuffed and Starved*; Berry, *Bringing It to the Table*.

16. Nielsen, Kaare M. "Biosafety Data as Confidential Business Information." *PLoS Biology* 11, no. 3 (2013): e1001499. http://journals.plos.org/plosbiology /article?id=10.1371/journal.pbio.1001499; Diels et al., "Association of Financial or Professional Conflict of Interest"; Krimsky and Gruber, *The GMO Deception*.

17. Quaddus, M. A., and Muhammed Abu B. Siddique. *Handbook of Sustainable Development Planning: Studies in Modeling and Decision Support*. Cheltenham, UK: Edward Elgar, 2013. 91–116; Picó, Yolanda. *Chemical Analysis of Food: Techniques and Applications*. Waltham, MA: Academic Press, 2012. 453–54; Krimsky and Gruber, *The GMO Deception*; Druker and Goodall, *Altered Genes*; Salatin, *Folks, This Ain't Normal*, 225–39; Shiva, *The Vandana Shiva Reader*; Gustafson, *We the Eaters*; Patel, *Stuffed and Starved*.

18. Krimsky and Gruber, *The GMO Deception*. After publicly voicing his concerns on the safety of GM potatoes, Pusztai was subject to a number of professional and personal attacks in what came to be known as the Pusztai Affair. For the original study, see Ewen, S. W. B, and A. Pusztai. "Effect of Diets Containing Genetically Modified Potatoes Expressing Galanthus Nivalis Lectin on Rat Small Intestine." *The Lancet* 354 (1999): 1353–54.

19. Snell, Chelsea, et al. "Assessment of the Health Impact of GM Plant Diets in Long-Term and Multigenerational Animal Feeding Trials: A Literature Review." *Food and Chemical Toxicology* 50, no. 3 (2012): 1134–48; GM Free Scotland. "Three Reviews of GM Safety." May 2012. http://gmfreescotland.blogspot .com/2012/05/three-reviews-of-gm-safety.html.

20. Domingo, José L., and Jordi Ginéi Bordonaba. "A Literature Review on the Safety Assessment of Genetically Modified Plants." *Environment International* 37, no. 4 (2011): 734–42; GM Free Scotland, "Three Reviews."

21. Hilbeck, Angelika, et al. "No Scientific Consensus on GMO Safety." *Environmental Sciences Europe* 27, no. 1 (2015): 1–6.

22. Samsel, Anthony, and Stephanie Seneff. "Glyphosate, Pathways to Modern Diseases III: Manganese, Neurological Diseases, and Associated Pathologies." *Surgical Neurology International* 6 (2015): 45; Seneff, Stephanie, Nancy Swanson,

and Chen Li. "Aluminum and Glyphosate Can Synergistically Induce Pineal Gland Pathology: Connection to Gut Dysbiosis and Neurological Disease." *Agricultural Sciences* 6, no. 1 (2015): 42.

23. Lee, R., et al. "Using Human-Severe Combined Immunodeficiency (hu-SCID) Mice as a Model for Testing Allergenicity of Genetically Modified Organisms (GMOs)." *Clinical and Translational Allergy* 3, no. 3 (2013): 18; Flanagan, Simon. *Handbook of Food Allergen Detection and Control.* Cambridge, MA: Waltham, 2015. 161–76.

24. Williams, A. L., R. E. Watson, and J. M. Desesso. "Developmental and Reproductive Outcomes in Humans and Animals after Glyphosate Exposure: A Critical Analysis." *Journal of Toxicology and Environmental Health, Part B* 15 (2012): 39–96.

25. Antoniou, M., et al. "Teratogenic Effects of Glyphosate-Based Herbicides: Divergence of Regulatory Decisions from Scientific Evidence." *Journal of Environmental and Analytical Toxicology* 4 (2012): 2161–525; Cattani D., et al. "Mechanisms Underlying the Neurotoxicity Induced by Glyphosate-Based Herbicide in Immature Rat Hippocampus: Involvement of Glutamate Excitotoxicity." *Toxicology* 320 (2014): 34–45; Mesnage, R. S. "The Need for a Closer Look at Pesticide Toxicity during GMO Assessment in Practical Food Safety: Contemporary Issues and Future Directions." In *Practical Food Safety: Contemporary Issues and Future Directions.* Bhat R., and V. M. Gómez-López, eds. Chichester, UK: John Wiley and Sons, Ltd., 2014; Vandenberg, L. N., et al. "Hormones and Endocrine-Disrupting Chemicals: Low-Dose Effects and Nonmonotonic Dose Responses." *Endocrinology Reviews* 33 (2012): 378–455; Swanson, Nancy L., et al. "Genetically Engineered Crops, Glyphosate and the Deterioration of Health in the United States of America." *Journal of Organic Systems* 9, no. 2 (2014): 6–37.

26. Fritschi, L., et al. "Carcinogenicity of Tetrachlorvinphos, Parathion, Malathion, Diazinon, and Glyphosate." *The Lancet Oncology.* 2015. http://www.the lancet.com/pdfs/journals/lanonc/PIIS1470-2045(15)70134-8.pdf.

27. Krimsky and Gruber, *The GMO Deception*; Druker and Goodall, *Altered Genes.*

28. Séralini, G. E., et al. "Long-Term Toxicity of a Roundup Herbicide and a Roundup-Tolerant Genetically Modified Maize." *Food and Chemical Toxicology* (2012): 4221–31; Krimsky and Gruber, *The GMO Deception*; Druker and Goodall, *Altered Genes*; GM Free Scotland, "Three Reviews."

29. Pirondini, Andrea, and Nelson Marmiroli. "Environmental Risk Assessment in GMO Analysis." *Rivista di Biologia* 101, no. 2 (2008): 215–46; Benbrook, Charles M. "Impacts of Genetically Engineered Crops on Pesticide Use in the US—The First Sixteen Years." *Environmental Sciences Europe* 24, no. 1 (2012): 1–13; Sirinathsinghji, Eva. "Study Confirms GM Crops Lead to Increased Pesticide Use." *Science in Society* 56 (2012): 8–10; Wagner, Norman, et al. "Questions Concerning the Potential Impact of Glyphosate-Based Herbicides on Amphibians." *Environmental Toxicology and Chemistry* 32, no. 8 (2013): 1688–1700; Meehan, T. D., et al. "Agricultural Landscape Simplification and Insecticide Use in the Midwestern United States." *Proceedings of the National Academy of Sciences*

108 (2011): 11500–505; Blesh, J., and L. E. Drinkwater. "The Impact of Nitrogen Source and Crop Rotation on Nitrogen Mass Balances in the Mississippi River Basin." *Ecological Applications* 23, no. 5 (2013): 1017–35; Davis, Adam S., et al. "Increasing Cropping System Diversity Balances Productivity, Profitability and Environmental Health." *PLoS One* 7, no. 10 (2012): e47149; Jacobsen, Sven-Erik, et al. "Feeding the World: Genetically Modified Crops Versus Agricultural Biodiversity." *Agronomy for Sustainable Development* 33, no. 4 (2013): 651–62; Krimsky and Gruber, *The GMO Deception*; Druker and Goodall, *Altered Genes*; Salatin, *Folks, This Ain't Normal,* 225–39; Shiva, *The Vandana Shiva Reader*; Gustafson, *We the Eaters*; Patel, *Stuffed and Starved*.

30. Gassmann, Aaron J., et al. "Field-Evolved Resistance by Western Corn Rootworm to Multiple Bacillus Thuringiensis Toxins in Transgenic Maize." *Proceedings of the National Academy of Sciences* 111, no. 14 (2014): 5141–46; Gassmann, Aaron J., et al. "Western Corn Rootworm and Bt Maize: Challenges of Pest Resistance in the Field." GM Crops & Food 3, no. 3 (2012): 235–44; Krimsky and Gruber, *The GMO Deception*.

31. Benbrook, "Impacts"; Krimsky and Gruber, *The GMO Deception*.

32. Klümper, Wilhelm, and Matin Qaim. "A Meta-Analysis of the Impacts of Genetically Modified Crops." *PLoS One* 9, no. 11 (2014): e111629; Heinemann, Jack. "Correlation Is Not Causation." *RightBiotech*. November 27, 2014. http ://rightbiotech.tumblr.com/post/103665842150/correlation-is-not-causation.

33. Krimsky and Gruber, *The GMO Deception*.

34. Krimsky and Gruber, *The GMO Deception*; Pirondini and Marmiroli, "Environmental Risk Assessment"; Benbrook, "Impacts"; Sirinathsinghji, "Study Confirms"; Wagner et al. "Questions Concerning the Potential Impact"; Meehan et al. "Agricultural Landscape Simplification"; Blesh and Drinkwater, "Impact of Nitrogen Source and Crop Rotation"; Davis et al. "Increasing Cropping System Diversity"; Jacobsen et al. "Feeding the World"; Druker and Goodall, *Altered Genes*; Salatin, *Folks, This Ain't Normal,* 225–39; Shiva, *The Vandana Shiva Reader*; Gustafson, *We the Eaters*; Patel, *Stuffed and Starved*.

35. Price, Becky, and Janet Cotter. "The GM Contamination Register: a Review of Recorded Contamination Incidents Associated with Genetically Modified Organisms (GMOs), 1997–2013." *International Journal of Food Contamination* 1, no. 1 (2014): 1–13; Smith, Amanda. "Sowing Wild Oats: Bystander Strict Liability in Tort Applied to Organic Farm Contamination by Genetically Modified Seed." *University of Louisville Law Review* 51 (2012): 629; Reed, Genna. "GMOs v. Organic: Is Coexistence Possible?" 142nd APHA Annual Meeting and Exposition, November 15–19, 2014; Chandler, Stephen F., and Trevor W. Stevenson. "Gene Flow and Risk Assessment in Genetically Modified Crops." In *Alien Gene Transfer in Crop Plants*, vol. 1. New York: Springer, 2014. 247–65; Du, Dorothy. "Rethinking Risks: Should Socioeconomic and Ethical Considerations be Incorporated into the Regulation of Genetically Modified Crops." *Harvard Journal of Law & Technology* 26 (2012): 376–401; Mitchell, Shené. "Organic Crops, Genetic Drift, and Commingling: Theories of Remedy and Defense." *Drake Journal of Agricultural Law* 18 (2013): 313–33; Krimsky and Gruber,

*The GMO Deception*; Pirondini and Marmiroli, "Environmental Risk Assessment"; Benbrook, "Impacts"; Sirinathsinghji, "Study Confirms"; Davis et al., "Increasing Cropping System Diversity"; Jacobsen et al., "Feeding the World"; Druker and Goodall, *Altered Genes*; Salatin, *Folks, This Ain't Normal*, 225–39; Shiva, *The Vandana Shiva Reader*; Gustafson, *We the Eaters*; Patel, *Stuffed and Starved*.

36. Ibid.

37. Gustafson, *We the Eaters*.

38. Krimsky and Gruber, *The GMO Deception*; Jacobsen et al. "Feeding the World"; Druker and Goodall, *Altered Genes*; Salatin, *Folks, This Ain't Normal*, 225–39; Shiva, *The Vandana Shiva Reader*; Gustafson, *We the Eaters*; Patel, *Stuffed and Starved*.

39. Gustafson, *We the Eaters*; Patel, *Stuffed and Starved*.

40. Hesterman, *Fair Food*, 13.

41. Gustafson, *We the Eaters*; Patel, *Stuffed and Starved*; Krimsky and Gruber, *The GMO Deception*; Jacobsen et al. "Feeding the World"; Druker and Goodall, *Altered Genes*; Salatin, *Folks, This Ain't Normal*, 225–39; Shiva, *The Vandana Shiva Reader*.

42. Shiva, *The Vandana Shiva Reader*; Druker and Goodall, *Altered Genes*; Krimsky and Gruber, *The GMO Deception*; Salatin, *Folks, This Ain't Normal*, 225–39; Gustafson, *We the Eaters*; Patel, *Stuffed and Starved*; Berry, *Bringing It to the Table*; Stuart, *Waste*; Feed Back, "Global Waste Scandal"; Berry, "17 Rules"; Taylor et al., *Food Fight*; Pollan, *In Defense of Food*; Pollan, *The Omnivore's Dilemma*.

43. Sen, Amartya. *Poverty and Famines: An Essay on Entitlement and Deprivation*. Oxford: Oxford University Press, 1982. 1; Gustafson, *We the Eaters*; Patel, *Stuffed and Starved*.

44. Shiva, *The Vandana Shiva Reader*; Druker and Goodall, *Altered Genes*; Krimsky and Gruber, *The GMO Deception*; Salatin, *Folks, This Ain't Normal*, 225–39; Gustafson, *We the Eaters*; Patel, *Stuffed and Starved*; Berry, *Bringing It to the Table*; Stuart, *Waste*; Feed Back, "Global Waste Scandal"; Berry, "17 Rules"; Taylor et al., *Food Fight*; Pollan, *In Defense of Food*; Pollan, *The Omnivore's Dilemma*; Sen, *Poverty and Famines*.

45. Ibid.

46. Benbrook, C. "Troubled Times Amid Commercial Success for Roundup Ready Soybeans: Glyphosate Efficacy is Slipping and Unstable Transgene Expression Erodes Plant Defences and Yields." AgBioTech InfoNet Technical Paper No. 4 (May 2001): 3. http://www.biotech-info.net/troubledtimes.html; Elmore, et al. "Glyphosate-Resistant Soybean Cultivar Yields Compared with Sister Lines." *Agron* 93 (2001): 408–12; quote from press release announcing study at http://ian rnews.unl.edu/static/0005161.shtml; Krimsky and Gruber, *The GMO Deception*.

47. IAASTD. *Agriculture at a Crossroads*. Washington, DC: Island Press, 2009. http://www.unep.org/dewa/agassessment/reports/IAASTD/EN/Agriculture%20 at%20a%20Crossroads_Synthesis%20Report%20%28English%29.pdf; Krimsky and Gruber, *The GMO Deception*.

48. Gurian-Sherman, Doug. "Failure to Yield: Evaluating the Performance of Genetically Engineered Crops." Union of Concerned Scientists. April 2009. http ://www.ucsusa.org/sites/default/files/legacy/assets/documents/food_and_agricu lture/failure-to-yield.pdf; Krimsky and Gruber, *The GMO Deception*.

49. Oerke, E. C. "Crop Losses to Pests." *The Journal of Agricultural Science* 144, no. 1 (2006): 31–43; Hesterman, *Fair Food*, 2–46.

50. Shiva, *The Vandana Shiva Reader*; Druker and Goodall, *Altered Genes*; Krimsky and Gruber, *The GMO Deception*; Salatin, *Folks, This Ain't Normal*, 225–39; Gustafson, *We the Eaters*; Patel, *Stuffed and Starved*; Berry, *Bringing It to the Table*; Berry, "17 Rules"; Taylor et al., *Food Fight*; Pollan, *In Defense of Food*; Pollan, *The Omnivore's Dilemma*; Sen, *Poverty and Famines*.

51. Nash, J. Madeleine. "This Rice Could Save a Million Kids a Year." *Time*. July 31, 2000. http://content.time.com/time/magazine/article/0,9171,997586,00. html; Patel, *Stuffed and Starved*.

52. Patel, *Stuffed and Starved*.

53. Nash, "This Rice"; Patel, *Stuffed and Starved*.

54. Hine, R., J. Pretty, and S. Twarog. *Organic Agriculture and Food Security in Africa*. New York and Geneva: UNEP-UNCTAD Capacity-Building Task Force on Trade, Environment and Development, 2008. http://bit.ly/KBCgY0.

55. The Rodale Institute. "The Farming Systems Trial." http://rodaleinstitut e.org/wp-content/uploads/2013/03/FSTbrochure.pdf.

56. Chivian, Eric, and Aaron Bernstein. *Genetically Modified Foods and Organic Farming. In Sustaining Life: How Human Health Depends on Biodiversity*. New York: Oxford University Press, 2008. 399–400, 402; Hesterman, *Fair Food*, 293.

57. Ponisio, Lauren C., et al. "Diversification Practices Reduce Organic to Conventional Yield Gap." *Proceedings of the Royal Society of London B: Biological Sciences* 282, no. 1799 (2015): 20141396.

58. Jacobsen et al., "Feeding the World"; Davis et al., "Increasing Cropping System Diversity."

59. Shiva, *The Vandana Shiva Reader*; Druker and Goodall, *Altered Genes*; Krimsky and Gruber, *The GMO Deception*; Salatin, *Folks, This Ain't Normal*, 225–39; Gustafson, *We the Eaters*; Patel, *Stuffed and Starved*; Berry, *Bringing It to the Table*; Berry, "17 Rules"; Taylor et al., *Food Fight*; Pollan, *In Defense of Food*; Pollan, *The Omnivore's Dilemma*; Sen, *Poverty and Famines*.

60. Ibid.

61. Fernandez-Cornejo, Jorge, and David Schimmelpfennig. "Have Seed Industry Changes Affected Research Effort?" *Amber Waves* 2, no. 1 (2004): 14–19; Patel, *Stuffed and Starved*.

62. Pollan, Michael, "Vote for the Dinner Party." *The New York Times Magazine*. October 10, 2012. http://michaelpollan.com/articles-archive/vote-for-the -dinner-party/.

63. Pollan, "Vote For the Dinner Party"; Shiva, *The Vandana Shiva Reader*; Druker and Goodall, *Altered Genes*; Krimsky and Gruber, *The GMO Deception*.

64. Ibid.; Druker and Goodall, *Altered Genes*; Krimsky and Gruber, *The GMO Deception*; Salatin, *Folks, This Ain't Normal*, 225–39; Gustafson, *We the Eaters*;

Patel, *Stuffed and Starved*; Berry, *Bringing It to the Table*; Berry, "17 Rules"; Taylor et al., *Food Fight*; Pollan, *In Defense of Food*; Pollan, *The Omnivore's Dilemma*; Sen, *Poverty and Famines*; Ronald, Pamela C., and Raoul W. Adamchak. *Tomorrow's Table: Organic Farming, Genetics, and the Future of Food*. New York: Oxford University Press, 2008. 137–51; Kenner et al., *Food, Inc.*

65. Hattori, Y., et al. "The Ethylene Response Factors SNORKEL1 and SNORKEL2 Allow Rice to Adapt to Deep Water." *Nature* 460 (2009): 1026–30; Krimsky and Gruber, *The GMO Deception*.

66. Ronald and Adamchak, *Tomorrow's Table*.

67. Benyus, Janine M. *Biomimicry: Innovation Inspired by Nature*. Pymble, NSW: HarperCollins e-books, 2009; Salatin, *Folks, This Ain't Normal*, 20.

68. Benyus, *Biomimicry*.

69. Salatin, *Folks, This Ain't Normal*; Butterfield, Jody, et al. *Holistic Management Handbook: Healthy Land, Healthy Profits*. Washington, DC: Island Press, 2006; Allen, Will, and Charles Wilson. *The Good Food Revolution: Growing Healthy Food, People, and Communities*. New York: Gotham Books, 2012. Kindle Edition; White, Joseph Courtney. *Grass, Soil, Hope: A Journey Through Carbon Country*. White River Junction: Chelsea Green Publishing, 2014. Kindle Edition; Chase, Lisa, and Vernon P. Grubinger. *Food, Farms, and Community: Exploring Food Systems*. Durham, NH: The University of New Hampshire Press, 2014. Kindle Edition; Barber, *The Third Plate*; Ackerman-Leist, *Rebuilding the Foodshed*; Niman, Nicolette Hahn. *Defending Beef: The Case for Sustainable Meat Production*. White River Junction: Chelsea Green Publishing, 2014. Kindle Edition; Bernstein, Sylvia. *Aquaponic Gardening: A Step-by-Step Guide to Raising Vegetables and Fish Together*. Gabriola, BC: New Society Publishers, 2011.

70. Salatin, *Folks, This Ain't Normal*, 20; Growing Power. "History." 2014. http://www.growingpower.org/about/history/.

71. Stafford, Beth. "UW-Milwaukee Spring Commencement 2012." Press release. University of Wisconsin-Milwaukee. May 9, 2012.

## Chapter 8: Mindset and Meal

1. American Psychological Association. "Stress in America (TM): Our Health at Risk." 2012. http://www.apa.org/news/press/releases/stress/2011/final-2011.pdf; American Institute of Stress. "Stress Is Killing You." n.d. http://www.stress.org/stress-is-killing-you/; Harvard Medical School's Mind-Body Institute. Published research by date. http://www.bensonhenryinstitute.org/index.php/our-research/published-research; The Institute of HeartMath. "Local and Nonlocal Effects of Coherent Heart Frequencies on Conformational Changes of DNA." 2001. http://appreciativeinquiry.case.edu/uploads/HeartMath%20article.pdf; Kinderman, P., et al. "Psychological Processes Mediate the Impact of Familial Risk. Social Circumstances and Life Events on Mental Health." *PLoS* (2013), http://journals.plos.org/plosone/article?id=10.1371/journal.pone.0076564; Powell, N. D., et al. "Social Stress Up-Regulates Inflammatory Gene Expression in the Leukocyte Transcriptome Via β-Adrenergic Induction of Myelopoiesis." *PNAS* (2013),

http://www.pnas.org/content/110/41/16574.full; Cohen, S., et al. "Psychological Stress and Disease." *JAMA* (2007): 1685–87; Cohen, S, et al. "Chronic Stress, Glucocorticoid Receptor Resistance, Inflammation, and Disease Risk." *PNAS* (2012): 5995–99; Seaward, B. "Are Your Wellness Programs Prepared for the Super Stress Super Storm." Wellness Council of America, 2010. http://www.brianluke seaward.com/downloads/SuperStress-WELCOA-Seaward.pdf; "Cancer Statistics and Views of Causes." *Science News* 115, no. 2 (January 13, 1979): 23; Nijhout, H. F. "Metaphors and the Role of Genes and Development." *BioEssays* 12 (1990): 444–46; Willett, W. C. "Balancing Lifestyle and Genomics Research for Disease Prevention." *Science* 296 (2002): 695–98; Pert, C. B. *Molecules of Emotion: Why You Feel the Way You Feel*. New York: Simon and Schuster, 1997; Lipton, B. *The Biology of Belief: Unleashing the Power of Consciousness, Matter and Miracles*. Santa Cruz, CA: Mountain of Love Productions, 2008; Church, D. *Genie in Your Genes*. Santa Rosa, CA: Energy Psychology Press, 2007.

2. Attwell, David, and Simon B. Laughlin. "An Energy Budget for Signaling in the Grey Matter of the Brain." *Journal of Cerebral Blood Flow & Metabolism* 21, no. 10 (2001): 1133–45; Peters, A., and D. Langemann. "Build-ups in the Supply Chain of the Brain: on the Neuroenergetic Cause of Obesity and Type 2 Diabetes Mellitus." *Front. Neuroenerg* 1 (2009): 2. doi:10.3389/neuro.14.002.2009; Hovda, David A., et al. "Metabolic Dysfunction Following Traumatic Brain Injury." In *Concussions in Athletics*. New York: Springer, 2014. 205–15.

3. Gustafson, *We the Eaters*, xiv; Pan et al. "Exporting Diabetes to Asia"; Yang, Lijun. "The Effect of Western Diet Culture on Chinese Diet Culture." In *International Conference on Education, Language, Art and Intercultural Communication* (ICELAIC-14). Amsterdam: Atlantis Press, 2014; Myles, Ian A. "Fast Food Fever: Reviewing the Impacts of the Western Diet on Immunity." *Nutrition Journal* 13, no. 1 (2014): 61; Taylor, Allyn L., Emily Whelan Parento, and Laura Schmidt. "The Increasing Weight of Regulation: Countries Combat the Global Obesity Epidemic." *Indiana Law Journal* 90 (2014): forthcoming; Vineis, Paolo, and Christopher P. Wild. "Global Cancer Patterns: Causes and Prevention." *The Lancet* 383, no. 9916 (2014): 549–57.

4. Hoffmann, Beth. "It's Convenience, Not Cost, That Makes Us Fat." *Forbes*. July 17, 2012. http://www.forbes.com/sites/bethhoffman/2012/07/17/its-conve nience-not-cost-that-makes-us-fat/; Puzic, Sonja. "How We Eat: The Rise of the Convenience Food Market." *CTV News*. August 20, 2014; Salatin, *Folks, This Ain't Normal*; Hesterman, *Fair Food*; Nestle and Peters, *Eat Drink Vote*, 128–35; Taylor et al., *Food Fight*; Gustafson, *We the Eaters*, 31–78; Pollan, *In Defense of Food*; Pollan, *The Omnivore's Dilemma*, 14–183; Faillace et al., *Farmageddon*; Cheney et al., *King Corn*; Berry, *Bringing It to the Table*; Nestle, *Food Politics*; Schlosser, *Fast Food Nation*; Imhoff, *CAFO Reader*; Kenner et al., *Food, Inc.*; Barber, *The Third Plate*; Graham and Ramsey, *The Happiness Diet*; Nestle, *What to Eat*, 67–305; Stuart, *Waste*.

5. Ibid.

6. Nijhout, "Metaphors and the Role of Genes"; Watters, Ethan. "DNA Is Not Destiny: The New Science of Epigenetics." *Discover Magazine*. November

22, 2006. http://discovermagazine.com/2006/nov/cover; "Ghost in Your Genes." *Nova*, 2008. http://www.pbs.org/wgbh/nova/genes/; Satel, Sally L., and Scott O. Lilienfeld. *Brainwashed: The Seductive Appeal of Mindless Neuroscience*. New York: Basic Books, 2013; Kinderman, Peter. *A Prescription for Psychiatry: Why We Need a Whole New Approach to Mental Health and Wellbeing*. Basingstoke: Palgrave Macmillan, 2014.

## Chapter 9: Taking Responsibility

1. Leaf, Caroline. *Switch On Your Brain: The Key to Peak Happiness, Thinking, and Health*. Grand Rapids: Baker, 2013, chap. 1; Leaf, Caroline. "Ridiculous." TED Talks. TEDxOaksChristianSchool. 2015. http://tedxtalks.ted.com/video /Ridiculous-Caroline-Leaf-TEDxOa;search%3Acaroline%20leaf; Leaf, Caroline. "Mind-Mapping: A Therapeutic Technique for Closed-Head Injury." Master's Thesis. Pretoria: University of Pretoria, 1990.

2. Reardon, Thomas, Peter Timmer, and Julio Berdegue. "The Rapid Rise of Supermarkets in Developing Countries." *Journal of Agricultural and Development Economics* 1, no. 2 (2004): 168–83; Gustafson, *We the Eaters*, v–xix.

3. Oxfam International. "Food Aid or Hidden Dumping?" 2005. https:// www.oxfam.org/sites/www.oxfam.org/files/bp71_food_aid.pdf; Gustafson, *We the Eaters*, v–xix; Edelman, Marc, et al. "Introduction: Critical Perspectives on Food Sovereignty." *Journal of Peasant Studies* 41, no. 6 (2014): 911–31; Shattuck, Annie, and Eric Holt-Giménez. "Moving from Food Crisis to Food Sovereignty." *Yale Human Rights and Development Journal* 13, no. 2 (2014): 421–34; Barrett, Christopher B., and Dan Maxwell. *Food Aid after Fifty Years: Recasting Its Role*. London: Routledge, 2007.

4. Wright, N. T. *Surprised by Scripture: Engaging Contemporary Issues*. San Francisco: HarperOne, 2014. 83–106; Salatin, *Folks, This Ain't Normal*, 179.

5. Ibid.

6. Kendrick, Malcolm. *Doctoring Data: How to Sort Out Medical Advice from Medical Nonsense*. London: Columbus Publishing, 2015. 9–11; Andersen, Klaus Kaae, and Tom Skyhøj Olsen. "The Obesity Paradox in Stroke: Lower Mortality and Lower Risk of Readmission for Recurrent Stroke in Obese Stroke Patients." *International Journal of Stroke* 10, no. 1 (2015): 99–104; Shil Hong, Eun, et al. "Counterintuitive Relationship Between Visceral Fat and All-Cause Mortality in an Elderly Asian Population." *Obesity* 23, no. 1 (2015): 220–27.

7. Ibid.

8. Society for the Study of Ingestive Behavior. "Dieting Young May Lead to Poor Health Outcomes Later: Trends in Dieting Strategies in Young Adult Women from 1982 to 2012." *ScienceDaily*, July 29, 2014. www.sciencedaily.com /releases/2014/07/140729224908.htm; Naish, John. "Why Dieting Makes You FAT: Research Shows Trying to Lose Weight Alters Your Brain and Hormones So You're Doomed to Pile It on Again." *Daily Mail*. April 23, 2012. http://www.daily mail.co.uk/health/article-2134162/Research-shows-trying-lose-weight-alters -brain-hormones-youre-doomed-pile-again.html.

## Chapter 10: The Meeting of the Minds

1. Leaf, Caroline, Brenda Louw, and Isabel Uys. "The Development of a Model for Geodesic Learning: The Geodesic Information Processing Model." *The South African Journal of Communication Disorders* 44 (1997): 53–70. http://drleaf.co m/download-dispatch/?fn=/TheDevelopmentOfAModelForGeodesicLearning .pdf; Leaf, *Switch On Your Brain*, 123–28; Leaf, Caroline. "The Mind-Mapping Approach: A Model and Framework for Geodesic Learning." PhD dissertation, University of Pretoria, March 1997.

2. "Dr. Leaf's Research." http://drleaf.com/about/dr-leafs-research/; "Dr. Leaf's Curriculum Vitae." http://drleaf.com/download-dispatch/?fn=/DrCarolineLeaf _CurriculumVitae1.pdf.

3. Ibid.

4. Craddock, Travis John Adrian, and Jack A. Tuszynski. "A Critical Assessment of the Information Processing Capabilities of Neuronal Microtubules Using Coherent Excitations." *Journal of Biological Physics* 36, no. 1 (2010): 53–70. Published online June 4, 2009. http://www.ncbi.nlm.nih.gov/pmc/articles/PMC2791807/.

5. Leaf, *Switch On Your Brain*, chap. 1; Leaf, "Ridiculous"; Leaf, "Mind-Mapping."

6. Fuchs, Eberhard, and Gabriele Flügge. "Adult Neuroplasticity: More Than 40 Years of Research." Neural Plasticity 2014 (2014): 1–10; Merzenich, Michael. "Growing Evidence of Brain Plasticity." TED Talk, February 2004. http://www .ted.com/talks/michael_merzenich_on_the_elastic_brain?language=en.

7. Pittenger, C., and E. Kandel. "A Genetic Switch for Long-Term Memory." *Comptes Rendus de l'Academie des Sciences-Series III-Sciences de la Vie* 321, no. 2 (1998): 91–96.

8. Kandel, Eric R. "The Molecular Biology of Memory: cAMP, PKA, CRE, CREB-1, CREB-2, and CPEB." *Molecular Brain* (2012): 1–12. http://www.bio medcentral.com/content/pdf/1756-6606-5-14.pdf; Smith, S. L., et al. "Dendritic Spikes Enhance Stimulus Selectivity in Cortical Neurons in Vivo." *Nature* 503, no. 7474 (2013): 115–20; Sheffield, Mark E. J., and Daniel A. Dombeck. "Calcium Transient Prevalence Across the Dendritic Arbour Predicts Place Field Properties." *Nature* 517 (January 8, 2015): 200–204.

9. Fodor, J. *The Modularity of Mind*. Cambridge, MA: MIT/Bradford, 1983; Neal, D. T., et al. "How Do Habits Guide Behavior? Perceived and Actual Triggers of Habits in Daily Life." *Journal of Experimental Social Psychology* 48, no. 2 (2012): 492–98; Phillippa, A. "How Are Habits Formed: Modelling Habit Formation in the Real World." *European Journal of Social Psychology* 40, no. 6 (2010): 998–1009; Gardner, B., P. Lally, and J. Wardle. "Making Health Habitual: the Psychology of 'Habit-Formation' and General Practice." *British Journal of General Practice* 62, no. 605 (2012): 664–66.

10. Leaf et al., "The Development of a Model for Geodesic Learning"; Leaf, *Switch On Your Brain*; Leaf, "The Mind-Mapping Approach."

11. Penrose, Roger. "Quantum Nonlocality and Complex Reality." Oxford University, 1992. In Tucker, Kenneth H., Jr. *The Renaissance of General Relativity*

*and Cosmology: A Survey to Celebrate the 65th Birthday of Dennis Sciama.* Cambridge University Press, 2005, 314–25; Penrose, Roger. "Twistor, Reality and Quantum Non Locality." August 4, 2014. This talk was held during the Summer School on the Foundations of Quantum Mechanics dedicated to John Bell in Sesto, Italy. https://www.youtube.com/watch?v=zQ8Bm33o0uI.

12. Leaf, Caroline. *The Gift in You: Discovering New Life Through Gifts Hidden in Your Mind.* Nashville: Nelson, 2009.

13. Gardner, H. *Frames of Mind.* New York: Basic Books, 1985; Iran-Nejad, A. "Active and Dynamic Self-Regulation of Learning Processes." *Review of Educational Research* 60, no. 4 (1990): 573–602; Satel and Lilienfeld, *Brainwashed.*

14. Markowsky, George. "Information Theory—Physiology." *Encylopaedia Britannica,* http://www.britannica.com/EBchecked/topic/287907/information-theory/214958/Physiology; Fan, Jin. "ITACC." *Front Hum Neurosci.* 8 (2014): 680.

15. Travis et al. "A Critical Assessment."

16. Elsevier. "Discovery of Quantum Vibrations in 'Microtubules' Inside Brain Neurons Corroborates Controversial 20-Year-Old Theory of Consciousness." Amsterdam, January 16, 2014. http://www.elsevier.com/about/press-releases/research-and-journals/discovery-of-quantum-vibrations-in-microtubules-inside-brain-neurons-corroborates-controversial-20-year-old-theory-of-consciousness; Bandyopadhyay, Anirban. Brain Mapping Symposium, April 24, 2014 at University of Arizona, Tucson, AZ, https://streaming.biocom.arizona.edu/event/?id=25224&play=1&format=hd.

17. Horga, Guillermo, and Tiago V. Maia. "Conscious and Unconscious Processes in Cognitive Control: A Theoretical Perspective and a Novel Empirical Approach." *Frontiers in Human Neuroscience* (July 4, 2012): 4.

18. Leaf, *Switch On Your Brain*; Hameroff, Stuart, and Roger Penrose. "Consciousness in the Universe: a Review of the 'Orch OR' Theory." *Physics of Life Reviews* 11, no. 1 (2014): 39–78; Hameroff, S., and R. Penrose. "In the Quantum World, the Future Affects the Past: Hindsight and Foresight Together More Accurately 'Predict' a Quantum System's State." *Science Daily*, February 9, 2015. http://www.sciencedaily.com/releases/2015/02/150209083011.htm; Tan, D., et al. "Prediction and Retrodiction for a Continuously Monitored Superconducting Qubit." *Physical Review Letters* (2015): 1–9. http://arxiv.org/pdf/1409.0510.pdf.

19. Hameroff and Penrose, "In the Quantum World."

20. Gardner, *Frames of Mind*; Iran-Nejad, "Active and Dynamic Self-Regulation"; Satel and Lilienfeld, *Brainwashed.*

21. Koch, Kristen, et al., "How Much the Eye Tells the Brain," *Current Biology* 16 (2006): 1428–34; Markowsky, "Information Theory"; Fan, "ITACC."

22. Leaf, *The Gift in You.*

23. Walker, H. K., W. D. Hall, and J. W. Hurst, eds. *Clinical Methods: The History, Physical, and Laboratory Examinations.* 3rd edition. Boston: Butterworths, 1990. Chap. 57.

24. Karim, Nader, Glenn E. Schafe, and Joseph E. Le Doux. "Fear Memories Require Protein Synthesis in the Amygdala for Reconsolidation after Retrieval." *Nature* 406 (August 17, 2000): 722–26.

25. Sharot, Tali. "The Optimism Bias: A Tour of the Irrationally Positive." TED Talk. June 14, 2011. http://www.ted.com/talks/tali_sharot_the_optimism _bias?language=en.

26. Nader et al., "Fear Memories."

27. Ibid.

28. Cleeremans, A., and J. C. Sarrazin. "Time, Action, and Consciousness." *Human Movement Science* 26, no. 2 (April 2007):180–202.

29. Misra, B., and E. C. G. Sudarshan. "The Zeno's Paradox in Quantum Theory." *Journal of Mathematical Physics* 18 (1977): 756. doi:10.1063/1.523304; Fischer, M. C., B. Gutiérrez-Medina, and M. G. Raizen. "Observation of the Quantum Zeno and Anti-Zeno Effects in an Unstable System." *Physical Review Letters* 87, no. 4 (July 23, 2001): 1–4. http://arxiv.org/pdf/quant-ph/0104035.pdf; Schwartz, Jeffrey M., Henry P. Stapp, and Mario Beauregard. "Quantum Physics in Neuroscience and Psychology: a Neurophysical Model of Mind–Brain Interaction." *Philosophical Transactions of the Royal Society of London B: Biological Sciences* 360, no. 1458 (2005): 1309–27.

30. Leaf et al., "The Development of a Model for Geodesic Learning"; The Senses—A Primer (Part I). The Dana Foundation. http://www.brainfacts.org /Sensing-Thinking-Behaving/Senses-and-Perception/Articles/2013/The-Senses -A-Primer-Part-I; The Senses— A Primer (Part II). The Dana Foundation. http://w ww.brainfacts.org/Sensing-Thinking-Behaving/Senses-and-Perception/Articles /2013/The-Senses-A-Primer-Part-II.

31. Kandel, "The Molecular Biology of Memory"; Lipton, B. H., K. G. Bensch, and M. A. Karasek. "Microvessel Endothelial Cell Transdifferentiation: Phenotypic Characterization." *Differentiation* 46, no. 2 (1991): 117–33; Lipton, B. H., K. G. Bensch, and M. A. Karasek. "Histamine-Modulated Transdifferentiation of Dermal Microvascular Endothelial Cells." *Experimental Cell Research* 199, no. 2 (1992): 279–91.

32. Schwartz et al., "Quantum Physics in Neuroscience and Psychology."

## Chapter 11: Toxic Schedules and Television: Twin Enemies of Our Minds

1. Wolff, Jonathan. "Technology Just Makes Us All Busier." *The Guardian.* November 7, 2011. http://gu.com/p/3359x/sbl.

2. Gleick, James. *Faster: The Acceleration of Just about Everything.* New York: Vintage, 2000.

3. The Directorate of Time at the US Naval Observatory is the official source of time used in the United States. http://tycho.usno.navy.mil/gif/timex.html.

4. Chang, Lin. "The Role of Stress on Physiological Responses and Clinical Symptoms in Irritable Bowel Syndrome." *Gastroenterology* 140, no. 3 (March 2011): 761–65; Glise, Kristina, Gunnar Ahlborg, and Ingibj H. Jonsdottir. "Prevalence and Course of Somatic Symptoms in Patients with Stress-Related Exhaustion: Does Sex or Age Matter." *BMC Psychiatry* 14, no. 1 (2014): 118; Keightley, Philip C., Natasha A. Koloski, and Nicholas J. Talley. "Pathways in Gut-Brain Communication: Evidence for Distinct Gut-to-Brain and Brain-to-Gut Syndromes." *Australian*

*and New Zealand Journal of Psychiatry* 49, no. 3 (2015): 207–14; Kennedy, P. J., G. Clarke, A. O'Neill, J. A. Groeger, E. M. M. Quigley, F. Shanahan, J. F. Cryan, and T. G. Dinan. "Cognitive Performance in Irritable Bowel Syndrome: Evidence of a Stress-Related Impairment in Visuospatial Memory." *Psychological Medicine* 44, no. 7 (2014): 1553–66.

5. Bittman, Mark. "Slow Food Quickens the Pace." *New York Times*, March 26, 2013. http://opinionator.blogs.nytimes.com/2013/03/26/slow-food-quickens -the-pace/?_r=0.

6. Schlosser, *Fast Food Nation*.

7. Gleick, *Faster*, Kindle location 226–30.

8. Gustafson, Ellen. "Obesity + Hunger = 1 Global Food Issue." Ted Talk. May 2010. https://www.ted.com/talks/ellen_gustafson_obesity_hunger_1_ global_food_issue#t-482099; Via, Michael. "The Malnutrition of Obesity: Micronutrient Deficiencies That Promote Diabetes." *Endocrinology* (2012): 103472; Gustafson, *We the Eaters*.

9. Nestle, Marion. "Soft Drink 'Pouring Rights': Marketing Empty Calories to Children." *Public Health Reports* 115, no. 4 (2000): 308–19; Nestle, *Food Politics*.

10. Saleem, Munazza, Aimal Hassan, Tahir Mahmood, Saba Mushtaq, Javeria Bhatti, and Matloob Azam. "Factors Associated with Excessive TV Viewing in School Children of Wah Cantt, Pakistan." *Rawal Medical Journal* 39, no. 3 (2014): 323–26; Christakis, D. A., F. J. Zimmerman, D. L. DiGiuseppe, and C. A. McCarty. "Early Television Exposure and Subsequent Attentional Problems in Children." *Pediatrics* 113, no. 4 (April 2004): 708–13; Lin, L. Y., R. J. Cherng, Y. J. Chen, and H. M. Yang. "Effects of Television Exposure on Developmental Skills among Young Children." *Infant Behavior and Development* 38 (February 2015): 20–26; Hamer, M., E. Stamatakis, and G. D. Mishra. "Television- and Screen-Based Activity and Mental Well-being in Adults." *American Journal of Preventive Medicine* 38, no. 4 (April 2010): 375–80; Costa, Silvia, William Johnson, and Russell M. Viner. "Health Effects of Media on Children and Adolescents." *Pediatrics* 125, no. 4 (April 2010): 756–67; Japas, Claudio, Synnly Knutsen, Salem Dehom, Hildemar Dos Santos, and Serena Tonstad. "Body Mass Index Gain between Ages 20 and 40 Years and Lifestyle Characteristics of Men at Ages 40–60 Years: The Adventist Health Study-2." *Obesity Research and Clinical Practice* 8, no. 6 (2014): e549–57; Shiue, Ivy. "Duration of Daily TV/Screen Watching with Cardiovascular, Respiratory, Mental and Psychiatric Health: Scottish Health Survey, 2012–2013." *International Journal of Cardiology* 186 (2015): 241–46.

11. Christakis et al., "Early Television Exposure."

12. Cherng et al., "Effects of Television Exposure."

13. Hamer et al., "Television- and Screen-Based Activity"; Strasburger, Victor C., Amy B. Jordan, and Ed Donnerstein. "Health Effects of Media on Children and Adolescents. " *Pediatrics* 125, no. 4 (2010): 756–67.

14. Abrams, Michael, and Dan Winters. "Can You See with Your Tongue? The Brain Is So Adaptable, Some Researchers Now Think, That Any of the Five Senses Can Be Rewired." *Discover Magazine*, June 1, 2003, http://discovermagazine

.com/2003/jun/feattongue; Bach-y-Rita, P. "Tactile Sensory Substitution Studies." *Annals of the New York Academy of Sciences* 1013 (May 2004): 83–91; Fuchs and Flügg, "Adult Neuroplasticity."

15. Pierce, R. Christopher, and Louk J. M. J. Vanderschuren. "Kicking the Habit: The Neural Basis of Ingrained Behaviors in Cocaine Addiction." *Neuroscience and Biobehavioral Reviews* 35, no. 2 (November 2010): 212–19.

16. American Academy of Pediatrics. "Familiarity with Television Fast-Food Ads Linked to Obesity." *ScienceDaily*. April 29, 2012. www.sciencedaily.com /releases/2012/04/120429085415.htm; Boyland, Emma J., Melissa Kavanagh-Safran, and Jason C. G. Halford. "Exposure to 'Healthy' Fast Food Meal Bundles in Television Advertisements Promotes Liking for Fast Food but Not Healthier Choices in Children." *British Journal of Nutrition* 113, no. 6 (2015): 1012–18; Uribe, Rodrigo, and Alejandra Fuentes-García. "The Effects of TV Unhealthy Food Brand Placement on Children. Its Separate and Joint Effect with Advertising." *Appetite* (2015): 165–72; Kraak, V. I., and M. Story. "An Accountability Evaluation for the Industry's Responsible Use of Brand Mascots and Licensed Media Characters to Market a Healthy Diet to American Children." *Obesity Reviews* (2015): 433–53; Cornwell, T. Bettina, Anna R. McAlister, and Nancy Polmear-Swendris. "Children's Knowledge of Packaged and Fast Food Brands and Their BMI. Why the Relationship Matters for Policy Makers." *Appetite* 81 (2014): 277–83.

17. Rusmevichientong, P., N. A. Streletskaya, W. Amatyakul, and H. M. Kaiser. "The Impact of Food Advertisements on Changing Eating Behaviors: An Experimental Study." *Food Policy* 44 (2014): 59–67.

18. Kemps, Eva, Marika Tiggemann, and Sarah Hollitt. "Exposure to Television Food Advertising Primes Food-related Cognitions and Triggers Motivation to Eat." *Psychology & Health* 29, no. 10 (2014): 1192. doi:10.1080/08870446.2014.918267.

19. Boyland, E. J., et al. "Food Commercials Increase Preference for Energy-Dense Foods, Particularly in Children Who Watch More Television." *Pediatrics* (2011): e93–e100. doi:10.1542/peds.2010-185; Mathias, Kevin C., et al. "Foods and Beverages Associated with Higher Intake of Sugar-Sweetened Beverages." *American Journal of Preventive Medicine* (2013): 351–57. doi:10.1016/j.amepre.2012.11.036.

20. Olafsdottir, Steingerdur, et al. "Young Children's Screen Habits Are Associated with Consumption of Sweetened Beverages Independently of Parental Norms." *International Journal of Public Health* (2013): 65–73. doi:10.1007/ s00038-013-0473-2.

21. Rudd Center for Food and Policy. "Food Marketing." 2015. http://www.uc onnruddcenter.org/food-marketing; World Health Organization. "A Framework for Implementing the Set of Recommendations on the Marketing of Foods and Non-alcoholic Beverages to Children." 2012. http://apps.who.int/iris/bitstream /10665/80148/1/9789241503242_eng.pdf?ua=1.

22. Rudd Center, "Food Marketing"; Bernhardt, Amy M., et al. "How Television Fast Food Marketing Aimed at Children Compares with Adult Advertisements." *PLoS One* 8, no. 8 (2013): e72479. doi:10.1371/journal.pone.0072479; American Academy of Pediatrics, "Familiarity with Television"; Boyland, Emma J., and

Jason C. G. Halford. "Television Advertising and Branding: Effects on Eating Behaviour and Food Preferences in Children." *Appetite* 62 (2013): 236–41; Uribe and Fuentes-Garcia, "Effects of TV"; Kraak and Story, "Influence of Food Companies' Brand Mascots"; Cornwell et al., "Children's Knowledge."

23. Ibid.; Rusmevichientong et al., "The Impact of Food Advertisements."

24. Story, Mary, and Simone French. "Food Advertising and Marketing Directed at Children and Adolescents in the US." *International Journal of Behavioral Nutrition and Physical Activity* 1 (2004): 3.

25. Leibowitz, J., et al. "A Review of Food Marketing to Children and Adolescents: Follow-Up Report." Washington, DC: Federal Trade Commission, 2012.

26. Rudd Center, "Food Marketing."

27. Scully, P., et al. "Food and Beverage Cues in UK and Irish Children— Television Programming." *Archives of Disease in Childhood* (2014). doi:10.1136/archdischild-2013-305430.

28. Scully et al., "Food and Beverage Cues"; Rudd Center, "Food Marketing"; Kunkel, Dale, Christopher McKinley, and Paul Wright. "The Impact of Industry Self-Regulation on the Nutritional Quality of Foods Advertised on Television to Children." *Children Now* (2010): 9–38; Ronit, Karsten, et al. "Obesity and Industry Self-Regulation of Food and Beverage Marketing: a Literature Review." *European Journal of Clinical Nutrition* 68, no. 7 (2014): 753–59; Reeve, Belinda. "Private Governance, Public Purpose? Assessing Transparency and Accountability in Self-Regulation of Food Advertising to Children." *Journal of Bioethical Inquiry* 10, no. 2 (2013): 149–63.

29. Caballero, Benjamin. "The Global Epidemic of Obesity: An Overview." *Epidemiologic Reviews* 29, no. 1 (2007): 1–5; Malhotra, A. "Obesity among Indian Adolescents: Some Emerging Trends." *Journal of Obesity and Metabolic Research* 1, no. 1 (2014): 46–48.

30. Ronit et al., "Obesity and Industry."

31. Dentzer, S. "The Child Abuse We Inflict Through Child Obesity." *Health Affairs* 29, no. 3 (2010): 342; Jackson, Sandra L., and Solveig A. Cunningham. "Social Competence and Obesity in Elementary School." *American Journal of Public Health* 105, no. 1 (2015): 153–58.

32. Lustig, Robert H. *Fat Chance: Beating the Odds Against Sugar, Processed Food, Obesity, and Disease.* New York: Plume, 2013.

33. Choudry, Souvik. "Fast Food for the Mind: Why I Don't Have a Facebook or Twitter Account." *Forbes,* April 2014, http://www.forbes.com/sites/sungardas/2014/04/08/fast-food-for-the-mind-why-i-dont-have-a-facebook-or-twitter-account.

34. Leiter, Melissa. "The Lifespan of Social Media Posts." Melissaleiter.com. June 19, 2014. http://www.melissaleiter.com/lifespan-of-social-media-posts/.

35. Craddock and Tuszynski, "A Critical Assessment."

36. Leaf, *Switch On Your Brain.*

37. Sussman, Steve, and Meghan B. Moran. "Hidden Addiction: Television." *Journal of Behav Addict.* 2, no. 3 (2013): 125–32; Bilimoria, P. M., T. K. Hensch, and D. Bavelier. "A Mouse Model for Too Much TV?" *Trends Cogn Sci* 16, no. 11

(2012): 529–31; Olsen, C. M. "Natural Rewards, Neuroplasticity, and Non-Drug Addictions." *Neuropharmacology* 61, no. 7 (2011): 1109–22.

38. Doidge, Norman. *The Brain That Changes Itself: Stories of Personal Triumph from the Frontiers of Brain Science*. New York: Penguin, 2007. Kindle Edition, 309.

39. Ibid.

40. Harris, Jennifer L., and Samantha K. Graff. "Protecting Young People from Junk Food Advertising: Implications of Psychological Research for First Amendment Law." *American Journal of Public Health* 102, no. 2 (2012): 214–22; Harris, Jennifer L., John A. Bargh, and Kelly D. Brownell. "Priming Effects of Television Food Advertising on Eating Behavior." *Health Psychol* 28, no. 4 (2009): 404–13.

41. Malik, Vasanti S., Matthias B. Schulze, and Frank B. Hu. "Intake of Sugar-Sweetened Beverages and Weight Gain: a Systematic Review." *The American Journal of Clinical Nutrition* 84, no. 2 (2006): 274–88.

42. Jackson, K., et al. "Amylin Deposition in the Brain: A Second Amyloid in Alzheimer Disease?" *Ann Neurol* 74, no. 4 (2013): 517–26; Vlassenko, Andrei G., and Marcus E. Raichle. "Brain Aerobic Glycolysis Functions and Alzheimer's Disease." *Clinical and Translational Imaging* (2014): 1–11.

43. Li, J., D. Liu, L. Sun, Y. Lu, and Z. Zhang. "Advanced Glycation End Products and Neurodegenerative Diseases: Mechanisms and Perspective." *Journal of the Neurological Sciences* 317, nos. 1, 2 (2012): 1–5.

44. Harding, J. L., et al. "Psychosocial Stress Is Positively Associated with Body Mass Index Gain over 5 Years: Evidence from the Longitudinal Ausdiab Study Obesity." *Obesity* 22, no. 1 (2014): 277–86; Arbex, Marcos Abdo, et al. "Air Pollution from Biomass Burning and Asthma Hospital Admissions in a Sugar Cane Plantation Area in Brazil." *Journal of Epidemiology and Community Health* (2007): 395–400.

45. Rothschild, H., and J. J. Mulvey. "An Increased Risk for Lung Cancer Mortality Associated with Sugarcane Farming." *Journal of the National Cancer Institute* 68, no. 5 (1982): 755–60; Silveira, Henrique César Santejo, et al. "Emissions Generated by Sugarcane Burning Promote Genotoxicity in Rural Workers: A Case Study in Barretos, Brazil." *Environmental Health* 12, no. 1 (2013): 87–92; Ould, David. "Trafficking and International Law." *The Political Economy of New Slavery* (2004): 55–74; Rahman, Majeed A. "Human Trafficking in the Era of Globalization: The Case of Trafficking in the Global Market Economy." *Transcience Journal* 2 (2011): 54–71; Martin, Michael T. "Documenting Modern-Day Slavery in the Dominican Republic: An Interview with Amy Serrano." *Camera Obscura* 25, no. 274 (2010): 161–71; Smucker, Glenn R., and Gerald F. Murray. "The Uses of Children: A Study of Trafficking in Haitian Children." USAID/Haiti Mission, 2004.

46. Leaf, Caroline. "The Switch On Your Brain 5-Step Learning Process." Dallas, TX: Switch on Your Brain USA LP, 2009.

47. Remondes, M., and E. M. Schuman. "Role for a Cortical Input to Hippocampal Area CA1 in the Consolidation of a Long-Term Memory." *Nature* 431, no. 7009 (2004): 699–703.

**Chapter 12: What's Eating You?**

1. Toussaint-Samat, Maguelonne. *A History of Food.* Chichester, West Sussex, UK: Wiley-Blackwell, 2009.

2. Filaretova, L. "The Hypothalamic-Pituitary-Adrenocortical System: Hormonal Brain-Gut Interaction and Gastroprotection." *Autonomic Neuroscience* 125 (2006): 86–93; Ahima, Rexford S., and Daniel A. Antwi. "Brain Regulation of Appetite and Satiety." *Endocrinology and Metabolism Clinics of North America* 37, no. 4 (2008): 811–23; Kojima, K., et al. "Relationship of Emotional Behaviors Induced by Electrical Stimulation of the Hypothalamus to Changes in EKG, Heart, Stomach, Adrenal Glands, and Thymus." *Psychosomatic Medicine* 58, no. 4 (1996): 383–91; Luna, Ruth Ann, and Jane A. Foster. "Gut Brain Axis: Diet Microbiota Interactions and Implications for Modulation of Anxiety and Depression." *Current Opinion in Biotechnology* 32 (2015): 35–41; Cryan, John F., and Timothy G. Dinan. "More than a Gut Feeling: the Microbiota Regulates Neurodevelopment and Behavior." *Neuropsychopharmacology* 40, no. 1 (2015): 241–42; Mayer, Emeran A. "Gut Feelings: The Emerging Biology of Gut-Brain Communication." *National Review of Neuroscience* 12, no. 8 (2011): 453–66; Macht, Michael. "Research Review How Emotions Affect Eating: A Five-Way Model." *Appetite* 50 (2008): 1–11.

3. Pert, Candace B. *Molecules of Emotion: The Science Behind Mind-Body Medicine.* New York: Scribner, 1999.

4. Steere, J., and P. J. Cooper. "The Effects on Eating of Dietary Restraint, Anxiety, and Hunger." *International Journal of Eating Disorders* 13, no. 2 (1993): 211–19; Lee, S. P., et al. "The Effect of Emotional Stress and Depression on the Prevalence of Digestive Diseases." *Journal of Neurogastroenterology and Motility* 21 (2015): 273–82.

5. Steere and Cooper, "Effects on Eating."

6. Selye, Hans. "Stress and the General Adaptation Syndrome." *BMJ* 1, no. 4667 (1950): 1383–92.

7. Friedman, Lawrence. "How the Mind-Gut Connection Affects Your Health. The 'Second Brain' in Your Stomach Can Cause or Relieve Illness and Stress. Here's How It Works." NextAvenue.org. June 24, 2013. http://www.nextavenue.org/how-mind-gut-connection-affects-your-health/; Luna and Foster, "Gut Brain Axis"; Cryan and Dinan, "More than a Gut Feeling"; Keightley, Philip C., Natasha A. Koloski, and Nicholas J. Talley. "Pathways in Gut-Brain Communication: Evidence for Distinct Gut-to-Brain and Brain-to-Gut Syndromes." *Australian and New Zealand Journal of Psychiatry* 49, no. 3 (2015): 207–14.

8. Ibid.; Arranga, Teri, Claire I. Viadro, and Lauren Underwood, eds. *Bugs, Bowels, and Behavior: The Groundbreaking Story of the Gut-Brain Connection.* New York: Skyhorse Publishing, June 1, 2013; Macht, "How Emotions Affect Eating"; Cannon, W. B. *The Wisdom of the Body.* New York: Norton, 1947.

9. McConalogue, K., and J. B. Furness. "Gastrointestinal Neurotransmitters." *Baillieres Clinical Endocrinology and Metabolism* 8, no. 1 (1994): 51–76.

10. Gershon, Michael. *The Second Brain: The Scientific Basis of Gut Instinct and a Groundbreaking New Understanding of Nervous Disorders of the Stomach*

*and Intestine.* New York: HarperCollins, 1998; Johns Hopkins Medicine. "It's High Time for the Gut-Brain." December 12, 2012. http://www.hopkinsmedicine .org/news/publications/inside_tract/inside_tract_fall_2012/its_high_time_for_ the_gut_brain.

11. Avallone R., et al. "Endogenous Benzodiazepine-Like Compounds and Diazepam Binding Inhibitor in Serum of Patients with Liver Cirrhosis with and without Overt Encephalopathy." *Gut* 42, no. 6 (1998): 861–67.

12. Orr, W., et al. "Sleep and Gastric Function in Irritable Bowel Syndrome: Derailing the Brain-Gut Axis." *Gut* 41, no. 3 (1997): 390–93.

13. Dotto, L. "Sleep Stages, Memory and Learning." *CMAJ* 154, no. 8 (1996): 1193–96.

14. Reardon, Sara. "Gut-Brain Link Grabs Neuroscientists Idea that Intestinal Bacteria Affect Mental Health Gains Ground." *Nature.* November 12, 2014. http ://www.nature.com/news/gut-brain-link-grabs-neuroscientists-1.16316.

15. Stewart, Charles. "William Beaumont, the Man and the Opportunity." In Roberts. *Clinical Methods: The History, Physical, and Laboratory Examinations.* 3rd edition. Ed. H. K. Walker, W. D. Hall, and J. W. Hurst. Boston: Butterworths, 1990.

16. Beaumont, William. *Complete Dictionary of Scientific Biography.* 2008. Encyclopedia.com. http://www.encyclopedia.com/doc/1G2-2830900321.html.

17. Friedman, "Mind-Gut Connection"; Mai, F. M. "Beaumont's Contribution to Gastric Psychophysiology: A Reappraisal." *Canadian Journal of Psychiatry* 33, no. 7 (1988): 650–53.

18. Gershon, *The Second Brain.*

19. Mayer, "Gut Feelings."

20. Gershon, *The Second Brain.*

21. Duke University. "Researchers Map Direct Gut-Brain Connection." *ScienceDaily.* www.sciencedaily.com/releases/2015/01/150106095120.htm (accessed April 23, 2015); ETH Zürich. "How the 'Gut Feeling' Shapes Fear." *ScienceDaily.* May 22, 2014. www.sciencedaily.com/releases/2014/05/140522104848.htm; Kavli Foundation. "Could Gut Microbes Help Treat Brain Disorders? Mounting Research Tightens Their Connection with the Brain." *ScienceDaily.* January 8, 2015. www.sciencedaily.com/releases/2015/01/150108125953.htm; Karolinska Institutet. "Gut Microbiota Influences Blood-Brain Barrier Permeability." *ScienceDaily.* November 19, 2014. www.sciencedaily.com/releases/2014/11/141119142205.htm.

22. Grundy, David, et al. "Fundamentals of Neurogastroenterology: Basic Science." *Gastroenterology* 130 (2006): 1391–1411.

23. Gershon, *The Second Brain.*

24. Furness, J. B., et al. "The Enteric Nervous System and Gastrointestinal Innervation: Integrated Local and Central Control." *Adv Exp Med Biol* 817 (2014): 39–71.

25. Sadler, Thomas W. *Langman's Medical Embryology.* Philadelphia: Lippincott Williams & Wilkins, 2011. 67.

26. Arranga et al., *Bugs, Bowels, and Behavior.*

27. Furness et al., "The Enteric Nervous System."

28. Ratcliffe, E. M., N. R. Farrar, and E. A. Fox. "Development of the Vagal Innervation of the Gut: Steering the Wandering Nerve." *Neurogastroenterology and Motility* 23, no. 10 (2011): 898–911.

29. Wang, G. J., et al. "Gastric Distention Activates Satiety Circuitry in the Human Brain." *Neuroimage* 39, no. 4 (2008): 1824–31.

30. Mayer, "Gut Feelings."

31. "H.R.4432—Safe and Accurate Food Labeling Act of 2014." 113th Congress (2013–2014). https://www.congress.gov/bill/113th-congress/house-bill/4432; Borra, S. "Consumer Perspectives on Food Labels." *American Journal of Clinical Nutrition* 83, no. 5 (2006): 1235S; Philipson, T. "Government Perspective: Food Labeling." *American Journal of Clinical Nutrition* 82, no. S1 (2005): 262S–64S; Mandle, Jessie, et al. "Nutrition Labelling: A Review of Research on Consumer and Industry Response in the Global South." *Global Health Action* 8 (2015): 10.3402/gha.v8.25912.

32. Kidwell, Blair, Jonathan Hasford, and David M. Hardesty. "Emotional Ability Training and Mindful Eating." *Journal of Marketing Research* (2014): 140723133331005. doi:10.1509/jmr.13.0188; Lofgren, Ingrid Elizabeth. "Mindful Eating: An Emerging Approach for Healthy Weight Management." *American Journal of Lifestyle Medicine* (2015): 1559827615569684; Smart, Rebekah, et al. "Women's Experience with a Mindful Eating Course on a University Campus: A Pilot Study." *Californian Journal of Health Promotion* 13, no. 1 (2015): 59–65; Olson, KayLoni L., and Charles F. Emery. "Mindfulness and Weight Loss: A Systematic Review." *Psychosomatic Medicine* 77, no. 1 (2015): 59–67.

33. Ibid.; Wansink, Brian. *Mindless Eating: Why We Eat More Than We Think.* New York: Bantam, 2006.

34. Kidwell, "Emotional Ability Training."

35. Drossman, Douglas A. *Rome II: The Functional Gastrointestinal Disorders: Diagnosis, Pathophysiology, and Treatment: A Multinational Consensus.* McLean: Degnon Associates, 2000.

36. Heffernan, Margaret. *Willful Blindness: Why We Ignore the Obvious at Our Peril.* New York: Walker, 2011.

37. "You Think Food Tastes Better If It's Expensive." *TIME.* May 1, 2014. http://time.com/84332/you-think-food-tastes-better-if-its-expensive/; Almenberg, Johan, and Anna Dreber. "When Does the Price Affect the Taste? Results from a Wine Experiment." *Journal of Wine Economics* 6, no. 1 (2011): 111–21; Veale, Roberta, and Pascale Quester. "Consumer Sensory Evaluations of Wine Quality: The Respective Influence of Price and Country of Origin." *Journal of Wine Economics* 3, no. 1 (2008): 10–29; Veale, Roberta, and Pascale Quester. "Tasting Quality: the Roles of Intrinsic and Extrinsic Cues." *Asia Pacific Journal of Marketing and Logistics* 21, no. 1 (2009): 195–207.

38. Just, David, Ozge Sigirci, and Brian Wansink. "Lower Buffet Prices Lead to Less Taste Satisfaction." *Journal of Sensory Studies* 29 (2014): 362–70.

39. Rozin, P., S. Dow, M. Moscovitch, and S. Rajaram. "What Causes Humans to Begin and End a Meal? A Role for Memory for What Has Been Eaten, as Evidenced by a Study of Multiple Meal Eating in Amnesic Patients." *Psychological Science* 9, no. 5 (1998): 392–96.

40. Winterich, Karen Page, and Kelly L. Haws. "Helpful Hopefulness: The Effect of Future Positive Emotions on Consumption." *Journal of Consumer Research* 38, no. 3 (2011): 505–24. doi: 10.1086/659873.

41. Morris, N. P. "The Neglect of Nutrition in Medical Education: A Firsthand Look." *Internal Medicine* 174, no. 6 (2014): 841–42; Nestle, Marion, and Robert B. Baron. "Nutrition in Medical Education: From Counting Hours to Measuring Competence." *Internal Medicine* 174, no. 6 (2014): 843–44.

42. Nee, Watchman. *The Spiritual Man*. Anaheim, CA: Living Stream Ministry, 1968.

43. Leaf, *The Gift in You*; Leaf, Perfectly You online program.

44. Nee, *The Spiritual Man*.

45. Sadler, *Langman's Medical Embryology*.

46. Leaf, Caroline. "'Spirit, Soul and Body' in Scientific Philosophy." http://dr leaf.com/about/scientific-philosophy/.

47. Stote, Kim S., et al. "A Controlled Trial of Reduced Meal Frequency without Caloric Restriction in Healthy, Normal-Weight, Middle-Aged Adults." *American Journal of Clinical Nutrition* 85, no. 4 (2007): 981–88.

48. Trepanowski, John F., and Richard J. Bloomer. "The Impact of Religious Fasting on Human Health." *Nutrition Journal* 9 (2010): 57.

49. Wegman, Martin P., et al. "Practicality of Intermittent Fasting in Humans and its Effect on Oxidative Stress and Genes Related to Aging and Metabolism." *Rejuvenation Research* (2014): 141229080855001. doi:10.1089/rej.2014.1624; Intermountain Medical Center. "Fasting Reduces Cholesterol Levels in Prediabetic People over Extended Period of Time, New Research Finds." June 14, 2014; Anson, R. M., et al. "Intermittent Fasting Dissociates Beneficial Effects of Dietary Restriction on Glucose Metabolism and Neuronal Resistance to Injury from Calorie Intake." *Proceedings of the National Academy of Science USA* 100, no. 10 (2003): 6216–20; Mattson M. P., and R. Wan. "Beneficial Effects of Intermittent Fasting and Caloric Restriction on the Cardiovascular and Cerebrovascular Systems." *J Nutr Biochem* 16, no. 3 (2005): 129–37; Halagappa, V. K., et al. "Intermittent Fasting and Caloric Restriction Ameliorate Age-Related Behavioral Deficits in the Triple-Transgenic Mouse Model of Alzheimer's Disease." *Neurobiol Dis* 26, no. 1 (2007): 212–20; Martin, B., M. P. Mattson, and S. Maudsley. "Caloric Restriction and Intermittent Fasting: Two Potential Diets for Successful Brain Aging." *Ageing Res Rev* 5, no. 3 (2006): 332–53. http://ajcn.nutrition.org/content/85/4/981 .short; Trepanowski, J. F., and R. J. Bloomer. "The Impact of Religious Fasting on Human Health." *Nutr J* 22, no. 9 (2010): 57; Weindruch, Richard, and Rajindar S. Sohal. "Caloric Intake and Aging." *New England Journal of Medicine* 337, no. 14 (1997): 986–94.

50. B. Martin et al., "Caloric Restriction"; Martin-Montalvo, A., and R. de Cabo. "Mitochondrial Metabolic Reprogramming Induced by Calorie Restriction." *Antioxid Redox Signal* 19, no. 3 (2013): 310–20.

51. Wang, J., et al. "Caloric Restriction Favorably Impacts Metabolic and Immune/Inflammatory Profiles in Obese Mice but Curcumin/Piperine Consumption Adds No Further Benefit." *Nutr Metab (Lond)* 10, no. 1 (2013): 29.

52. Mattson and Wan, "Beneficial Effects"; Maswood, Navin, et al. "Caloric Restriction Increases Neurotrophic Factor Levels and Attenuates Neurochemical and Behavioral Deficits in a Primate Model of Parkinson's Disease." *Proceedings of the National Academy of Sciences* 101, no. 52 (2004): 18171–76.

53. Srivastava, S., and M. C. Haigis. "Role of Sirtuins and Calorie Restriction in Neuroprotection: Implications in Alzheimer's and Parkinson's Diseases." *Curr Pharm Des* 17, no. 31 (2011): 3418–33.

54. Acheson, Ann, et al. "A BDNF Autocrine Loop in Adult Sensory Neurons Prevents Cell Death." *Nature* 374 (1995): 450–53; Huang, Eric J., and Louis F. Reichardt. "Neurotrophins: Roles in Neuronal Development and Function." *Annual Review of Neuroscience* 24 (2001): 677.

55. Mattson and Wan, "Beneficial Effects."

56. Halagappa et al., "Intermittent Fasting."

57. B. Martin et al., "Caloric Restriction."

58. Trepanowski and Bloomer, "Impact of Religious Fasting."

59. Ibid.; Bloomer, Richard J., et al. "Effect of a 21 Day Daniel Fast on Metabolic and Cardiovascular Disease Risk Factors in Men and Women." *Lipids in Health and Disease* 9, no. 1 (2010): 94.

60. McKnight, Scot. *Fasting: The Ancient Practices*. Nashville: Thomas Nelson, 2010. Kindle Edition.

61. Murray, Andrew. *With Christ in the School of Prayer*. Springdale, PA: Whitaker House, 1981. 101; McKnight, *Fasting*.

62. McKnight, *Fasting*.

## Chapter 13: This Is Your Brain on Brain Scans

1. Kinderman, Peter. "Why We Need to Abandon the Disease Model of Mental Health Care. Scientific American." MIND Guest Blog. November 17, 2014. http://blogs.scientificamerican.com/mind-guest-blog/2014/11/17/why-we-need-to-abandon-the-disease-model-of-mental-health-care/.

2. Dossey, L. "Counterclockwise: When Biology Is Not Destiny." *Explore (NY)* 11, no. 2 (2015): 75–81; Diamond, Adele, and Dima Amso. "Contributions of Neuroscience to Our Understanding of Cognitive Development." *Curr Dir Psychol Sci* 17, no. 2 (2008): 136–41.

3. Langer, E., and J. Rodin. "The Effects of Choice and Enhanced Personality on the Aged: a Field Experience in an Institutional Setting." *Journal of Personality & Social Psychology* 34 (1976): 191–98.

4. Beauregard, Mario. *Brain Wars: The Scientific Battle over the Existence of the Mind and the Proof that Will Change the Way We Live Our Lives*. New York: HarperCollins, 2013.

5. Leaf, *Switch On Your Brain*; Leaf, "Ridiculous"; Leaf, "Mind-Mapping: A Therapeutic Technique."

6. Beauregard, *Brain Wars*.

7. Machado, Armando. "Toward a Richer View of the Scientific Method: The Role of Conceptual Analysis." *American Psychologist* 62, no. 7 (2007): 671–81.

8. Satel and Lilienfeld, *Brainwashed*; Hall, Wayne, Adrian Carter, and Cynthia Forlini. "The Brain Disease Model of Addiction: Is It Supported by the Evidence and Has It Delivered on its Promises?" *The Lancet Psychiatry* 2, no. 1 (2015): 105–10; Lilienfeld, Scott O., Steven Jay Lynn, and Rachel J. Ammirati. "Science Versus Pseudoscience." *The Encyclopedia of Clinical Psychology*. Wiley Online Library, 2015.

9. Bandettini, Peter A. "What's New in Neuroimaging Methods?" *Ann N Y Acad Sci*. 1156 (2009): 260–93; Columbia Center for New Media Teaching and Learning. "Neuroimaging, Visualizing Brain Structure and Function." http://ccn mtl.columbia.edu/projects/neuroethics/module1/foundationtext/.

10. Satel and Lilienfeld, *Brainwashed*.

11. Ibid.

12. Ibid.

## Chapter 14: Confused Emotions, Destructive Behaviors

1. Kandel, "The Molecular Biology of Memory"; Nader, Karim, Glenn E. Schafe, and Joseph E. Le Doux. "Fear Memories Require Protein Synthesis in the Amygdala for Reconsolidation after Retrieval." *Nature* 406 (2000): 722–26; Smith, S. L., I. T. Smith, T. Branco, M. Tusser. "Dendritic Spikes Enhance Stimulus Selectivity in Cortical Neurons In Vivo." *Nature* 503 (2013):115–20; Sheffield, Mark E. J., and Daniel A. Dombeck. "Calcium Transient Prevalence Across the Dendritic Arbour Predicts Place Field Properties." *Nature* 517 (2015): 200–204; Fodor, J. *The Modularity of Mind*. Cambridge, MA: MIT/Bradford, 1983; Jog, M. S., et al. "Building Neural Representations of Habits." *Science* 286 (1999): 1745–49; Gardner, B., P. Lally, and J. Wardle. "Making Health Habitual: The Psychology Of 'Habit-Formation' and General Practice." *Br J Gen Pract* 62 (2012): 664–66.

2. Leaf, Caroline. *Switch On Your Brain*. Grand Rapids: Baker, 2013.

3. "How Healthy Behaviour Supports Children's Wellbeing." Gov.uk. https ://www.gov.uk/government/publications/how-healthy-behaviour-supports -childrens-wellbeing; Mitchell, J. A., et al. "Sedentary Behaviour and Obesity in a Large Cohort of Children." *Obesity* 17, no. 8 (2009): 1596–1602; Smith, L., B. Gardner, and M. Hamer. "Childhood Correlates of Adult TV Viewing Time: A 32-Year Follow-Up of the 1970 British Cohort Study." *Journal of Epidemiology and Community Health* (2014): 1–5.

4. McEwen, Bruce S. *The End of Stress as We Know It*. New York: Dana Press, 2012. Kindle Edition, locations 2964–69; Richards, Marcus, and Felicia A. Huppert. "Do Positive Children Become Positive Adults? Evidence from a Longitudinal Birth Cohort Study." *J Posit Psychol* 6, no. 1 (2011): 75–87.

5. Leaf, Caroline. "Who Switched Off My Brain?: Controlling Toxic Thoughts and Emotions." Southlake: Inprov Ltd., 2008.

6. Ricca, V., et al. "Emotional Eating in Anorexia Nervosa and Bulimia Nervosa." *Compr Psychiatry* 53, no. 3 (2012): 245–51.

7. Sullivan, Patrick F. "Mortality in Anorexia Nervosa." *American Journal of Psychiatry* 152, no. 7 (1995): 1073–74.

8. Selby, E. A., et al. "Nothing Tastes as Good as Thin Feels: Low Positive Emotion Differentiation and Weight-Loss Activities in Anorexia Nervosa." *Clinical Psychological Science* 2, no. 4 (2013): 514. doi:10.1177/2167702613512794.

9. Titova, O. E., et al. "Anorexia Nervosa Is Linked to Reduced Brain Structure in Reward and Somatosensory Regions: A Meta-Analysis of VBM Studies." *BMC Psychiatry* 13 (2013): 110; Maguire, E. A., et al. "Navigation-Related Structural Change in the Hippocampi of Taxi Drivers." *Proc Natl Acad Sci USA* 97, no. 8 (2000): 4398–403.

10. Goodman, A. "Neurobiology of Addiction. An Integrative Review." *Biochem Pharmacol* 75, no. 1 (2008): 266–322.

11. Smith, D. E. "The Process Addictions and the New ASAM Definition of Addiction." *J Psychoactive Drugs* 44, no. 1 (2012): 1–4.

12. Garber, A. K., et al. "Is Fast Food Addictive? Food Craving and Food 'Addiction': A Critical Review of the Evidence from a Biopsychosocial Perspective." *Curr Drug Abuse Rev* 4, no. 3 (2011): 146–62; Kaye, Walter H., et al. "Does a Shared Neurobiology for Foods and Drugs of Abuse Contribute to Extremes of Food Ingestion in Anorexia and Bulimia Nervosa?" *Biological Psychiatry* 73, no. 9 (2013): 836–42; Brownell, Kelly D., and Kenneth E. Warner. "The Perils of Ignoring History: Big Tobacco Played Dirty and Millions Died. How Similar Is Big Food?" *Milbank Quarterly* 87, no. 1 (2009): 259–94.

13. Gearhardt, A. N., et al. "Neural Correlates of Food Addiction." *Arch Gen Psychiatry* 68, no. 8 (2011): 808–16.

14. Lustig, *Fat Chance*; Moss, Michael. "The Extraordinary Science of Addictive Junk Food." *New York Times Magazine*, Feb. 20, 2013, http://www.nytimes.com/2013/02/24/magazine/the-extraordinary-science-of-junk-food.html?_r=0; Moss, *Salt, Sugar, Fat*, 339–40.

15. Guy, Allison. "How Food Scientists Engineer the 'Bliss Point.'" *Next Nature*. February 26, 2013. http://www.nextnature.net/2013/02/how-food-scientists-engineer-the-bliss-point-in-junk-food/; Moss, *Salt, Sugar, Fat*; Moss, "The Extraordinary Science of Addictive Junk Food"; Ferrier, Peyton. "Food in Popular Literature." *Choices* 29, no. 1 (2014): 1–6; Fell-Carlson, Deborah L. "Safety: What's Health Got to Do With It?" ASSE Professional Development Conference and Exposition. American Society of Safety Engineers, 2014; Roshan, N. M., and B. Sakeenabi. "Practical Problems in Use of Sugar Substitutes in Preventive Dentistry." *Journal of International Society of Preventive & Community Dentistry* 1, no. 1 (2011): 1.

16. Avena, N. M., P. Rada, and B. G. Hoebel. "Evidence for Sugar Addiction: Behavioral and Neurochemical Effects of Intermittent, Excessive Sugar Intake." *Neurosci Biobehav Rev* 32, no. 1 (2008): 20–39.

17. Willett, Walter. *Eat, Drink, and Be Healthy: The Harvard Medical School Guide to Healthy Eating*. New York: Free Press, 2011. Kindle Edition, locations 1896–98.

18. Monteiro, C. A., et al. "Increasing Consumption of Ultra-Processed Foods and Likely Impact on Human Health: Evidence from Brazil." *Public Health Nutr* 14, no. 1 (2011): 5–13.

19. Gearhardt, A. N., et al. "The Addiction Potential of Hyperpalatable Foods." *Curr Drug Abuse Rev* 4, no. 3 (2011): 140–45.

20. Ibid., 217; see also Brownell, K., and M. Gold. "Food products. Addiction. Also in the mind. [Commentary]." *World Nutrition* 3, no. 9 (2012): 392–405. www.wphna.org.

21. Rada, P., N. M. Avena, and B. G. Hoebel. "Daily Bingeing on Sugar Repeatedly Releases Dopamine in the Accumbens Shell." *Neuroscience* 134, no. 3 (2005): 737–44.

22. Moss, *Salt, Sugar, Fat*; Baik, J. H. "Dopamine Signaling in Food Addiction: Role of Dopamine D2 Receptors." *BMB Rep* 46, no. 11 (2013): 519–26.

23. Doidge, Norman. "Hypnosis, Neuroplasticity, and the Plastic Paradox." *American Journal of Clinical Hypnosis* 57, no. 3 (2015): 349–54.

24. Doidge, Norman. *The Brain That Changes Itself*.

25. Satel and Lilienfeld, *Brainwashed*.

26. American Society of Addiction Medicine. "Definition of Addiction." http://www.asam.org/for-the-public/definition-of-addiction.

27. Peele, Stanton. *Truth about Addiction and Recovery*. New York: Simon and Schuster, 2014; Peele, Stanton. *The Meaning of Addiction: Compulsive Experience and Its Interpretation*. Lexington: Lexington Books/DC Heath and Com, 1985; Doherty, Brian. "Addiction: Easier to Beat Than Its Reputation." October 1, 2014. http://reason.com/blog/2014/10/01/addiction-easier-to-beat-than-its-reputa; Satel and Lilienfeld, *Brainwashed*.

28. Satel and Lilienfeld, *Brainwashed*, chap. 6.

29. Quenqua, Douglas. "Rethinking Addiction's Roots, and Its Treatment." *New York Times*. July 10, 2011. http://www.nytimes.com/2011/07/11/health/11 addictions.html; see also Kalivas, Peter W., and Nora D. Volkow. "The Neural Basis of Addiction: A Pathology of Motivation and Choice." *American Journal of Psychiatry* 162, no. 8 (2005): 1403–13; Koob, George F., and Nora D. Volkow. "Neurocircuitry of Addiction." *Neuropsychopharmacology* 35, no. 1 (2010): 217–38.

30. Lubman, D. I., and C. Pantelis. "Addiction, a Condition of Compulsive Behaviour? Neuroimaging and Neuropsychological Evidence of Inhibitory Dysregulation." *Addiction* 99, no. 12 (2004): 1491–502; Satel and Lilienfeld, "Addiction and the Brain-Disease Fallacy." Frontiers in Psychiatry 4 (2013): 1–11.

31. Kaati, G., L. O. Bygren, and M. Pembrey. "Transgenerational Response to Nutrition, Early Life Circumstances and Longevity." *Eur J Hum Genet* 15, no. 7 (2007): 784–90.

32. Doidge, *Brain That Changes Itself*.

33. Berns, Gregory S., et al. "Short- and Long-Term Effects of a Novel on Connectivity in the Brain." *Brain Connectivity* 3, no. 6 (2013): 590–600; Doidge, *Brain That Changes Itself*; Temple, Elise, et al. "Neural Deficits in Children with Dyslexia Ameliorated by Behavioral Remediation: Evidence from Functional MRI." *Proceedings of the National Academy of Sciences* 100, no. 5 (2003): 2860–65.

34. Peele, *Truth about Addiction and Recovery*; Peele, *The Meaning of Addiction*; Hasin, Deborah S., et al. "Prevalence, Correlates, Disability, and Comorbidity of DSM-IV Alcohol Abuse and Dependence in the United States: Results

from the National Epidemiologic Survey on Alcohol and Related Conditions." *Archives of General Psychiatry* 64, no. 7 (2007): 830–42; Doherty, "Addiction"; Satel and Lilienfeld, "Addiction and the Brain-Disease Fallacy"; Peele, Stanton. "Government Says You Can't Overcome Addiction, Contrary to What Government Research Shows. Why Does the National Institute on Drug Abuse Contradict Its Own Research?" Reason.com. February 1, 2014. https://reason.com/archive s/2014/02/01/the-government-wants-you-to-know-you-can; Grant, B. F., D. A. Dawson, and S. P. Chou. "National Longitudinal Alcohol Epidemiologic Survey (NLAES) Reinterview Study: Major Findings." Rockville, MD: National Institute on Alcohol Abuse and Alcoholism, 1994.

35. Satel and Lilienfeld, "Addiction and the Brain-Disease Fallacy."

36. Lewis, C. S. *The Weight of Glory and Other Addresses*. New York: Macmillan, 1949. 26.

## Chapter 15: Me, Myself, and My Epigenetic Environment

1. Cairns, John, Julie Overbaugh, and Stephan Miller. "The Origin of Mutants." *Nature* 335 (1988): 142–45.

2. Esteller, Manel. *Epigenetics in Biology and Medicine*. Boca Raton, FL: CRC Press, 2009. 245–47; Felsenfeld, G. "A Brief History of Epigenetics." *Cold Spring Harbor Perspectives in Biology* 6, no. 1. (2014): 1–10.

3. Cairns et al., "Origin of Mutants"; Nijhout, H. F. "Metaphors and the Role of Genes in Development." *Bioessays* 12, no. 9 (1990): 441–46; Lipton, B. H. "A Fine Structural Analysis of Normal and Modulated Cells in Myogenic Culture." *Developmental Biology* 60 (1977a): 26–47; Lipton, B. H. "Collagen Synthesis by Normal and Bromodeoxyuridine-Treated Cells in Myogenic Culture." *Developmental Biology* 61 (1977b): 153–65; Lipton, B. H., K. G. Bensch, et al. "Microvessel Endothelial Cell Transdifferentiation: Phenotypic Characterization." *Differentiation* 46 (1991): 117–33; Lipton, B. H., K. G. Bensch, et al. "Histamine-Modulated Transdifferentiation of Dermal Microvascular Endothelial Cells." *Experimental Cell Research* 199 (1992): 279–91; Appenzeller, T. "Test Tube Evolution Catches Time in a Bottle." *Science* 284, no. 5423 (1999): 2108–10.

4. Bassing, C. H., W. Swat, and F. W. Alt. "The Mechanism and Regulation of Chromosomal V(D)J Recombination." *Cell* 109 (2002): S45–S55; Berg, Jeremy M., John L. Tymoczko, and Lubert Stryer. "Diversity Is Generated by Gene Rearrangements." *Biochemistry*. 5th ed. New York: W. H. Freeman, 2002. Section 33.4.

5. Stiles, J. "Brain Development and the Nature Versus Nurture Debate." *Prog Brain Res* 189 (2011): 3–22.

6. Jaenisch, Rudolf, and Adrian Bird. "Epigenetic Regulation of Gene Expression: How the Genome Integrates Intrinsic and Environmental Signals." *Nature Genetics* 33 (2003): 245–54.

7. Hernandez, L. M., and D. G. Blazer, eds. *Genes, Behavior, and the Social Environment: Moving Beyond the Nature/Nurture Debate*. Institute of Medicine (US) Committee on Assessing Interactions Among Social, Behavioral, and Genetic Factors in Health. Washington, DC: National Academies Press, 2006.

8. Dolinoy, Dana C. "The Agouti Mouse Model: An Epigenetic Biosensor for Nutritional and Environmental Alterations on the Fetal Epigenome." *Nutrition Reviews* 66, no. 1 (2008): S7–S11; Adams, Jill U. "Obesity, Epigenetics, and Gene Regulation." *Nature Education* 1, no. 1 (2008): 128; Watters, Ethan. "DNA Is Not Destiny: The New Science of Epigenetics: Discoveries in Epigenetics are Rewriting the Rules of Disease, Heredity, and Identity." Discovermagazine.com. November 22, 2006.

9. Leaf, *The Gift in You*.

10. Holliday, Robin. "Epigenetics: a Historical Overview." *Epigenetics* 1, no. 2 (2006): 76–80; Bird, Adrian. "Perceptions of Epigenetics." *Nature* 447, no. 7143 (2007): 396–98.

11. Day, J. J., and J. D. Sweatt. "Epigenetic Mechanisms in Cognition." *Neuron* 70, no. 5 (2011): 813–29.

12. Tollefsbol, Trygve, ed. *Handbook of Epigenetics: The New Molecular and Medical Genetics*. Amsterdam: Elsevier/Academic Press, 2011.

13. Ganesan, A., et al. "Epigenetic Therapy: Histone Acetylation, DNA Methylation and Anti-Cancer Drug Discovery." *Curr Cancer Drug Targets* 9, no. 8 (2009): 963–81.

14. Weinhold, Bob. "Epigenetics: The Science of Change." *Environmental Health Perspectives* 114, no. 3 (2006): A160–A167; *Ghost in Your Genes* [DVD]. Retrieved May 9, 2010, from http: www.pbs/wgbh/nova/transcripts/3413_genes .html.

15. Mihelic, Matthew. "Model of Biological Quantum Logic in DNA." *Life (Basel)* 3, no. 3 (2013): 474–81; Rieper, Elisabeth. "Classical and Quantum Information in DNA." Google Workshop on Quantum Biology. https://www.youtube. com/watch?v=2nqHOnVTxJE; Rieper, Elisabeth, Janet Anders, and Vlatko Vedral. "Quantum Physics: Quantum Entanglement between the Electron Clouds of Nucleic Acids in DNA." http://arxiv.org/abs/1006.4053.

16. Antell, D. E., and E. M. Taczanowski. "How Environment and Lifestyle Choices Influence the Aging Process." *Ann Plast Surg* 43, no. 6 (1999): 585–88; Irigaray, P., et al. "Lifestyle-Related Factors and Environmental Agents Causing Cancer: An Overview." *Biomed Pharmacother* 61, no. 10 (2007): 640–58.

17. Kim, Go-Woon, et al. "Dietary, Metabolic, and Potentially Environmental Modulation of the Lysine Acetylation Machinery." *Int J Cell Biol* 2010 (2010): 1–14.

18. Perry, Tilden Wayne, and Michael J. Cecava. *Beef Cattle Feeding and Nutrition*. San Diego: Academic Press, 1995. 156; MacKinnon, Eli. "Candy Not Corn for Cows in Drought." Livescience.com. August 23, 2012. http://www.live science.com/22627-candy-fed-cows.html; Weise, Elizabeth. "Consumers May Have a Beef with Cattle Feed." *USA TODAY*. June 9, 2003. http://usatoday30.usa today.com/news/health/2003-06-09-beef-cover_x.htm.

19. Patterson, E., et al. "Health Implications of High Dietary Omega-6 Polyunsaturated Fatty Acids." *J Nutr Metab* 2012 (2012): 1–16; De Lorgeril, M. "Essential Polyunsaturated Fatty Acids, Inflammation, Atherosclerosis and Cardiovascular Diseases." *Subcell Biochem* 42 (2007): 283–97.

20. Hagi, A., et al. "Effects of the Omega-6:Omega-3 Fatty Acid Ratio of Fat Emulsions on the Fatty Acid Composition in Cell Membranes and the Anti-Inflammatory Action." *JPEN J Parenter Enteral Nutr* 34, no. 3 (2010): 263–70.

21. Simopoulos, A. P. "The Importance of the Omega-6/Omega-3 Fatty Acid Ratio in Cardiovascular Disease and Other Chronic Diseases." *Exp Biol Med* 233, no. 6 (2008): 674–88.

22. Daley et al., "A Review of Fatty Acid Profiles."

23. McAfee, A. J., et al. "Red Meat from Animals Offered a Grass Diet Increases Plasma and Platelet N-3 PUFA in Healthy Consumers." *British Journal of Nutrition* 105 (2011): 80–89.

24. Kumar, B., A. Manuja, and P. Aich. "Stress and Its Impact on Farm Animals." *Front Biosci* (Elite Ed) 4 (2012): 1759–67.

25. Gardner, G. E., P. McGilchrist, and D. W. Pethick. "Ruminant Glycogen Metabolism." *Animal Production Science* 54, no. 10 (2014): 1575–83; Ferguson, D. M., and R. D. Warner. "Have We Underestimated the Impact of Pre-Slaughter Stress on Meat Quality in Ruminants?" *Meat Science* 80, no. 1 (2008): 12–19; Grandin, Temple. "Transferring Results of Behavioral Research to Industry to Improve Animal Welfare on the Farm, Ranch and the Slaughter Plant." *Applied Animal Behaviour Science* 81, no. 3 (2003): 215–28.

26. Daley et al., "A Review of Fatty Acid Profiles"; Realini, C. E., et al. "Effect of Pasture vs. Concentrate Feeding with or without Antioxidants on Carcass Characteristics, Fatty Acid Composition, and Quality of Uruguayan Beef." *Meat Science* 66, no. 3 (2004): 567–77; Realini, C. E., S. K. Duckett, and W. R. Windham. "Effect of Vitamin C Addition to Ground Beef from Grass-Fed or Grain-Fed Sources on Color and Lipid Stability, and Prediction of Fatty Acid Composition by Near-Infrared Reflectance Analysis." *Meat Science* 68, no. 1 (2004): 35–43.

27. Pollan, *In Defense of Food.*

28. Pottenger, Francis Marion Jr. *Pottenger's Cats: A Study in Nutrition.* La Mesa, CA: Price-Pottenger Nutrition Foundation, 1995.

29. Godfrey, K. M., et al. "Epigenetic Gene Promoter Methylation at Birth Is Associated with Child's Later Adiposity." *Diabetes* 60, no. 5 (2011): 1528–34; Trevizol, F., et al. "Cross-generational Trans Fat Intake Facilitates Mania-Like Behavior: Oxidative and Molecular Markers in Brain Cortex." *Neuroscience* 12, no. 286 (2015): 353–63.

30. Price-Pottenger Nutrition Foundation. "Pottenger's Cats: Early Epigenetics and Implications for Your Health." November 13, 2014. http://blog.ppnf.org/pottengers-cats-early-epigenetics-and-implications-for-your-health/; Alexander, Denis R. "Guarding Our Genome: The Impact of Epigenetics." In *The Language of Genetics: An Introduction.* West Conshohocken, PA: Templeton Foundation Press, 2011; Choudhuri, Supratim. "From Waddington's Epigenetic Landscape to Small Noncoding RNA: Some Important Milestones in the History of Epigenetics Research." *Toxicology Mechanisms and Methods* (2011): 252–74. http://www.ncbi.nlm.nih.gov/pubmed/21495865; Graham, Gray, Deborah Kesten, and Larry Scherwitz. *Pottenger's Prophecy: How Food Resets Genes for Wellness*

*or Illness*. Amherst, MA: White River Press, 2011; Pottenger, *Pottenger's Cats: A Study in Nutrition*.

31. Waterland, R. A., and R. L. Jirtle. "Transposable Elements: Targets for Early Nutritional Effects on Epigenetic Gene Regulation." *Mol Cell Biol* 23, no. 15 (2003): 5293–300.

32. Wilson, B. D., et al. "Structure and Function of Asp, the Human Homolog of the Mouse Agouti Gene." *Hum Mol Genet* 4, no. 2 (1995): 223–30.

33. Yen, T. T., et al. "Obesity, Diabetes, and Neoplasia in Yellow A(vy)/- Mice: Ectopic Expression of the Agouti Gene." *FASEB J* 8, no. 8 (1994): 479–88.

34. Jirtle, Randy L., and Frederick L. Tyson, eds. "Environmental Epigenomics in Health and Disease: Epigenetics and Disease Origins." *Epigenetics and Human Health*. May 17, 2013.

35. Waterland and Jirtle, "Transposable Elements."

36. Razin, A., and H. Cedar. "DNA Methylation and Gene Expression." *Microbiol Review* 55, no. 3 (1991): 451–58.

37. Waterland and Jirtle, "Transposable Elements."

38. Godfrey et al., "Epigenetic Gene Promoter."

39. Dominguez-Salas, Paula, et al. "Maternal Nutrition at Conception Modulates DNA Methylation of Human Metastable Epialleles." *Nature Communications* 5 (2014). doi: 10.1038/ncomms4746.

40. Godfrey et al., "Epigenetic Gene Promoter"; Haast, R. A., and A. J. Kiliaan. "Impact of Fatty Acids on Brain Circulation, Structure and Function." *Prostaglandins Leukot Essent Fatty Acids* 92 (2015): 3–14.

41. Nixon, Robin. "What Women Eat May Affect Kids, Grandkids: Eating a High-Fat Diet During Pregnancy Can Increase the Risk of Cancer in Future Children and Grandchildren—Even If They Eat Well—A New Study Conducted in Rats Suggests." *MSNBC*. April 28, 2010. http://www.nbcnews.com/id/36836653/ns/health-diet_and_nutrition/from/ET#.Ve8ZVrSJnww; de Assis, Sonia, et al. "High-Fat or Ethinyl-Oestradiol Intake During Pregnancy Increases Mammary Cancer Risk in Several Generations of Offspring." *Nature Communications* 3 (2012): 1053; Scarino, Maria Laura. "A Sideways Glance. Do You Remember Your Grandmother's Food? How Epigenetic Changes Transmit Consequences of Nutritional Exposure from One Generation to the Next." *Genes & Nutrition* 3, no. 1 (2008): 1–3.

42. Marsh, Geoff. "Fat Fathers Affect Daughters' Health: Female Offspring of Male Rats on Bad Diets Are More Likely to Develop Diabetes-Like Disease." *Nature*. October 20, 2010. http://www.nature.com/news/2010/101020/full/news.2010.553.html; Ng, Sheau-Fang, et al. "Chronic High-Fat Diet in Fathers Programs β-Cell Dysfunction in Female Rat Offspring." *Nature* 467, no.7318 (2010): 963–66; Gaetani, Sancia. "A Sideways Glance: Lamarck Strikes Back? Fathers Pass on to Progeny Characteristics They Develop during Their Lives." *Genes & Nutrition* 7, no. 4 (2012): 471–73.

43. Fullston, T., et al. "Paternal Obesity Initiates Metabolic Disturbances in Two Generations of Mice with Incomplete Penetrance to the F2 Generation and Alters the Transcriptional Profile of Testis and Sperm MicroRNA Content." *FASEB J* 27, no. 10 (2013): 4226–43.

44. University of Edinburgh. "Obese Mums May Pass Health Risks on to Grandchildren." *ScienceDaily.* www.sciencedaily.com/releases/2013/06/13060 5104430.htm, accessed May 6, 2015; King, Vicky, et al. "Maternal Obesity Has Little Effect on the Immediate Offspring but Impacts on the Next Generation." *Endocrinology* 154, no. 7 (2013): 2514–24.

45. Radford, Elizabeth J., et al. "In Utero Undernourishment Perturbs the Adult Sperm Methylome and Intergenerational Metabolism." *Science.* July 10, 2014. doi: 10.1126/science.1255903.

46. Saavedra-Rodredra, Lorena, and Larry A. Feig. "Chronic Social Instability Induces Anxiety and Defective Social Interactions Across Generations." *Biological Psychiatry* 73, no. 1 (2013): 44–53; see also Champagne, Frances A. "Effects of Stress Across Generations: Why Sex Matters." *Biological Psychiatry* 73, no. 1 (2013): 2–4.

47. Weaver, Ian C. G., et al. "Epigenetic Programming by Maternal Behavior." *Nature Neuroscience* 7 (2004): 847–54.

48. Dietz, D. M., et al. "Paternal Transmission of Stress-Induced Pathologies." *Biol Psychiatry* 70 (2011): 408–14.

49. Bolton, J. L., and S. D. Bilbo. "Developmental Programming of Brain and Behavior by Perinatal Diet: Focus on Inflammatory Mechanisms." *Dialogues Clin Neurosci* 16, no. 3 (2014): 307–20. http://www.nature.com/neuro/journal/v17/n1/abs/nn.3594.html; Dias, B. G., and K. J. Ressler. "Parental Olfactory Experience Influences Behavior and Neural Structure in Subsequent Generations." *Nat Neurosci* 17, no. 1 (2014): 89–96; Anway, M. D. "Epigenetic Transgenerational Actions of Endocrine Disruptors and Male Fertility." *Science* 308 (2005): 1466–69; Weaver et al., "Epigenetic Programming."

50. Edinburgh, "Obese Mums"; King et al. "Maternal Obesity Has Little Effect."

51. Weaver et al., "Epigenetic Programming."

52. Antell and Taczanowski, "How Environment and Lifestyle Choices Influence the Aging Process"; Irigaray et al., "Lifestyle-Related Factors and Environmental Agents."

## Chapter 16: The Whole Beef and Nothing but the Beef

1. Gandy, Joan, Angela Madden, and Michelle Holdsworth. "Macronutrients and Energy Balance." Chap. 5 in *Oxford Handbook of Nutrition and Dietetics.* Oxford: Oxford University Press, 2006.

2. National Institute of General Medical Sciences. "Proteins Are the Body's Worker Molecules." Chap. 1 in *The Structures of Life.* http://publications.nigms.nih.gov/structlife/chapter1.html.

3. Sims, C. E., and N. L. Allbritton. "Analysis of Single Mammalian Cells On-Chip." *Lab Chip* 7, no. 4 (2007): 423–40.

4. Ferrier, Denise R. *Biochemistry.* Lippincott Illustrated Reviews Series. May 24, 2013. Chap. 3, "Globular Proteins."

5. Ferrier, "Enzymes," chap. 5 in *Biochemistry.*

6. Gandy et al., "Macronutrients and Energy Balance"; Akuyam, S. A. "A Review of Some Metabolic Changes in Protein-Energy Malnutrition." *Niger Postgrad Med J* 14, no. 2 (2007): 155–62.

7. Costanzo, Linda S. *Physiology with Student Consult Online Access*. Philadelphia: Saunders Elsevier, 2014. Chap. 9.

8. Ferrier, "Cholesterol, Lipoprotein, and Steroid Metabolism," chap. 18 in *Biochemistry*.

9. Gandy et al., "Macronutrients and Energy Balance."

10. Purves D., G. J. Augustine, and D. Fitzpatrick et al., eds. "Neurotransmitter Synthesis." *Neuroscience*. 2nd ed. Sunderland, MA: Sinauer Associates, 2001. http ://www.ncbi.nlm.nih.gov/books/NBK11110/; Purves et al. "Two Major Categories of Neurotransmitters." http://www.ncbi.nlm.nih.gov/books/NBK10960/.

11. Purves et al. "What Defines a Neurotransmitter?" In *Neuroscience*. http ://www.ncbi.nlm.nih.gov/books/NBK10957/.

12. Kuhar, M. J., P. R. Couceyro, and P. D. Lambert. "Biosynthesis of Catecholamines." In *Basic Neurochemistry: Molecular, Cellular and Medical Aspects*. 6th ed. G. J. Siegel et al., eds. Philadelphia: Lippincott-Raven, 1999. http://www.ncbi .nlm.nih.gov/books/NBK27988/.

13. Purves et al. "The Biogenic Amines." In *Neuroscience*. http://www.ncbi .nlm.nih.gov/books/NBK11035/.

14. Purves et al. "GABA and Glycine." In *Neuroscience*. http://www.ncbi.nlm .nih.gov/books/NBK11084/; Kalueff, A. V., and D. J. Nutt. "Role of GABA in Anxiety and Depression." *Depress Anxiety* 24, no. 7 (2007): 495–517.

15. Frazer, A., and J. G. Hensler. "Serotonin." In Siegel et al., *Neurochemistry*. http://www.ncbi.nlm.nih.gov/books/NBK28150/; Banerjee, P., M. Mehta, and B. Kanjilal. "The 5-HT1A Receptor: A Signaling Hub Linked to Emotional Balance." Chap. 7 in *Serotonin Receptors in Neurobiology*. Ed. A. Chattopadhyay. Boca Raton, FL: CRC Press, 2007. http://www.ncbi.nlm.nih.gov/books/NBK5212/.

16. Purves et al. "The Circadian Cycle of Sleep and Wakefulness." In *Neuroscience*. http://www.ncbi.nlm.nih.gov/books/NBK10839/.

17. Purves et al. "Peptide Neurotransmitters." In *Neuroscience*. http://www .ncbi.nlm.nih.gov/books/NBK10873/.

18. Purves et al. "What Defines a Neurotransmitter?" In *Neuroscience*. http ://www.ncbi.nlm.nih.gov/books/NBK10957/.

19. Purves et al. "Long-Term Synaptic Potentiation." In *Neuroscience*. http ://www.ncbi.nlm.nih.gov/books/NBK10878/.

20. Purves et al. "Neurotransmitter Release and Removal." In *Neuroscience*. http://www.ncbi.nlm.nih.gov/books/NBK11106/.

21. Sathyanarayana Rao, T. S., et al. "Understanding Nutrition, Depression and Mental Illnesses." *Indian Journal of Psychiatry* 50, no. 2 (2008): 77–82.

22. Ibid.

23. Ibid., 77.

24. Pillai, R. R., and A. V. Kurpad. "Amino Acid Requirements in Children and the Elderly Population." *British Journal of Nutrition* 108, no. S2 (2012): S44–49; Ferrier, "Amino Acids," chap. 1 in *Biochemistry*.

25. National Research Council (US) Subcommittee on the Tenth Edition of the Recommended Dietary Allowances. "Protein and Amino Acids." Chap. 6 in *Recommended Dietary Allowances: 10th Edition.* Washington, DC: National Academies Press, 1989. http://www.ncbi.nlm.nih.gov/books/NBK234922/.

26. Gandy et al., "Macronutrients and Energy Balance," 60; Parker-Pope, Tara. "Switching to Grass-Fed Beef." *The New York Times.* March 11, 2010. http://well.blogs.nytimes.com/2010/03/11/switching-to-grass-fed-beef/?_r=0; Daley et al., "A Review of Fatty Acid Profiles."

27. Tome, D. "Criteria and Markers for Protein Quality Assessment: A Review." *Br J Nutr* 108, no. S2 (2012): S222–29; Mine, Y. "Egg Proteins and Peptides in Human Health—Chemistry, Bioactivity and Production." *Curr Pharm Des* 13, no. 9 (2007): 875–84; Price, Catherine. "Sorting Through the Claims of the Boastful Egg." *The New York Times.* September 16, 2008. http://www.nytimes.com/2008/09/17/dining/17eggs.html?pagewanted=all.

28. Hossain, M. I., et al. "Lentil-Based High Protein Diet Is Comparable to Animal-Based Diet in Respect to Nitrogen Absorption and Nitrogen Balance in Malnourished Children Recovering from Shigellosis." *Asia Pac J Clin Nutr* 18, no. 1 (2009): 8–14.

29. Villa, P., et al. "Fasting and Post-Methionine Homocysteine Levels in Alzheimer's Disease and Vascular Dementia." *Int J Vitam Nutr Res* 2009 79, no. 3 (2009): 166–72; Refsum, H., et al. "Homocysteine and Cardiovascular Disease." *Annu Rev Med* 49 (1998): 31–62; Minger, *Death by Food Pyramid,* 182–83.

30. Watanabe, F. "Vitamin B12 Sources and Bioavailability." *Exp Biol Med (Maywood)* 232, no. 10 (2007): 1266–74.

31. Lonn, E., et al. "Homocysteine Lowering with Folic Acid and B Vitamins in Vascular Disease." *New England Journal of Medicine* 354, no. 15 (2006): 1567–77; Murphy, Sabina A. "Heart Outcomes Prevention Evaluation (HOPE-2)." *The American College of Cardiology's Cardiosource.* http://www.medscape.com/viewarticle/533038; Minger, *Death by Food Pyramid,* 182–83.

32. Brind, Joel, et al. "Dietary Glycine Supplementation Mimics Lifespan Extension by Dietary Methionine Restriction in Fisher 344 Rats." *The FASEB Journal* 25, no. 1. MeetingAbstracts (2011): 528.2; Sugiyama, K., Y. Kushima, and K. Muramatsu. "Effect of Dietary Glycine on Methionine Metabolism in Rats Fed a High-Methionine Diet." *J Nutr Sci Vitaminol* 33, no. 3 (1987): 195–205; Minger, *Death by Food Pyramid,* 182–83.

33. O'Dea, K. "Traditional Diet and Food Preferences of Australian Aboriginal Hunter-Gatherers." *Philos Trans R Soc Lond B Biol Sci* 334, no. 1270 (1991): 233–40. Discussion 240-1; Minger, *Death by Food Pyramid,* 182–83.

34. Ibid.; Viegas, Jennifer. "Predators Pick Body Parts for Balanced Diet." *Discovery News.* May 27, 2010. http://news.discovery.com/animals/insects/predators-carnivores-spiders.htm; Mayntz, David, et al. "Balancing of Protein and Lipid Intake by a Mammalian Carnivore, the Mink, Mustela Vison." *Animal Behaviour* 77, no. 2 (2009): 349–55; Raubenheimer, David, et al. "Nutrient-Specific Compensation Following Diapause in a Predator: Implications for Intraguild Predation."

*Ecology* 88, no. 10 (2007): 2598–608; Forbes, J. Michael. "Dietary Awareness." *Applied Animal Behaviour Science* 57, no. 3 (1998): 287–97.

35. Planck, Max. *Wissenschaftliche Selbstbiographie. Mit einem Bildnis und der von Max von Laue gehaltenen Traueransprache.* Leipzig: Johann Ambrosius Barth Verlag, 1948. 22. In *Scientific Autobiography and Other Papers.* Trans. F. Gaynor. New York: Philosophical Library, 1949. 33–34. Cited in T. S. Kuhn, *The Structure of Scientific Revolutions.*

36. Masterjohn, Chris. "Heart Disease." *The Daily Lipid.* http://blog.cho lesterol-and-health.com/search/label/Heart%20Disease; Chen, Vincent C. W., et al. "The Effect of Resistance Exercise Combined with Cholesterol Intake on Serum Lipid Profile in Elderly Men and Women." *The FASEB Journal* 26, no. 1 (2012): 1142–43; Colpo, Anthony. "LDL Cholesterol: 'Bad' Cholesterol, or Bad Science?" *Journal of American Physicians and Surgeons* 10, no. 3 (2005): 83–89; Diep, Francie. "Cholesterol Conundrum: Changing HDL and LDL Levels Does Not Always Alter Heart Disease or Stroke Risk." *Scientific American.* October 12, 2011. http://www.scientificamerican.com/article/cholesterol-conundrum/; Minger, *Death by Food Pyramid,* 82–210; Kummerow, Fred A., and Jean M. Kummerow. *Cholesterol Is Not the Culprit: A Guide to Preventing Heart Disease.* Summerfield, FL: Spacedoc Media LLC, 2014. Kindle Edition; Ravnskov, Uffe. *Ignore the Awkward!: How the Cholesterol Myths Are Kept Alive.* Charleston, SC: CreateSpace, 2010. Kindle Edition.

37. Ibid.; Berg, J. M., J. L. Tymoczko, and L. Stryer. *Biochemistry.* 5th edition. New York: W. H. Freeman, 2002. Section 26.3, "The Complex Regulation of Cholesterol Biosynthesis Takes Place at Several Levels." http://www.ncbi.nlm .nih.gov/books/NBK22336/.

38. Ibid.; Berg et al., "Important Derivatives of Cholesterol Include Bile Salts and Steroid Hormones." *Biochemistry.* Section 26.4, http://www.ncbi.nlm.nih .gov/books/NBK22339/.

39. Ibid.; Campbell-McBride, Natasha. "Cholesterol: Friend or Foe?" Weston A. Price Foundation. May 4, 2008. www.westonaprice.org; Smith, L. L. "Another Cholesterol Hypothesis: Cholesterol as Antioxidant." *Free Radic Biol Med* 11, no. 1 (1991): 47–61; Girao, H., C. Mota, and P. Pereira. "Cholesterol May Act as an Antioxidant in Lens Membranes." *Curr Eye Res* 18, no. 6 (1999): 448–54; Maxwell, S. R., O. Wiklund, and G. Bondjers. "Measurement of Antioxidant Activity in Lipoproteins Using Enhanced Chemiluminescence." *Atherosclerosis* 111, no. 1 (1994): 79–89; Enig, Mary G. *Know Your Fats: The Complete Primer for Understanding the Nutrition of Fats, Oils and Cholesterol.* Silver Spring, MD: Bethesda Press, 2000; Kontush, A., and J. M. Chapman. "Antiatherogenic Function of HDL Particle Subpopulations: Focus on Antioxidative Activities." *Curr Opin Lipidol* 21 (2010): 312–18.

40. Ibid.

41. Berg et al. "Important Derivatives of Cholesterol Include Bile Salts and Steroid Hormones."

42. Ibid.; Campbell-McBride, "Cholesterol: Friend or Foe?"; Masterjohn, Chris. "Fat and Cholesterol." *The Daily Lipid.* http://blog.cholesterol-and-health.com;

Kummerow and Kummerow, *Cholesterol Is Not the Culprit*; Ravnskov, *Ignore the Awkward*.

43. Masterjohn, "Fat and Cholesterol"; Chen et al., "The Effect of Resistance Exercise"; Colpo, "LDL Cholesterol"; Diep, "Cholesterol Conundrum"; Minger, *Death by Food Pyramid*, 82–210; Kummerow and Kummerow, *Cholesterol Is Not the Culprit*; Ravnskov, *Ignore the Awkward*.

44. Analogy from Minger, *Death by Food Pyramid*, 86–87; Masterjohn, "Fat and Cholesterol"; see also Linna, Meri, et al. "Circulating Oxidised LDL Lipids, When Proportioned to HDL-C, Emerged as a Risk Factor of All-Cause Mortality in a Population-Based Survival Study." *Age and Ageing* 42, no. 1 (2013): 110–13; Meisinger, C., et al. "Plasma Oxidized Low-Density Lipoprotein, A Strong Predictor for Acute Coronary Heart Disease Events in Apparently Healthy, Middle-Aged Men from the General Population." *Circulation* 112 (2005): 651–57; Ahotupa, M., et al. "Baseline Diene Conjugation in LDL Lipids as a Direct Measure of In Vivo LDL Oxidation." *Clin Biochem* 31 (1998): 257–61; Ahotupa, M., et al. "Lipoprotein-Specific Transport of Circulating Lipid Peroxides." *Ann Med* 42 (2010): 521–29.

45. Bae, Jong-Myon, et al. "Low Cholesterol Is Associated with Mortality from Cardiovascular Diseases: A Dynamic Cohort Study in Korean Adults." *J Korean Med Sci* 27, no. 1 (2012): 58–63; Nago, N., S. Ishikawa, T. Goto, and K. Kayaba. "Low Cholesterol Is Associated with Mortality from Stroke, Heart Disease, and Cancer: the Jichi Medical School Cohort Study." *J Epidemiol* 21, no. 1 (2011): 67–74; Morgan, R. E., et al. "Plasma Cholesterol and Depressive Symptoms in Older Men." *The Lancet* 341, no. 8837 (1993): 75–79; Golomb, B. A., H. Stattin, and S. Mednick. "Low Cholesterol and Violent Crime." *Journal of Psychiatric Research* 34, nos. 4, 5 (2000): 301–9; Steegmans, Paul H. A., et al. "Higher Prevalence of Depressive Symptoms in Middle-Aged Men with Low Serum Cholesterol Levels." *Psychosomatic Medicine* 62, no. 2 (2000): 205–11; Minger, *Death by Food Pyramid*, 82–210; Masterjohn, "Fat and Cholesterol."

46. Ibid.; Elias, P. K., et al. "Serum Cholesterol and Cognitive Performance in the Framingham Heart Study." *Psychosomatic Medicine* 67, no. 1 (2005): 24–30; Minger, *Death by Food Pyramid*.

47. Nago, N., et al. "Low Cholesterol Is Associated with Mortality"; Minger, *Death by Food Pyramid*, 82–210; Masterjohn, "Fat and Cholesterol."

48. American College of Cardiology. "Low LDL Cholesterol Is Related to Cancer Risk." *ScienceDaily*. March 26, 2012. www.sciencedaily.com/releases /2012/03/120326113713.htm; Minger, *Death by Food Pyramid*, 82–210; Masterjohn, "Fat and Cholesterol."

49. Minger, *Death by Food Pyramid*, 82–210; Masterjohn, "Fat and Cholesterol."

50. Steegmans et al., "Higher Prevalence"; Morgan et al., "Plasma Cholesterol"; Minger, *Death by Food Pyramid*, 82–210; Masterjohn, "Fat and Cholesterol."

51. Kunugi, H., et al. "Low Serum Cholesterol in Suicide Attempters." *Biol Psychiatry* 41, no. 2 (1997): 196–200; Minger, *Death by Food Pyramid*, 82–210; Masterjohn, "Fat and Cholesterol."

52. Valappil, Ashraf V., et al. "Low Cholesterol as a Risk Factor for Primary Intracerebral Hemorrhage: A Case-Control Study." *Annals of the Indian Academy*

*of Neurology* 15, no. 1 (2012): 19–22; Wang, X., et al. "Cholesterol Levels and Risk of Hemorrhagic Stroke: A Systematic Review and Meta-analysis." *Stroke* 44, no. 7 (2013): 1833–39; Minger, *Death by Food Pyramid*, 82–210; Masterjohn, "Fat and Cholesterol."

53. Ravnskov, U. "High Cholesterol May Protect Against Infections and Atherosclerosis." *QJM* 96, no. 12 (2003): 927–34; Muldoon, M. F., et al. "Immune System Differences in Men with Hypo- or Hypercholesterolemia." *Clinical Immunology and Immunopathology* 84 (1997): 145–49; Minger, *Death by Food Pyramid*, 82–210; Masterjohn, "Fat and Cholesterol."

54. Ehnholm, Christian. *Cellular Lipid Metabolism*. Berlin: Springer, 2009. 132; Minger, *Death by Food Pyramid*, 82–210; Masterjohn, "Fat and Cholesterol."

55. Dietschy, John M. "Biol Central Nervous System: Cholesterol Turnover, Brain Development and Neurodegeneration." *Chem* 390, no. 4 (2009): 287–93; Minger, *Death by Food Pyramid*, 82–210; Masterjohn, "Fat and Cholesterol."

56. Elias et al., "Serum Cholesterol"; Minger, *Death by Food Pyramid*, 82–210; Masterjohn, "Fat and Cholesterol."

57. Andrade, Jason, et al. "Ancel Keys and the Lipid Hypothesis: from Early Breakthroughs to Current Management of Dyslipidemia." *BCMJ* 51, no. 2 (2009): 66–72; Minger, *Death by Food Pyramid*, 82–210; Masterjohn, "Fat and Cholesterol."

58. Gotto, Antonio M., Jr. "Jeremiah Metzger Lecture: Cholesterol, Inflammation and Atherosclerotic Cardiovascular Disease: Is It All LDL?" *Trans Am Clin Climatol Assoc.* 122 (2011): 256–89; Minger, *Death by Food Pyramid*, 82–210; Masterjohn, "Fat and Cholesterol."

59. Keys, A. "Atherosclerosis: A Problem in Newer Public Health." *J Mt Sinai Hosp N Y* 20, no. 2 (1953): 118–39; Minger, *Death by Food Pyramid*, 82–210; Masterjohn, "Fat and Cholesterol."

60. Masterjohn, Chris. "Let Us Honor Ancel Keys, Our Patron, As We Cherry Pick Studies to Bash Fructose (Revised and Extended)." *The Daily Lipid*. April 28, 2011. http://blog.cholesterol-and-health.com/2011/04/let-us-honor-ancel-keys -our-patron-as.html; Ravnskov, Uffe. *The Cholesterol Myths: Exposing the Fallacy That Cholesterol and Saturated Fat Cause Heart Disease*. Washington, DC: NewTrends Pub, 2002; Yerushalmy, Jacob, and Herman Hilleboe. "Fat in the Diet and Mortality from Heart Disease: A Methodologic Note." *New York State Journal of Medicine* 57, no. 14 (1957): 2343–54; Minger, *Death by Food Pyramid*, chap. 7; Weinberg, Sylvan Lee. "The Diet-Heart Hypothesis: A Critique." *Journal of the American College of Cardiology* 43, no. 5 (2004): 731–33; Feinman, Richard, and Sara Keough. "Ethics in Medical Research. The Low Fat-Diet-Heart Hypothesis. First, How Much Harm Has Been Done?" *Ethics in Biology, Engineering and Medicine: An International Journal* 5 (2014): 149–59; Noakes, Timothy David. "The Women's Health Initiative Randomized Controlled Dietary Modification Trial: An Inconvenient Finding and the Diet-Heart Hypothesis." *SAMJ: South African Medical Journal* 103, no. 11 (2013): 824–25; Schwab, Ursula, and Matti Uusitupa. "Diet Heart Controversies–Quality of Fat Matters." *Nutrition, Metabolism and Cardiovascular Diseases* 25 (2015): 617–22; Goldberg, Ira J., Robert H.

Eckel, and Ruth McPherson. "Triglycerides and Heart Disease Still a Hypothesis?" *Arteriosclerosis, Thrombosis, and Vascular Biology* 31, no. 8 (2011): 1716–25.

61. Ibid.

62. Ibid.; Menotti, A., and P. E. Puddu. "How the Seven Countries Study Contributed to the Definition and Development of the Mediterranean Diet Concept: a 50-Year Journey." *Nutrition, Metabolism and Cardiovascular Diseases* 25, no. 3 (2015): 245–52; Blackburn, H. "Seven Countries Study." University of Minnesota School of Public Health. 2015. http://sph.umn.edu/site/docs/epi/SPH%20Seven%20Countries%20Study.pdf.

63. Ibid.

64. Posner, Barbara Millen, et al. "Diet, Menopause, and Serum Cholesterol Levels in Women: The Framingham Study." *American Heart Journal* 125, no. 2 (1993): 483–89; Kannel, William B., and Tavia Gordon. "The Framingham Diet Study: Diet and the Regulation of Serum Cholesterol." Section 24 in *The Framingham Study: An Epidemiological Investigation of Cardiovascular Diseases*. Washington, DC: US Government Printing Office, 1970; Dawber, Thomas R., et al. "Eggs, Serum Cholesterol, and Coronary Heart Disease." *American Journal of Clinical Nutrition* 36, no. 4 (1982): 617–25; Minger, *Death by Food Pyramid*, 144–45.

65. Kannel and Gordon, "The Framingham Diet Study"; Minger, *Death by Food Pyramid*, 144.

66. Sorlie, Paul D., and Manning Feinleib. "The Serum Cholesterol-Cancer Relationship: An Analysis of Time Trends in the Framingham Study." *Journal of the National Cancer Institute* 69, no. 5 (1982): 989–96; Kreger, Bernard E., et al. "Serum Cholesterol Level, Body Mass Index, and the Risk of Colon Cancer: The Framingham Study." *Cancer* 70, no. 5 (1992): 1038–43; Elias et al. "Serum Cholesterol; Minger, *Death by Food Pyramid*, 146.

67. Lawrence, G. D. "Dietary Fats and Health: Dietary Recommendations in the Context of Scientific Evidence." *Adv Nutr* 4, no. 3 (2013): 294–302.

68. Cooper, G. M. "Cell Membranes." In *The Cell: A Molecular Approach*. 2nd ed. Sunderland, MA: Sinauer Associates, 2000. http://www.ncbi.nlm.nih.gov/books/NBK9928/; Berg et al. Section 12.3, "There Are Three Common Types of Membrane Lipids." http://www.ncbi.nlm.nih.gov/books/NBK22361/; Agranoff, B. W., J. A. Benjamins, and A. K. Hajra. "Analysis of Brain Lipids." In Siegel et al., *Basic Neurochemistry*. http://www.ncbi.nlm.nih.gov/books/NBK28239/; Berg et al. Section 26.4, "Important Derivatives of Cholesterol Include Bile Salts and Steroid Hormones." http://www.ncbi.nlm.nih.gov/books/NBK22339/.

69. Agranoff, B. W., J. A. Benjamins, and A. K. Hajra. "Properties of Brain Lipids." In Siegel et al., *Basic Neurochemistry*. http://www.ncbi.nlm.nih.gov/books/NBK28219/; Yehuda, S., S. Rabinovitz, and D. I. Mostofsky. "Essential Fatty Acids Are Mediators of Brain Biochemistry and Cognitive Functions." *J Neurosci Res* 56, no. 6 (1999): 565–70.

70. Chang, C. Y., D. S. Ke, and J. Y. Chen. "Essential Fatty Acids and Human Brain." *Acta Neurol Taiwan* 18, no. 4 (2009): 231–41.

71. Ferrier, *Biochemistry*, chap. 27, section V; Gandy et al., "Macronutrients and Energy Balance," chap. 5.

72. Barnard, N. D., A. E. Bunner, and U. Agarwal. "Saturated and Trans Fats and Dementia: A Systematic Review." *Neurobiology of Aging* 35, no. S2 (2015): S65–73; Haast, R. A., and A. J. Kiliaan. "Impact of Fatty Acids on Brain Circulation, Structure and Function." *Prostaglandins Leukot Essent Fatty Acids* 92 (2015): 3–14.

73. Bureš, D., et al. "Quality Attributes and Composition of Meat from Red Deer (Cervus Elaphus), Fallow Deer (Dama Dama) and Aberdeen Angus and Holstein Cattle (Bos Taurus)." *J Sci Food Agric* 95 (2014): 2299–2306. doi:10.1002/jsfa.6950; Daley et al., "A Review of Fatty Acid Profiles"; Leheska, J. M., et al. "Effects of Conventional and Grass-Feeding Systems on the Nutrient Composition of Beef." *Journal of Animal Science* 86, no. 12 (2008): 3575–85; McAfee, A. J., et al. "Red Meat from Animals Offered a Grass Diet Increases Plasma and Platelet N-3 PUFA in Healthy Consumers." *British Journal of Nutrition* 105, no. 1 (2011): 80–89; Alfaia, Cristina P. M., et al. "Effect of the Feeding System on Intramuscular Fatty Acids and Conjugated Linoleic Acid Isomers of Beef Cattle, with Emphasis on Their Nutritional Value and Discriminatory Ability." *Food Chemistry* 114, no. 3 (2009): 939–46.

74. Ibid.; Masterjohn.

75. Ibid.; Pollan, *In Defense of Food*.

76. Hickenbottom, S. J., et al. "Variability in Conversion of Beta-Carotene to Vitamin A in Men as Measured by Using a Double-Tracer Study Design." *Am J Clin Nutr* 75, no. 5 (2002): 900–907; Lin, Y., et al. "Variability of the Conversion of Beta-Carotene to Vitamin A in Women Measured by Using a Double-Tracer Study Design." *Am J Clin Nutr* 71, no. 6 (2000): 1545–54.

77. Okano, T., et al. "Conversion of Phylloquinone (Vitamin K1) into Menaquinone-4 (Vitamin K2) in Mice: Two Possible Routes for Menaquinone-4 Accumulation in Cerebra of Mice." *J Biol Chem* 283, no. 17 (2008): 11270–79; Masterjohn, Christopher. "On the Trail of the Elusive X-Factor: A Sixty-Two-Year-Old Mystery Finally Solved." Weston A. Price Foundation. February 14, 2008. http://www.westonaprice.org/health-topics/abcs-of-nutrition/on-the-trail-of-the-elusive-x-factor-a-sixty-two-year-old-mystery-finally-solved/#three.

78. Vermeer, Cees. "Vitamin K: The Effect on Health Beyond Coagulation—An Overview." *Food Nutr Res* 56 (2012): 10.3402/fnr.v56i0.5329; Masterjohn, "On the Trail of the Elusive X-Factor."

79. Vermeer, C., et al. "Beyond Deficiency: Potential Benefits of Increased Intakes of Vitamin K for Bone and Vascular Health." *European Journal of Nutrition* 43 (2004): 325–35; Masterjohn, "On the Trail of the Elusive X-Factor."

80. Masterjohn, Christopher. "Good Fats, Bad Fats: Separating Fact from Fiction." March 24, 2012. http://www.westonaprice.org/health-topics/good-fats-bad-fats-separating-fact-from-fiction/; Price, Weston A. *Nutrition and Physical Degeneration: A Comparison of Primitive and Modern Diets and Their Effects.* Oxford: Benediction Classics, 2010.

81. Ibid.; Minger, *Death by Food Pyramid*, 215–44.

82. Ibid.; see also Popkin, Barry M., Linda S. Adair, and Shu Wen Ng. "Now and Then: The Global Nutrition Transition: The Pandemic of Obesity in Developing Countries." *Nutr Rev.* 70, no. 1 (2012): 3–21.

83. Pearce, Morton Lee, and Seymour Dayton. "Incidence of Cancer in Men on a Diet High in Polyunsaturated Fat." *The Lancet* 297, no. 7697 (1971): 464–67; Minger, *Death by Food Pyramid*, chap. 9; Masterjohn, *The Daily Lipid*.

84. Leren, P. "The Effect of Plasma-Cholesterol-Lowering Diet in Male Survivors of Myocardial Infarction. A Controlled Clinical Trial." *Bull N Y Acad Med.* 44, no. 8 (1968): 1012–20; Minger, *Death by Food Pyramid*, chap. 9; Masterjohn, *The Daily Lipid*.

85. G. F. Watts, et al. "Effects on Coronary Artery Disease of Lipid-Lowering Diet, or Diet Plus Cholestyramine, in the St. Thomas' Atherosclerosis Regression Study (STARS)." *The Lancet* 339, no. 8793 (1992): 563–69; Burr, M. L., et al. "Diet and Reinfarction Trial (DART): Design, Recruitment, and Compliance." *European Heart Journal* 10, no. 6 (1989): 558–67; Minger, *Death by Food Pyramid,* chap. 9; Masterjohn, *The Daily Lipid*.

86. Minger, *Death by Food Pyramid*, chap. 9; Masterjohn, *The Daily Lipid*.

87. Turpeinen, O., et al. "Dietary Prevention of Coronary Heart Disease: Long-Term Experiment." *American Journal of Clinical Nutrition* 21 (1968): 255–76; Turpeinen, O., et al. "Dietary Prevention of Coronary Heart Disease: The Finnish Mental Hospital Study." *International Journal of Epidemiology* 8, no. 2 (1979): 99–118; Minger, *Death by Food Pyramid*, chap. 9; Masterjohn, *The Daily Lipid*.

88. Turpeinen et al., "Dietary Prevention of Coronary Heart Disease: Long-Term Experiment."; Turpeinen et al., "Dietary Prevention of Coronary Heart Disease: The Finnish Mental Hospital Study."; Minger, *Death by Food Pyramid,* chap. 9.

89. Mente, A., et al. "A Systematic Review of the Evidence Supporting a Causal Link between Dietary Factors and Coronary Heart Disease." *Arch Intern Med* 169, no. 7 (2009): 659–69; Masterjohn, *The Daily Lipid*.

90. Hooper, L., et al. "Reduced or Modified Dietary Fat for Preventing Cardiovascular Disease." *Cochrane Database Syst Rev* no. 3 (2001): CD002137; Masterjohn, *The Daily Lipid*.

91. Mozaffarian, Dariush, Renata Micha, and Sarah Wallace. "Effects on Coronary Heart Disease of Increasing Polyunsaturated Fat in Place of Saturated Fat: A Systematic Review and Meta-Analysis of Randomized Controlled Trials." *PLoS Med* 7, no. 3 (2010): e1000252; Masterjohn, Christopher. "AJCN Publishes a New PUFA Study That Should Make Us Long for the Old Days." Weston A. Price Foundation. May 17, 2012. http://www.westonaprice.org/blogs/cmasterjohn/ajcn-publishes-a-new-pufa-study-that-should-make-us-long-for-the-old-days/.

92. "Low-Carb Experts: Chris Masterjohn, PhD." Segment Two (8:55). https://www.youtube.com/watch?v=vbBXy5xssY0.

93. Okereke, Olivia I., et al. "Dietary Fat Types and 4-Year Cognitive Change in Community-Dwelling Older Women." *Annals of Neurology* 72 (2012). 124–34; Brigham and Women's Hospital. "With Fat: What's Good or Bad for the Heart, May Be the Same for the Brain." *ScienceDaily*. May 18, 2012. www.sciencedaily.com/releases/2012/05/120518081358.htm; Bakalar, Nicholas. "Some Fats May Harm the Brain More." *The New York Times*. May 21, 2012. http://well.blogs.nytimes.com/2012/05/21/some-fats-may-harm-the-brain-more/?_r=0; Kotz,

Deborah. "Tweaking Dietary Fat Intake Could Help Slow Brain Aging, Study Suggests." *The Boston Globe.* May 18, 2012. http://www.boston.com/dailydo se/2012/05/18/tweaking-dietary-fat-intake-could-help-slow-brain-aging-study -suggests/OO7tmvxhB2E8V0algT7DlL/story.html; English, Cameron. "Saturated Fat Is Not Bad for Your Brain, and You've Been Lied To." *Policy.Mic.* May 22, 2012. http://mic.com/articles/8673/saturated-fat-is-not-bad-for-your-brain-and -you-ve-been-lied-to.

94. Rimer, B. K. "Correlation Is Not Causation." *Am J Public Health* 88, no. 5 (1998): 832–35; Greenhalgh, Trisha. *How to Read a Paper: The Basics of Evidence Based Medicine.* Oxford; Malden, MA: BMJ, 2006; Goldacre, Ben. *Bad Science.* London: Fourth Estate, 2009; Minger, *Death by Food Pyramid,* 67–81.

95. Roberts, R. O., et al. "Relative Intake of Macronutrients Impacts Risk of Mild Cognitive Impairment or Dementia." *J Alzheimers Dis* 32, no. 2 (2012): 329–39.

96. Goritz, C., et al. "Role of Glia-Derived Cholesterol in Synaptogenesis: New Revelations in the Synapse-Glia Affair." *J Physiol Paris* 96 (2002): 257–63; Mielke, M. M., et al. "High Total Cholesterol Levels in Late Life Associated with a Reduced Risk of Dementia." *Neurology* 64 (2005): 1689–95; West, R., et al. "Better Memory Functioning Associated with Higher Total and Low-Density Lipoprotein Cholesterol Levels in Very Elderly Subjects without the Apolipoprotein E4 Allele." *Am J Geriatr Psychiatry* 16 (2008): 781–85.

97. Howland, D. S., et al. "Modulation of Secreted Beta-Amyloid Precursor Protein and Amyloid Beta-Peptide in Brain by Cholesterol." *J Biol Chem* 273 (1998): 16576–82.

98. Volk, B. M., et al. "Effects of Step-Wise Increases in Dietary Carbohydrate on Circulating Saturated Fatty Acids and Palmitoleic Acid in Adults with Metabolic Syndrome." *PLoS One* 9, no. 11 (2014): e113605.

99. Volk et al., "Effects of Step-Wise Increases"; Jakobsen, M. U., et al. "Major Types of Dietary Fat and Risk of Coronary Heart Disease: A Pooled Analysis of 11 Cohort Studies." *Am J Clin Nutr* 89, no. 5 (2009): 1425–32; Goritz, C., et al. "Role of Glia-Derived Cholesterol in Synaptogenesis: New Revelations in the Synapse-Glia Affair." *J Physiol Paris* 96 (2002): 257–63; Mielke et al., "High Total Cholesterol Levels"; Roberts, R. O., et al. "Relative Intake of Macronutrients Impacts Risk"; West et al., "Better Memory Functioning."

100. Venäläinen, T., et al. "Cross-Sectional Associations of Food Consumption with Plasma Fatty Acid Composition and Estimated Desaturase Activities in Finnish Children." *Lipids* 49, no. 5 (2014): 467–79.

101. Greene, C. M., et al. "Maintenance of the LDL Cholesterol: HDL Cholesterol Ratio in an Elderly Population Given a Dietary Cholesterol Challenge." *J Nutr* 135, no. 12 (2005): 2793–98.

102. Hu, F. B., et al. "A Prospective Study of Egg Consumption and Risk of Cardiovascular Disease in Men and Women." *JAMA* 281, no. 15 (1999): 1387–94.

103. Song, W. O., and J. M. Kerver. "Nutritional Contribution of Eggs to American Diets." *J Am Coll Nutr* 19, no. S5 (2000): 556S—62S; Gandy et al., chap. 5; Kummerow and Kummerow, *Cholesterol Is Not the Culprit.*

104. "Dr. Mercola Interviews Dr. Kummerow About Cholesterol." YouTube video, 16:54. Uploaded by Mercola. May 7, 2014. https://www.youtube.com/watch?v=Lkk7GgfLAa0.

105. Kummerow and Kummerow, *Cholesterol Is Not the Culprit*, 21.

106. Andrade et al., "Ancel Keys and the Lipid Hypothesis."

107. "Dr. Mercola Interviews Dr. Kummerow About Cholesterol."

108. Finking, G., and H. Hanke. "Nikolaj Nikolajewitsch Anitschkow (1885–1964) Established the Cholesterol-Fed Rabbit as a Model for Atherosclerosis Research." *Atherosclerosis* 135, no. 1 (1997): 1–7.

109. Rimer, "Correlation Is Not Causation"; Greenhalgh, *How to Read a Paper*; Goldacre, *Bad Science*; Minger, *Death by Food Pyramid*, 67–81; Nestle, *Food Politics*.

110. Ibid.; Goldacre, Ben. *I Think You'll Find It's a Bit More Complicated Than That*. New York: Fourth Estate, 2014.

111. Moyer, Michael. "The Salt Wars Rage On: A Chat with Nutrition Professor Marion Nestle." *Scientific American*. July 14, 2011. http://www.scientificamerican.com/article/the-salt-wars-rage-on-a-c/.

112. Morris, N. P. "The Neglect of Nutrition in Medical Education: A Firsthand Look." *Intern Med* 174, no. 6 (2014): 841–42; Nestle, *Food Politics*.

113. Feinman, Richard D. "Saturated Fat and Health: Recent Advances in Research." *Lipids* 45, no. 10 (2010): 891–92.

114. Kuipers, R. S., et al. "Saturated Fat, Carbohydrates and Cardiovascular Disease." *Neth J Med* 69, no. 9 (2011): 372–78; Minger, *Death by Food Pyramid*, chaps. 8–9.

115. Harcombe, Zoo, et al. "Evidence from Randomised Controlled Trials Did Not Support the Introduction of Dietary Fat Guidelines in 1977 and 1983: a Systematic Review and Meta-analysis." *Open Heart* 2, no. 1 (2015): e000196.

116. Masterjohn, "A New PUFA Study That Should Make Us Long for the Old Days."

117. Dhaka, Vandana, et al. "Trans Fats—Sources, Health Risks and Alternative Approach: A Review." *Journal of Food Science and Technology* 48, no. 5 (2011): 534–41; Kummerow and Kummerow, *Cholesterol Is Not the Culprit*, 41–64.

118. Ibid.; Meyer, J. M., et al. "Minimally Oxidized LDL Inhibits Macrophage Selective Cholesteryl Ester Uptake and Native LDL-Induced Foam Cell Formation." *The Journal of Lipid Research* 55, no. 8 (2014): 1648. doi: 10.1194/jlr.M044644; Texas A&M University. "'Bad' Cholesterol Not as Bad as People Think, Study Shows." *ScienceDaily*. May 8, 2011. www.sciencedaily.com/releases/2011/05/110505142730.htm; Perlmutter, David, and Kristin Loberg. *Grain Brain: The Surprising Truth about Wheat, Carbs, and Sugar—Your Brain's Silent Killers*. New York: Little, Brown, 2013.

119. Barclay, Eliza. "When Zero Doesn't Mean Zero: Trans Fats Linger in Food." NPR.org. August 28, 2014. http://www.npr.org/blogs/thesalt/2014/08/28/343971652/trans-fats-linger-stubbornly-in-the-food-supply.

120. Graham and Ramsey, *The Happiness Diet*, locations 604–5; Chowdhury, Rajiv, et al. "Association of Dietary, Circulating, and Supplement Fatty Acids with

Coronary Risk." *Annals of Internal Medicine* 160, no. 6 (2014): 398–406. doi: 10.7326/M13-1788; University of Eastern Finland. "High Serum Fatty Acid Protects Against Brain Abnormalities." *ScienceDaily.* October 17, 2013. www.science daily.com/releases/2013/10/131017080106.htm; Pottala, J.V., et al. "Higher RBC EPA DHA Corresponds with Larger Total Brain and Hippocampal Volumes: WHIMS-MRI Study." *Neurology* 82, no. 5 (2014): 435–42. doi: 10.1212/WNL.0000000000000080.

121. Kummerow and Kummerow, *Cholesterol Is Not the Culprit,* 53.

122. Ibid., 26; Zhou, Q., Y. Zhou, and Kummerow, F. A. "High-dose Lovastatin Decreased Basal Prostacyclin Production in Cultured Endothelial Cells." *Prostaglandins Other Lipid Mediat* 89, nos. 1, 2 (2009): 1–7.

123. Ibid.; American Heart Association. "Trans Fat Consumption Linked to Diminished Memory in Working-Aged Adults." *ScienceDaily.* November 18, 2014. www.sciencedaily.com/releases/2014/11/141118105406.htm; Granholm, Ann-Charlotte, et al. "Effects of a Saturated Fat and High Cholesterol Diet on Memory and Hippocampal Morphology in the Middle-Aged Rat." *Journal of Alzheimer's Disease* 14, no. 2 (2008): 133–45; Teixeira, A. M., et al. "Exercise Affects Memory Acquisition, Anxiety-Like Symptoms and Activity of Membrane-Bound Enzyme in Brain of Rats Fed with Different Dietary Fats: Impairments of Trans Fat." *Neuroscience* 195 (2011): 80–88; Collison, Kate S., et al. "Dietary Trans-Fat Combined with Monosodium Glutamate Induces Dyslipidemia and Impairs Spatial Memory." *Physiology & Behavior* 99, no. 3 (2010): 334–42; Willett, W. C. "Dietary Fats and Coronary Heart Disease." *Journal of Internal Medicine* 272, no. 1 (2012): 13–24.

124. Kummerow and Kummerow, *Cholesterol Is Not the Culprit.*

125. Andrew. "Professor Starts New Research Track as He Turns 100." *The Daily Illini.* October 6, 2014. http://www.dailyillini.com/news/article_6db9b5d6-4cec-11e4-a756-0017a43b2370.html.

126. Severson, Kim. "The Basics: A Question of Fat, and of Taste." *The New York Times.* October 1, 2006. http://www.nytimes.com/2006/10/01/weekin review/01basic.html; Eng, Monica. "Has Your Food Gone Rancid? Consumers May Have Kitchen Full of Dangerous Products and Not Know It." *The Chicago Tribune.* March 7, 2012. http://articles.chicagotribune.com/2012-03-07/features /sc-food-0302-rancidity-20120307_1_trans-fats-polyunsaturated-oils-food-chain; Moss, *Salt, Sugar, Fat.*

127. Hite, A. H., et al. "In the Face of Contradictory Evidence: Report of the Dietary Guidelines for Americans Committee." *Nutrition* 26, no. 10 (2010): 915–24.

## Chapter 17: Sugar: The Forbidden Fruit?

1. Carey, Nessa. *The Epigenetics Revolution: How Modern Biology Is Rewriting Our Understanding of Genetics, Disease, and Inheritance.* New York: Columbia University Press, 2012.

2. Ibid.; Blakeslee, Sandra. "A Pregnant Mother's Diet May Turn the Genes Around." *The New York Times*. October 7, 2003. http://www.nytimes.com/2003 /10/07/science/a-pregnant-mother-s-diet-may-turn-the-genes-around.html.

3. Avena et al. "Evidence for Sugar Addiction"; Brownell, Kelly D., and Mark S. Gold. *Food and Addiction: A Comprehensive Handbook*. Oxford: Oxford University Press, 2012. Kindle Edition, locations 17648–49.

4. Mains, R. E., and B. A. Eipper. "The Neuropeptides." In Siegel et al., *Basic Neurochemistry*.

5. Zioudrou, C., R. A. Streaty, and W. A. Klee. "Opioid Peptides Derived from Food Proteins. The Exorphins." *J Biol Chem* 254, no. 7 (1979): 2446–49.

6. Teschemacher, H. "Opioid Receptor Ligands Derived from Food Proteins." *Curr Pharm Des* 9, no. 16 (2003): 1331–44.

7. Cohen, M. R., et al. "Naloxone Reduces Food Intake in Humans." *Psychosomatic Medicine* 47, no. 2 (1985): 132–38; Drewnowski, A., et al. "Naloxone, an Opiate Blocker, Reduces the Consumption of Sweet High-Fat Foods in Obese and Lean Female Binge Eaters." *American Journal of Clinical Nutrition* 61, no. 6 (1995): 1206–12.

8. Guyenet, Stephan. "The Case for the Food Reward Hypothesis of Obesity, Part II." *Wholehealthsource*. October 7, 2011. http://wholehealthsource.blogspot .com/2011/10/case-for-food-reward-hypothesis-of_07.html.

9. Moss, *Salt, Sugar, Fat*.

10. Ibid.

11. Ibid.

12. McGee, Harold. *On Food and Cooking: The Science and Lore of the Kitchen*. New York: Scribner, 2004; Chaudhari, N., A. M. Landin, and S. D. Roper. "A Metabotropic Glutamate Receptor Variant Functions as a Taste Receptor." *Nature Neuroscience* 3, no. 2 (2000): 113–19; Nelson, G., et al. "An Amino-Acid Taste Receptor." *Nature* 416, no. 6877 (2002): 199–202; Zhang, Y., et al. "Coding Sweet, Bitter, and Umami Tastes: Different Receptor Cells Sharing Signaling Pathways." *Cell* 112, no. 3 (2003): 293–301; Moss, *Salt, Sugar, Fat*.

13. Gustafson, *We the Eaters*.

14. Ravichandran, Balaji, and Robert Lustig. "The No Candy Man." *BMJ* 346, no. 7904 (2013): 20–21.

15. Moss, *Salt, Sugar, Fat*.

16. Davis, C. "From Passive Overeating to 'Food Addiction': A Spectrum of Compulsion and Severity." *SRN Obes* 2013 (2013): 1–20.

17. Moss, *Salt, Sugar, Fat*.

18. Lustig, Robert H., et al. "Public Health: The Toxic Truth about Sugar." *Nature* 482 (2012): 27–29; Kim, J., et al. "Functional Roles of Fructose." *Proc Natl Acad Sci USA* 109, no. 25 (2012): E1619–28; Ishimoto, T., et al. "Opposing Effects of Fructokinase C and A Isoforms on Fructose-Induced Metabolic Syndrome in Mice." *Proc Natl Acad Sci USA* 109, no. 11 (2012): 4320–25; Kyriazis, G. A., M. M. Soundarapandian, and B. Tyrberg. "Sweet Taste Receptor Signaling in Beta Cells Mediates Fructose-Induced Potentiation of Glucose-Stimulated Insulin Secretion." *Proc Natl Acad Sci USA* 109, no. 8 (2012): E524–32; Touger-Decker, R.,

and C. van Loveren. "Sugars and Dental Caries." *Am J Clin Nutr* 78, no. 4 (2003): 881S–92S.

19. Cha, S. H., et al. "Differential Effects of Central Fructose and Glucose on Hypothalamic Malonyl-Coa and Food Intake." *Proc Natl Acad Sci USA* 105, no. 44 (2008): 16871–75.

20. Page, Kathleen A., et al. "Effects of Fructose vs Glucose on Regional Cerebral Blood Flow in Brain Regions Involved with Appetite and Reward Pathways." *Journal of the American Medical Association*. Preliminary Communication. January 2, 2013.

21. American College of Neuropsychopharmacology. "Fructose and Glucose: Brain Reward Circuits Respond Differently to Two Kinds of Sugar." *ScienceDaily*. December 10, 2014. www.sciencedaily.com/releases/2014/12/141210080734.htm.

22. Cha et al., "Differential Effects."

23. American College of Neuropsychopharmacology, "Fructose and Glucose."

24. Page et al., "Effects of Fructose."

25. American College of Neuropsychopharmacology, "Fructose and Glucose."

26. Zhang, Wei, Mark A. Cline, and Elizabeth R. Gilbert. "Hypothalamus-Adipose Tissue Crosstalk: Neuropeptide Y and the Regulation of Energy Metabolism." *Nutrition & Metabolism* 11, no. 1 (2014): 27; Page, Kathleen A., and Robert S. Sherwin. "The Brain: Our Food-Traffic Controller." *New York Times*. April 26, 2013. http://www.nytimes.com/2013/04/28/opinion/sunday/the-brain-our-food-traffic-controller.html.

27. Page et al., "Effects of Fructose."

28. Purnell, J. Q., et al. "Brain Functional Magnetic Resonance Imaging Response to Glucose and Fructose Infusions in Humans." *Diabetes, Obesity and Metabolism* 13, no. 3 (2011): 229. doi:10.1111/j.1463-1326.2010.01340.x; Stranahan, Alexis M., et al. "Diet-Induced Insulin Resistance Impairs Hippocampal Synaptic Plasticity and Cognition in Middle-Aged Rats." *Hippocampus* 18, no. 11 (2008): 1085–88.

29. Leaf, "The Mind-Mapping Approach"; Leaf, *Switch On Your Brain*.

30. Page et al., "Effects of Fructose."

31. Stranahan et al., "Diet-induced Insulin Resistance."

32. Purnell et al., "Brain Functional Magnetic Resonance Imaging."

33. Lustig et al., "Public Health"; Stranahan et al., "Diet-Induced Insulin Resistance."

34. Ibid.

35. Conlee, R. K., R. M. Lawler, and P. E. Ross. "Effects of Glucose or Fructose Feeding on Glycogen Repletion in Muscle and Liver after Exercise or Fasting." *Ann Nutr Metab* 31, no. 2 (1987): 126–32.

36. Lustig et al., "Public Health"; Sanda, Bill. "The Double Danger of High Fructose Corn Syrup." *Wise Traditions in Food, Farming, and Healing Arts* (Winter 2003). http://www.westonaprice.org/health-topics/the-double-danger-of-high-fructose-corn-syrup/.

37. Lustig et al., "Public Health."

38. Faeh, David, et al. "Effect of Fructose Overfeeding and Fish Oil Administration on Hepatic De Novo Lipogenesis and Insulin Sensitivity in Healthy Men." *Diabetes* 54, no. 7 (2005): 1907–13.

39. Ouyang, Xiaosen, et al. "Fructose Consumption as a Risk Factor for Non-Alcoholic Fatty Liver Disease." *Journal of Hepatology* 48, no. 6 (2008): 993–99; Purnell, J. Q., and D. A. Fair. "Fructose Ingestion and Cerebral, Metabolic, and Satiety Responses." *JAMA* 309, no. 1 (2013): 85–86.

40. Bomback, Andrew S., et al. "Sugar-Sweetened Soda Consumption, Hyperuricemia, and Kidney Disease." *Kidney International* 77, no. 7 (2010): 609–16; Flavin, Dana. "Metabolic Danger of High-Fructose Corn Syrup." *Life Extension Magazine* (2008): http://www.lifeextension.com/magazine/2008/12/metabolic-dangers-of-high-fructose-corn-syrup/page-01.

41. White, J. S. "Straight Talk about High-Fructose Corn Syrup: What It Is and What It Ain't." *Am J Clin Nutr* 88, no. 6 (2008): 1716S–21S; Rippe, J. M., and T. J. Angelopoulos. "Sucrose, High-Fructose Corn Syrup, and Fructose, Their Metabolism and Potential Health Effects: What Do We Really Know." *Adv Nutr* 4, no. 2 (2013): 236–45. doi: 10.3945/an.112.002824.

42. Boukraâ, Laïd. *Honey in Traditional and Modern Medicine*. Boca Raton, FL: CRC Press, 2014.

43. Watson, Claire. "Benefits of Raw Organic Honey." *SFGate*. http://healthyeating.sfgate.com/benefits-raw-organic-honey-9105.html.

44. Moskowitz, Howard R. "The Sweetness and Pleasantness of Sugars." *The American Journal of Psychology* 84 (1971): 387–405; Shambaugh, P., V. Worthington, and J. H. Herbert. "Differential Effects of Honey, Sucrose, and Fructose on Blood Sugar Levels." *Journal of Manipulative and Physiological Therapeutics* 13, no. 6 (1989): 322–25.

45. Ouyang et al., "Fructose Consumption as a Risk Factor"; McGrane, M. M. *Carbohydrate Metabolism: Synthesis and Oxidation*. Philadelphia, PA: Elsevier, 2009. 258–77.

46. Page and Sherwin, *The Brain*.

47. Rippe and Angelopoulos, "Sucrose, High-Fructose Corn Syrup, and Fructose."

48. Ibid.; Schmidt, Ann Marie, et al. "RAGE: a Novel Cellular Receptor for Advanced Glycation End Products." *Diabetes* 45, no. S3 (1996): S77–S80.

49. Singh, R., et al. "Advanced Glycation End-Products: a Review." *Diabetologia* 44, no. 2 (2001): 129–46.

50. Ibid.; Vitek, Michael P., et al. "Advanced Glycation End Products Contribute to Amyloidosis in Alzheimer Disease." *Proceedings of the National Academy of Sciences* 91, no. 11 (1994): 4766–70; Lustig, Robert. "Fructose: The Poison Index." TheGuardian.com. October 21, 2013. http://www.theguardian.com/commentisfree/2013/oct/21/fructose-poison-sugar-industry-pseudoscience; Lustig, Robert H. *Fat Chance: Beating the Odds against Sugar, Processed Food, Obesity, and Disease*. New York: Hudson Street Press, 2013. Kindle Editon.

51. Ibid.

52. Ibid.; Appleton, Nancy, and G. N. Jacobs. *Suicide by Sugar: A Startling Look at Our #1 National Addiction.* Garden City Park, NY: Square One Publishers, 2008.

53. Singh et al., "Advanced Glycation End-Products."

54. Ibid.; Vitek et al., "Advanced Glycation End Products"; Ramasamy, Ravichandran, et al. "Advanced Glycation End Products and RAGE: a Common Thread in Aging, Diabetes, Neurodegeneration, and Inflammation." *Glycobiology* 15, no. 7 (2005): 16R–28R.

55. Lapolla, A., et al. "Evaluation of Advanced Glycation End Products and Carbonyl Compounds in Patients with Different Conditions of Oxidative Stress." *Mol Nutr Food Res* 49, no. 7 (2005): 685–90.

56. Syed, I. A. "Glycated Haemoglobin: Past, Present, and Future Are We Ready for the Change." *J Pak Med Assoc* 61, no. 4 (2011): 383–88.

57. Singh et al., "Advanced Glycation End-Products."

58. Niiya, Y., et al. "Susceptibility of Brain Microvascular Endothelial Cells to Advanced Glycation End Products-Induced Tissue Factor Upregulation Is Associated with Intracellular Reactive Oxygen Species." *Brain Res* 1108, no. 1 (2006): 179–87.

59. Coker, L. H., and L. E. Wagenknecht. "Advanced Glycation End Products, Diabetes, and the Brain." *Neurology* 77, no. 14 (2011): 1326–27; Luevano-Contreras, Claudia, and Karen Chapman-Novakofski. "Dietary Advanced Glycation End Products and Aging." *Nutrients* 2, no. 12 (2010): 1247–65.

60. Lapolla et al., "Evaluation of Advanced Glycation End Products."

61. Bisbal, Catherine, Karen Lambert, and Antoine Avignon. "Antioxidants and Glucose Metabolism Disorders." *Current Opinion in Clinical Nutrition & Metabolic Care* 13, no. 4 (2010): 439–46.

62. Page et al., "Effects of Fructose vs Glucose on Regional Cerebral Blood Flow."

63. Yaffe, K., et al. "Glycosylated Hemoglobin Level and Development of Mild Cognitive Impairment or Dementia in Older Women." *J Nutr Health Aging* 10, no. 4 (2006): 293–95; Bächle, C. et al. "Associations Between HbA1c and Depressive Symptoms in Young Adults with Early-Onset Type 1 Diabetes." *Psychoneuroendocrinology* 55 (2015): 48–58.

64. Lustig, Robert H. "Fructose: It's 'Alcohol Without the Buzz.'" *Adv Nutr* 4, no. 2 (2013): 226–35; Lustig, *Fat Chance.*

65. Andrews, Zane B., and Tamas L. Horvath. "Tasteless Food Reward." *Neuron* 57, no. 6 (2008): 806–8; Lindqvist, Andreas, Annemie Baelemans, and Charlotte Erlanson-Albertsson. "Effects of Sucrose, Glucose and Fructose on Peripheral and Central Appetite Signals." *Regulatory Peptides* 150, no. 1 (2008): 26–32.

66. Leaf, *Mind-Mapping*; Leaf, "The Mind-Mapping Approach."

67. Page et al., "Effects of Fructose"; Stanhope, Kimber L., Jean-Marc Schwarz, and Peter J. Havel. "Adverse Metabolic Effects of Dietary Fructose: Results from Recent Epidemiological, Clinical, and Mechanistic Studies." *Current Opinion in Lipidology* 24, no. 3 (2013): 198.

68. Lowette, Katrien, et al. "Effects of High-Fructose Diets on Central Appetite Signaling and Cognitive Function." *Frontiers in Nutrition* 2 (2015): 5; Isganaitis, Elvira, and Robert H. Lustig. "Fast Food, Central Nervous System Insulin Resistance, and Obesity." *Arteriosclerosis, Thrombosis, and Vascular Biology* 25, no. 12 (2005): 2451–62.

69. Andrews and Horvath, "Tasteless Food Reward."

70. Satel, Sally L., and Frederick K. Goodwin. "Is Drug Addiction a Brain Disease?" Ethics and Public Policy Center, 1998.

71. Tiffany, Demke. "Principles of Neurotheology by Andrew B. Newberg." *Zygon* 46, no. 3 (2011): 763–64.

72. Smith, Spencer L., et al. "Dendritic Spikes Enhance Stimulus Selectivity in Cortical Neurons In Vivo." *Nature* 503, no. 7474 (2013): 115–120. doi: 10.1038/nature12600.

73. Vyas, Ajai, et al. "Chronic Stress Induces Contrasting Patterns of Dendritic Remodeling in Hippocampal and Amygdaloid Neurons." *The Journal of Neuroscience* 22, no. 15 (2002): 6810–18.

74. Hartley, Tom, et al. "The Hippocampus Is Required for Short-Term Topographical Memory in Humans." *Hippocampus* 17, no. 1 (2007): 34–48; Cave, Carolyn Backer, and Larry R. Squire. "Intact Verbal and Nonverbal Short-Term Memory Following Damage to the Human Hippocampus." *Hippocampus* 2, no. 2 (1992): 151–63.

75. Molteni, Raffaella, et al. "A High-Fat, Refined Sugar Diet Reduces Hippocampal Brain-Derived Neurotrophic Factor, Neuronal Plasticity, and Learning." *Neuroscience* 112, no. 4 (2002): 803–14.

76. McEwen, *End of Stress As We Know It*, locations 2074–75.

77. Hsu, Ted M., and Scott E. Kanoski. "Blood-Brain Barrier Disruption: Mechanistic Links Between Western Diet Consumption and Dementia." *Frontiers in Aging Neuroscience* 6 (2014): 88; Barron, Anna M., et al. "Sex-Specific Effects of High Fat Diet on Indices of Metabolic Syndrome in 3xtg-AD Mice: Implications for Alzheimer's Disease." *PloS One* 8, no. 10 (2013): e78554.

78. Lee, J., W. Duan, and M. P. Mattson. "Evidence that Brain-Derived Neurotrophic Factor Is Required for Basal Neurogenesis and Mediates, in Part, the Enhancement of Neurogenesis by Dietary Restriction in the Hippocampus of Adult Mice." *J Neurochem* 82, no. 6 (2002): 1367–75; Monteggia, L. M., et al. "Essential Role of Brain-Derived Neurotrophic Factor in Adult Hippocampal Function." *Natl Acad Sci USA* 101, no. 29 (2004): 10827–32; Rossi, C., et al. "Brain-Derived Neurotrophic Factor (BDNF) Is Required for the Enhancement of Hippocampal Neurogenesis Following Environmental Enrichment." *Eur J Neurosci* 24, no. 7 (2006): 1850–56.

79. Hsu and Kanoski, "Blood-Brain Barrier Disruption."

80. Kanoski, S. E., et al. "The Effects of Energy-Rich Diets on Discrimination Reversal Learning and on BDNF in the Hippocampus and Prefrontal Cortex of the Rat." *Behav Brain Res* 182, no. 1 (2007): 57–66; Alloway, Tracy Packiam, and Ross G. Alloway, eds. "Working Memory: The Connected Intelligence." *Frontiers of Cognitive Psychology*. December 6, 2012. 167.

81. Kanoski, S. E., and T. L. Davidson. "Different Patterns of Memory Impairments Accompany Short- and Longer-Term Maintenance on a High-Energy Diet." *J. Exp. Psychol. Anim. Behav. Process* 36 (2010): 313–19.

82. Ibid.

83. Clouard, Caroline, et al. "Combined Compared to Dissociated Oral and Intestinal Sucrose Stimuli Induce Different Brain Hedonic Processes." *Frontiers in Psychology* 5 (2014): 861; Brewerton, Timothy D. "Are Eating Disorders Addictions?" In Timothy D. Brewerton and Amy Baker Dennis, eds., *Eating Disorders, Addictions and Substance Use Disorders*. Berlin: Springer, 2014. 267–300.

84. Kanoski and Davidson, "Different Patterns of Memory Impairments."

85. Page et al., "Effects of Fructose."

86. Leuner, B., and E. Gould. "Structural Plasticity and Hippocampal Function." *Annual Review of Psychology* 61 (2010): 1–35.

87. Duarte, Ana I., Paula I. Moreira, and Catarina R. Oliveira. "Insulin in Central Nervous System: More than Just a Peripheral Hormone." *Journal of Aging Research* 2012 (2012): 1–21; Cardoso, Susana, et al. "Impact of STZ-Induced Hyperglycemia and Insulin-Induced Hypoglycemia in Plasma Amino Acids and Cortical Synaptosomal Neurotransmitters." *Synapse* 65, no. 6 (2011): 457–66; Duarte, Ana Isabel, et al. "Insulin Affects Synaptosomal GABA and Glutamate Transport under Oxidative Stress Conditions." *Brain Research* 977, no. 1 (2003): 23–30; Moreira, Paula I., et al. "An Integrative View of the Role of Oxidative Stress, Mitochondria and Insulin in Alzheimer's Disease." *Journal of Alzheimer's Disease* 16, no. 4 (2009): 741–61; Bomfim, Theresa R., et al. "An Anti-Diabetes Agent Protects the Mouse Brain from Defective Insulin Signaling Caused by Alzheimer's Disease–Associated Aβ Oligomers." *The Journal of Clinical Investigation* 122, no. 4 (2012): 1339; Yarchoan, Mark, and Steven E. Arnold. "Repurposing Diabetes Drugs for Brain Insulin Resistance in Alzheimer's Disease." *Diabetes* 63, no. 7 (2014): 2253–61.

88. Nathan, David M., et al. "Medical Management of Hyperglycemia in Type 2 Diabetes: A Consensus Algorithm for the Initiation and Adjustment of Therapy, A Consensus Statement of the American Diabetes Association and the European Association for the Study of Diabetes." *Diabetes Care* 32, no. 1 (2009): 193–203.

89. Basu, Sanjay, et al. "The Relationship of Sugar to Population-Level Diabetes Prevalence: An Econometric Analysis of Repeated Cross-Sectional Data." *PLoS One* 8, no. 2 (2013): e57873.

90. Gupta, A., R. Gupta, and B. Lal. "Effect of Trigonella Foenum-Graecum (Fenugreek) Seeds on Glycaemic Control and Insulin Resistance in Type 2 Diabetes Mellitus: A Double Blind Placebo Controlled Study." *The Journal of the Association of Physicians of India* 49 (2001): 1057; Lustig, *Fat Chance*, i; Lustig, Robert H. *Sugar Has 56 Names: A Shopper's Guide*. New York: Penguin, 2013. Kindle Edition, location 53; see also Qi, Qibin, et al. "Sugar-Sweetened Beverages and Genetic Risk of Obesity." *New England Journal of Medicine* 367, no. 15 (2012): 1387–96; Ambrosini, Gina, et al. "Fat, Sugar or Both? A Prospective Analysis of Dietary Patterns and Adiposity in Children." *The FASEB Journal* 29, no. S1 (2015): 746–54; Slattery, Martha L., et al. "Dietary Sugar and Colon Cancer."

*Cancer Epidemiology Biomarkers & Prevention* 6, no. 9 (1997): 677–85; Genkinger, Jeanine M., et al. "Coffee, Tea, and Sugar-Sweetened Carbonated Soft Drink Intake and Pancreatic Cancer Risk: A Pooled Analysis of 14 Cohort Studies." *Cancer Epidemiology Biomarkers & Prevention* 21, no. 2 (2012): 305–18; Rhee, E. J., et al. "Hyperinsulinemia and the Development of Nonalcoholic Fatty Liver Disease in Nondiabetic Adults." *Am J Med* 124, no. 1 (2011): 69–76.

91. Suzanne, M., and Jack R. Wands. "Alzheimer's Disease Is Type 3 Diabetes—Evidence Reviewed." *Journal of Diabetes Science and Technology* 2, no. 6 (2008): 1101–13.

92. Harvard School of Public Health. "Carbohydrates and Blood Sugar." 2015. http://www.hsph.harvard.edu/nutritionsource/carbohydrates/carbohydrates-and-blood-sugar/.

93. Lambert, Victoria. "Sweet Poison: Why Sugar Is Ruining Our Health." *The Telegraph*. December 2014. http://www.telegraph.co.uk/foodanddrink/healthyeating /9987825/Sweet-poison-why-sugar-is-ruining-our-health.html; Monteiro, Carlos Augusto, et al. "Increasing Consumption of Ultra-Processed Foods and Likely Impact on Human Health: Evidence from Brazil." *Public Health Nutrition* 14, no. 1 (2011): 5–13; Brummer, Yolanda, et al. "Glycemic Response to Extruded Oat Bran Cereals Processed to Vary in Molecular Weight." *Cereal Chemistry* 89, no. 5 (2012): 255–61; Smith, Erin, Charles Benbrook, and Donald R. Davis. "A Closer Look at What's in Our Daily Bread." *The Organic Center* (2012): https://www.organic -center.org/reportfiles/Part1_YourDailyBread.pdf; Moubarac, Jean-Claude, et al. "Consumption of Ultra-Processed Foods and Likely Impact on Human Health: Evidence from Canada." *Public Health Nutrition* 16, no. 12 (2013): 2240–48.

94. Heller, R. F. "Hyperinsulinemic Obesity and Carbohydrate Addiction: The Missing Link Is the Carbohydrate Frequency Factor." *Med Hypotheses* 42, no. 5 (1994): 307–12.

95. Agrawal, R., and F. Gomez-Pinilla. "'Metabolic syndrome' in the Brain: Deficiency in Omega-3 Fatty Acid Exacerbates Dysfunctions in Insulin Receptor Signalling and Cognition." *The Journal of Physiology* 590, no. 10 (2012): 2485. doi: 10.1113/jphysiol.2012.230078.

96. Kamal, A., et al. "Hippocampal Synaptic Plasticity in Streptozotocin-Diabetic Rats: Impairment of Long-Term Potentiation and Facilitation of Long-Term Depression." *Neuroscience* 90, no. 3 (1999): 737–45; Ramakrishnan, R., et al. "PKC-Alpha Mediated Alterations of Indoleamine Contents in Diabetic Rat Brain." *Brain Res Bull.* 64, no. 2 (2004): 189–94; Oh, S. H., et al. "Chorea Associated with Non-Ketotic Hyperglycemia and Hyperintensity Basal Ganglia Lesion on T1-Weighted Brain MRI Study: A Meta-Analysis of 53 Cases Including Four Present Cases." *J Neurol Sci.* 200, nos. 1, 2 (2002): 57–62.

97. Agrawal and Gomez-Pinilla, "'Metabolic Syndrome' in the Brain."

98. Schwartz, M. W., and D. Porte Jr. "Diabetes, Obesity, and the Brain." *Science* 307, no. 5708 (2005): 375–79.

99. Payne, Anita H., and Dale B. Hales. "Overview of Steroidogenic Enzymes in the Pathway from Cholesterol to Active Steroid Hormones." *Endocrine Reviews* 25, no. 6 (2004): 947–70.

317

100. Abraham, S. B., et al. "Cortisol, Obesity, and the Metabolic Syndrome: A Cross-Sectional Study of Obese Subjects and Review of the Literature." *Obesity* 21, no. 1 (2013): E105–17; Djurhuus, C. B., et al. "Effects of Cortisol on Lipolysis and Regional Interstitial Glycerol Levels in Humans." *Am J Physiol Endocrinol Metab.* 283, no. 1 (2002): E172–77; Bradley, A. J., and T. G. Dinan. "A Systematic Review of Hypothalamic-Pituitary-Adrenal Axis Function in Schizophrenia: Implications for Mortality." *J Psychopharmacol* 24, no. S4 (2010): 91–118; Fukuda, Sanae, and Kanehisa Morimoto. "Lifestyle, Stress and Cortisol Response: Review I: Mental Stress." *Environ Health Prev Med* 6, no. 1 (2001): 9–14.

101. Lasley, Elizabeth, and Bruce S. McEwen. *End of Stress As We Know It*, locations 1922–23.

102. Emory Health Sciences. "High-Fructose Diet in Adolescence May Exacerbate Depressive-Like Behavior." *ScienceDaily*. 18 November 2014. www.science daily.com/releases/2014/11/141118141852.htm; Lakhan, Shaheen E., and Annette Kirchgessner. "The Emerging Role of Dietary Fructose in Obesity and Cognitive Decline." *Nutr J* 12, no. 114 (2013): 1475–2891.

103. Van Stegeren, Anda H., et al. "Endogenous Cortisol Level Interacts with Noradrenergic Activation in the Human Amygdala." *Neurobiology of Learning and Memory* 87, no. 1 (2007): 57–66; Abercrombie, Heather C., Nicole S. Speck, and Roxanne M. Monticelli. "Endogenous Cortisol Elevations Are Related to Memory Facilitation Only in Individuals Who Are Emotionally Aroused." *Psychoneuroendocrinology* 31, no. 2 (2006): 187–96; Newcomer, John W., et al. "Decreased Memory Performance in Healthy Humans Induced by Stress-Level Cortisol Treatment." *Archives of General Psychiatry* 56, no. 6 (1999): 527–33.

104. Ruby, Perrine, and Jean Decety. "How Would You Feel versus How Do You Think She Would Feel? A Neuroimaging Study of Perspective-Taking with Social Emotions." *Journal of Cognitive Neuroscience* 16, no. 6 (2004): 988–99; Sander, David, Jordan Grafman, and Tiziana Zalla. "The Human Amygdala: An Evolved System for Relevance Detection." *Reviews in the Neurosciences* 14, no. 4 (2003): 303–16.

105. Lasley and McEwen, *The End of Stress As We Know It*; Anderberg, R. H., et al. "Dopamine Signaling in the Amygdala, Increased by Food Ingestion and GLP-1, Regulates Feeding Behavior." *Physiol Behav* 136 (2014): 135–44.

106. Sainsbury, A., G. J. Cooney, and H. Herzog. "Hypothalamic Regulation of Energy Homeostasis." *Best Pract Res Clin Endocrinol Metab* 16, no. 4 (2002): 623–37.

107. Keller, A., et al. "Does the Perception that Stress Affects Health Matter? The Association with Health and Mortality." *Health Psychol* 31, no. 5 (2012): 677–84; Poulin, M. J., et al. "Giving to Others and the Association Between Stress and Mortality." *Am J Public Health* 103, no. 9 (2013): 1649–55.

108. Plotsky, Paul M., and Michael J. Meaney. "Early, Postnatal Experience Alters Hypothalamic Corticotropin-Releasing Factor (CRF) mRNA, Median Eminence CRF Content and Stress-Induced Release in Adult Rats." *Molecular Brain Research* 18, no. 3 (1993): 195–200; Leonard, Brian E. "The HPA and Immune Axes in Stress: The Involvement of the Serotonergic System." *European Psychiatry* 20 (2005): S302–S306.

109. Dallman, Mary F., et al. "Chronic Stress and Obesity: A New View of 'Comfort Food.'" *Proceedings of the National Academy of Sciences* 100, no. 20 (2003): 11696–701; Dallman, Mary F., et al. "Stress, Feedback and Facilitation in the Hypothalamo-Pituitary-Adrenal Axis." *Journal of Neuroendocrinology* 4, no. 5 (1992): 517–26.

110. Keller, "Does the Perception That Stress Affects Health Matter?," 677.

111. Jamieson, Jeremy P., Wendy Berry Mendes, and Matthew K. Nock. "Improving Acute Stress Responses the Power of Reappraisal." *Current Directions in Psychological Science* 22, no. 1 (2013): 51–56.

112. Björntorp, Per. "Abdominal Obesity and the Metabolic Syndrome." *Annals of Medicine* 24, no. 6 (1992): 465–68; Epel, Elissa S., et al. "Stress and Body Shape: Stress-Induced Cortisol Secretion Is Consistently Greater among Women with Central Fat." *Psychosomatic Medicine* 62, no. 5 (2000): 623–32; Lo, Joan C., et al. "'Buffalo hump' in men with HIV-1 infection." *The Lancet* 351, no. 9106 (1998): 867–70.

113. Newell-Price, J., et al. "Cushing's Syndrome." *The Lancet* 367, no. 9522 (2006): 1605–17.

114. McEwen, Bruce S. "Stressed or Stressed Out: What Is the Difference?" *J Psychiatry Neurosci* 30, no. 5 (2005): 315–18.

115. Bray, G. A., S. J. Nielsen, and B. M. Popkin. "Consumption of High-Fructose Corn Syrup in Beverages May Play a Role in the Epidemic of Obesity." *Am J Clin Nutr.* 79, no. 4 (2004): 537–43. http://ajcn.nutrition.org/content/79/4/537.short.

116. Ludwig, David S., Karen E. Peterson, and Steven L. Gortmaker. "Relation Between Consumption of Sugar-Sweetened Drinks and Childhood Obesity: A Prospective, Observational Analysis." *The Lancet* 357, no. 9255 (2001): 505–8. http://www.sciencedirect.com/science/article/pii/S0140673600040411.

117. Tuormaa, Tuula E. "The Adverse Effects of Food Additives on Health: A Review of the Literature with a Special Emphasis on Childhood Hyperactivity." *Journal of Orthomolecular Medicine* 9 (1994): 225–43; Ludwig et al., "Relation between Consumption of Sugar-Sweetened Drinks."

118. Moss, *Salt, Sugar, Fat*, location 584–85.

119. Ferri, C. P., et al. "Global Prevalence of Dementia: A Delphi Consensus Study." *The Lancet* 366 (2005): 2112–17. doi: 10.1016/s0140-6736(05)67889-0; Kelley, B. J., and R. C. Petersen. "Alzheimer's Disease and Mild Cognitive Impairment." *Neurol. Clin.* 25 (2007): 577–609. doi:10.1016/j.ncl.2007.03.008.

120. Arranga et al., *Bugs, Bowels, and Behavior*.

121. Ogden, C. L., et al. "The Epidemiology of Obesity." *Gastroenterology* 132, no. 6 (2007): 2087–102; Cornier, M. A., et al. "The Metabolic Syndrome." *Endocr Rev.* 29, no. 7 (2008): 777–822; Notarianni, Elena. "Hypercortisolemia and Glucocorticoid Receptor-Signaling Insufficiency in Alzheimer's Disease Initiation and Development." *Current Alzheimer Research* 10, no. 7 (2013): 714–31.

122. Ogden, C. L., et al. "Prevalence of Childhood and Adult Obesity in the United States, 2011–2012." *JAMA* 311, no. 8 (2014): 806–14; Wolf, Philip A., et al. "Relation of Obesity to Cognitive Function: Importance of Central Obesity

and Synergistic Influence of Concomitant Hypertension. The Framingham Heart Study." *Current Alzheimer Research* 4, no. 2 (2007): 111–16; Gunstad, John, et al. "Longitudinal Examination of Obesity and Cognitive Function: Results from the Baltimore Longitudinal Study of Aging." *Neuroepidemiology* 34, no. 4 (2010): 222. See below as well.

123. For example, Lakhan, Shaheen E., and Annette Kirchgessner. "The Emerging Role of Dietary Fructose in Obesity and Cognitive Decline." *Nutr J* 12, no. 114 (2013): 1475–2891; Berrino, F. "Western Diet and Alzheimer's Disease." *Epidemiologia e prevenzione* 26, no. 3 (2001): 107–15; Gustaw-Rothenberg, Katarzyna. "Dietary Patterns Associated with Alzheimer's Disease: Population Based Study." *International Journal of Environmental Research and Public Health* 6, no. 4 (2009): 1335–40; Mahar, Pamela A., and David R. Schubert. "Metabolic Links between Diabetes and Alzheimer's Disease." *Expert Review of Neurotherapeutics* 9, no. 5 (2009): 617–30; Stephan, B. C. M., et al. "Increased Fructose Intake as a Risk Factor for Dementia." *The Journals of Gerontology Series A: Biological Sciences and Medical Sciences* (2010): glq079; Stranahan et al., "Diet-Induced Insulin Resistance."

124. Hsu and Kanoski, "Blood-Brain Barrier Disruption."

125. Ballabh, P., A. Braun, and M. Nedergaard. "The Blood-Brain Barrier: An Overview: Structure, Regulation, and Clinical Implications." *Neurobiol Dis.* 16, no. 1 (2004): 1–13.

126. Ibid.

127. Crossgrove, Janelle S., G. Jane Li, and Wei Zheng. "The Choroid Plexus Removes β-amyloid from Brain Cerebrospinal Fluid." *Experimental Biology and Medicine* 230, no. 10 (2005): 771–76; Desai, Brinda S., et al. "Blood-Brain Barrier Pathology in Alzheimer's and Parkinson's Disease: Implications for Drug Therapy." *Cell Transplantation* 16, no. 3 (2007): 285–99; Gaillard, Pieter J., Corine C. Visser, and Albertus G. de Boer. "Targeted Delivery across the Blood-Brain Barrier." *Expert Opinion on Drug Delivery* 2, no. 2 (2005): 299–309.

128. Hsu and Kanoski, "Blood-Brain Barrier Disruption."

129. Ibid.

130. McEwen, Bruce S. "Protective and Damaging Effects of Stress Mediators: Central Role of the Brain." *Dialogues Clin Neurosci* 8, no. 4 (2006): 367–81; Gomez-Pinilla, Fernando, and Kristina Kostenkova. "The Influence of Diet and Physical Activity on Brain Repair and Neurosurgical Outcome." *Surg Neurol* 70 (2011): 333–36; Molteni, R., et al. "Exercise Reverses the Harmful Effects of Consumption of a High-Fat Diet on Synaptic and Behavioral Plasticity Associated to the Action of Brain-Derived Neurotrophic Factor." *Neuroscience* 123, no. 2 (2004): 429–40.

131. Kulkarni, A. A., B. A. Swinburn, and J. Utter. "Associations between Diet Quality and Mental Health in Socially Disadvantaged New Zealand Adolescents." *European Journal of Clinical Nutrition* 69, no. 1 (2015): 79–83; Jacka, Felice N., et al. "A Prospective Study of Diet Quality and Mental Health in Adolescents." *PLoS One* 6, no. 9 (2011): e24805; Zainuddin, Muhammad, Syahrul Anwar, and Sandrine Thuret. "Nutrition, Adult Hippocampal Neurogenesis and Mental Health." *British*

*Medical Bulletin* 103, no. 1 (2012): 89–114; McMartin, Seanna E., Felice N. Jacka, and Ian Colman. "The Association between Fruit and Vegetable Consumption and Mental Health Disorders: Evidence from Five Waves of a National Survey of Canadians." *Preventive Medicine* 56, no. 3 (2013): 225–30; Jacka, Felice N., et al. "The Association between Habitual Diet Quality and the Common Mental Disorders in Community-Dwelling Adults: the Hordaland Health Study." *Psychosomatic Medicine* 73, no. 6 (2011): 483–90; Holt, Steve. "This Is Your Brain on Food: The Link between Eating Well and Mental Health." *TakePart.com*. April 3, 2014. http://www.takepart.com/article/2014/04/03/powerful-connection-between -food-and-brain.

132. Holt, "This Is Your Brain on Food"; see also Rucklidge, Julian J., Jeanette Johnstone, and Bonnie J. Kaplan. "Magic Bullet Thinking—Why Do We Continue to Perpetuate This Fallacy?" *The British Journal of Psychiatry* 203, no. 2 (2013): 154.

133. Davison, K. M., and B. J. Kaplan. "Nutrient Intakes are Correlated with Overall Psychiatric Functioning in Adults with Mood Disorders." *Canadian Journal of Psychiatry* 57, no. 2 (2012): 85–92.

134. Rucklidge, J. J., and B. J. Kaplan. "Broad-Spectrum Micronutrient Treatment for Attention-Deficit/Hyperactivity Disorder: Rationale and Evidence to Date." *CNS Drugs* 28, no. 9 (2014): 775–85.

135. Michael Berk, a professor of psychiatry at the Deakin University School of Medicine in Australia, and his collaborators; Jacka et al., "Association between Habitual Diet Quality."

136. Rucklidge and Kaplan, "Broad-Spectrum Micronutrient Treatment."

### Chapter 18: To Eat Gluten or Not to Eat Gluten: That Is the Question

1. Moore, Lauren Renée. "'But We're Not Hypochondriacs': The Changing Shape of Gluten-Free Dieting and the Contested Illness Experience." *Social Science & Medicine* 105 (2014): 76–83.

2. Biesiekierski, J. R., et al. "No Effects of Gluten in Patients with Self-Reported Non-Celiac Gluten Sensitivity after Dietary Reduction of Fermentable, Poorly Absorbed, Short-Chain Carbohydrates." *Gastroenterology* 145, no. 2 (2013): 320–28.e1–3. doi: 10.1053/j.gastro.2013.04.051. Epub, May 4, 2013.

3. Dieterich, Walburga, et al. "Identification of Tissue Transglutaminase as the Autoantigen of Celiac Disease." *Nature Medicine* 3, no. 7 (1997): 797–801; Fasano, Alessio, et al. "Prevalence of Celiac Disease in At-Risk and Not-At-Risk Groups in the United States: A Large Multicenter Study." *Archives of Internal Medicine* 163, no. 3 (2003): 286–92; Fasano, Alessio, and Carlo Catassi. "Current Approaches to Diagnosis and Treatment of Celiac Disease: An Evolving Spectrum." *Gastroenterology* 120, no. 3 (2001): 636–51.

4. Lundin, Knut E. A., and Armin Alaedini. "Non-Celiac Gluten Sensitivity." *Gastrointestinal Endoscopy Clinics of North America* 22, no. 4 (2012): 723–34; Catassi, Carlo, et al. "Non-Celiac Gluten Sensitivity: The New Frontier of Gluten Related Disorders." *Nutrients* 5, no. 10 (2013): 3839–53; Holmes, Geoffrey. "Non

Coeliac Gluten Sensitivity." *Gastroenterology and Hepatology from Bed to Bench* 6, no. 3 (2013): 115.

5. Biesiekierski, J. R., J. G. Muir, and P. R. Gibson. "Is Gluten a Cause of Gastrointestinal Symptoms in People without Celiac Disease?" *Curr Allergy Asthma Rep.* 13, no. 6 (2013): 631–38. doi: 10.1007/s11882-013-0386-4.

6. Ibid.

7. Biesiekierski et al., "Is Gluten a Cause of Gastrointestinal Symptoms?"; Biesiekierski et al. "No Effects of Gluten in Patients with Self-Reported Non-Celiac Gluten Sensitivity."

8. Biesiekierski et al., "No Effects of Gluten in Patients With Self-Reported Non-Celiac Gluten Sensitivity."

9. Carroccio, Antonio, et al. "Non-Celiac Wheat Sensitivity Diagnosed by Double-Blind Placebo-Controlled Challenge: Exploring a New Clinical Entity." *The American Journal of Gastroenterology* 107, no. 12 (2012): 1898–1906; Hoffmanová, I., and D. Sánchez. "Non-Celiac Gluten Sensitivity." *Vnitrni Lekarstvi* 61, no. 3 (2014): 219–27.

10. Pomeroy, Ross. "Non-Celiac Gluten Sensitivity May Not Exist." *Real Clear Science.* May 14, 2014. http://www.realclearscience.com/blog/2014/05/gluten_se nsitivity_may_not_exist.html; Biesiekierski et al., "Gluten Causes Gastrointestinal Symptoms in Subjects without Celiac Disease: A Double-Blind Randomized Placebo-Controlled Trial." *The American Journal of Gastroenterology* 106, no. 3 (2011): 508–14.

11. Biesiekierski et al., "Is Gluten a Cause of Gastrointestinal Symptoms?"; Biesiekierski et al., "No Effects of Gluten in Patients with Self-Reported Non-Celiac Gluten Sensitivity"; Ellis, A., and B. D. Linaker. "Non-Coeliac Gluten Sensitivity?" *The Lancet* 311, no. 8078 (1978): 1358–59.

12. Ibid.; Pomeroy, "Non-Celiac Gluten Sensitivity May Not Exist."

13. Ibid.

14. For example, see Perlmutter and Loberg, *Grain Brain*; and Davis, William. *Wheat Belly: Lose the Wheat, Lose the Weight, and Find Your Path Back to Health.* Emmaus, PA: Rodale, 2011.

15. Pollan, Michael. *Cooked: A Natural History of Transformation.* New York: Penguin Books, 2014. Kindle Edition, 224.

16. Stevenson, Leo, et al. "Wheat Bran: Its Composition and Benefits to Health, a European Perspective." *Int J Food Sci Nutr* 63, no. 8 (2012): 1001–13. Published online June 20, 2012.

17. McGee, Harold. *On Food and Cooking*; Fallon, Sally, and Mary Enig. *Nourishing Traditions. The Cookbook That Challenges Politically Correct Nutrition and the Diet Dictocrats.* Brandywine, MD: NewTrends Publishing, 2001.

18. Fan, M. S., et al. "Evidence of Decreasing Mineral Density in Wheat Grain over the Last 160 Years." *J Trace Elem Med Biol* 22, no. 4 (2008): 315–24; Masterjohn, Chris. "What No One Is Saying about Zonulin—Is Celiac about More Than Genes and Gluten?" *Cholesterol and Health.* April 5, 2011. http://bl og.cholesterol-and-health.com/2011/04/what-no-one-is-saying-about-zonulin-is .html; Masterjohn, Chris. "Wheat Belly—The Toll of Hubris on Human Health."

*Cholesterol and Health*. October 12, 2011. http://blog.cholesterol-and-health.com /2011/10/wheat-belly-toll-of-hubris-on-human.html; Cochran, Amanda. "Modern Wheat a 'Perfect, Chronic Poison,' Doctor Says." *CBS News*. June 21, 2013. http ://www.cbsnews.com/news/modern-wheat-a-perfect-chronic-poison-doctor-says/.

19. Cranton, Elmer M. "Modern Bread, the Broken Staff of Life." *Total Health Secrets*. 2005. http://www.totalhealthsecrets.com/ENGLISH/resources/article Detail.php?articles_id=70.

20. Willett, Walter. *Eat, Drink, and Be Healthy: The Harvard Medical School Guide to Healthy Eating*. New York: Free Press, 2011. Kindle Edition, locations 1892–96.

21. Ibid.

22. Ibid.

23. Schroeder, Henry A. "Losses of Vitamins and Trace Minerals Resulting from Processing and Preservation of Foods." *The American Journal of Clinical Nutrition* 24, no. 5 (1971): 562–73.

24. Willett, *Eat, Drink, and Be Healthy*, fig. 16.

25. Patel, Chirag R. *Brain Foods*. Downers Grove, IL: Your Natural Youth, 2013. Kindle Edition, locations 528–34

26. Ibid., locations 489–98.

27. *Oregon State University Extension Service Master Gardener Handbook*. February 2, 2003. http://extension.oregonstate.edu/mg/botany/hormones.html; Patel, *Brain Foods*, locations 528–34.

28. Cordain et al., "Origins and Evolution of the Western Diet."

29. Celiac Disease Foundation. "What Is Celiac Disease?" http://celiac.org /celiac-disease/what-is-celiac-disease/.

30. Drago, S., et al. "Gliadin, Zonulin and Gut Permeability: Effects on Celiac and Non-Celiac Intestinal Mucosa and Intestinal Cell Lines." *Scand J Gastroenterol*. 41, no. 4 (2006): 408–19.

31. Matsudomi, Naotoshi, Akio Kato, and Kunihiko Kobayashi. "Conformation and Surface Properties of Deamidated Gluten." *Agricultural and Biological Chemistry* 46, no. 6 (1982): 1583–86; Kanerva, Päivi, et al. "Deamidation of Gluten Proteins and Peptides Decreases the Antibody Affinity in Gluten Analysis Assays." *Journal of Cereal Science* 53, no. 3 (2011): 335–39; Masterjohn, "What No One Is Saying about Zonulin"; Masterjohn, "Wheat Belly."

32. Ibid.

33. Carroccio et al., "Non-Celiac Wheat Sensitivity."

### Chapter 19: Sleep In, Then Move It

1. Leaf, *Who Switched Off My Brain?*

2. Chapman, Colin D., et al. "Acute Sleep Deprivation Increases Food Purchasing in Men." *Obesity* 21 (2013): E555–E560. doi:10.1002/oby.20579.

3. American Academy of Sleep Medicine. "MRI Scans Show How Sleep Loss Affects the Ability to Choose Proper Foods." *ScienceDaily*. June 10, 2012. www .sciencedaily.com/releases/2012/06/120610151445.htm; Knutson, Kristen L.

"Does Inadequate Sleep Play a Role in Vulnerability to Obesity?" *American Journal of Human Biology* 24, no. 3 (2012): 361. doi:10.1002/ajhb.22219; Spiegel, Karine, et al. "Leptin Levels Are Dependent on Sleep Duration: Relationships with Sympathovagal Balance, Carbohydrate Regulation, Cortisol, and Thyrotropin." *The Journal of Clinical Endocrinology & Metabolism* 89, no. 11 (2004): 5762–71.

4. Benedict, C., et al. "Acute Sleep Deprivation Increases Serum Levels of Neuron-Specific Enolase (NSE) and S100 Calcium Binding Protein B (S-100B) in Healthy Young Men." *Sleep* 37 (December 2013): 195–98; University of California San Diego School of Medicine. "Brain Activity Is Visibly Altered Following Sleep Deprivation." *ScienceDaily*. February 10, 2000. www.sciencedaily.com/releases/2000/02/000209215957.htm.

5. American Academy of Sleep Medicine. "MRI Scans Show How Sleep Loss Affects the Ability to Choose Proper Foods." *ScienceDaily*. June 10, 2012. www.sciencedaily.com/releases/2012/06/120610151445.htm; Knutson, "Does Inadequate Sleep Play a Role in Vulnerability to Obesity?"

6. Hogue, David A. "Sensing the Other in Worship: Mirror Neurons and the Empathizing Brain." *Liturgy* 21, no. 3 (2006): 31–39; Newberg, Andrew, and Mark Robert Waldman. *How God Changes Your Brain: Breakthrough Findings from a Leading Neuroscientist.* New York: Ballantine, 2009; Ironson, G., et al. "The Ironson-Woods Spirituality/Religiousness Index Is Associated with Long Survival, Health Behaviors, Less Distress, and Low Cortisol in People with HIV/AIDS." *Ann Behav Med.* 24, no. 1 (2002): 34–48; Hagerty, Barbara Bradley. *Fingerprints of God: What Science Is Learning about the Brain and Spiritual Experience.* New York: Riverhead, 2009.

7. Roenneberg, Till, et al. "Social Jetlag and Obesity." *Current Biology* 22 (2012): 939–43. doi:10.1016/j.cub.2012.03.038.

8. St-Onge, Marie-Pierre, et al. "Short Sleep Duration, Glucose Dysregulation and Hormonal Regulation of Appetite in Men and Women." *Sleep* 35 (2012): 1503–10.

9. Benedict, Christian, et al. "Acute Sleep Deprivation Enhances the Brain's Response to Hedonic Food Stimuli: An fMRI Study." *The Journal of Clinical Endocrinology & Metabolism* 97, no. 3 (2012): E443–E447. doi:10.1210/jc.2011–2759.

10. "MRI Scans Show How Sleep Loss Affects the Ability to Choose Proper Foods"; Knutson, "Does Inadequate Sleep Play a Role in Vulnerability to Obesity?"; Chapman et al., "Acute Sleep Deprivation Increases Food Purchasing in Men."

11. Guiney, Hayley, and Liana Machado. "Benefits of Regular Aerobic Exercise for Executive Functioning in Healthy Populations." *Psychonomic Bulletin & Review* 20 (2012): 73–86. doi:10.3758/s13423-012-0345-4.

12. Chapman, Sandra B., et al. "Shorter Term Aerobic Exercise Improves Brain, Cognition, and Cardiovascular Fitness in Aging." *Frontiers in Aging Neuroscience* 5 (2013): 1–9. doi:10.3389/fnagi.2013.00075.

13. Wrann, Christiane D., et al. "Exercise Induces Hippocampal BDNF through a PGC-1α/FNDC5 Pathway." *Cell Metabolism* 18 (2013): 649–59. doi:10.1016/j.cmet.2013.09.008; Chapman et al., "Shorter Term Aerobic Exercise Improves Brain."

14. Wrann et al., "Exercise Induces Hippocampal BDNF"; Jiménez-Maldonado, A., et al. "Chronic Exercise Increases Plasma Brain-Derived Neurotrophic Factor Levels, Pancreatic Islet Size, and Insulin Tolerance in a TrkB-Dependent Manner." *PLoS One* 9 (2014): e115177. doi: 10.1371/journal.pone.0115177; The PLoS One Staff. "Correction: Chronic Exercise Increases Plasma Brain-Derived Neurotrophic Factor Levels, Pancreatic Islet Size, and Insulin Tolerance in a TrkB-Dependent Manner." *PLoS One* 10 (2015): e0119047. doi: 10.1371/journal.pone.0119047; Takada, Shingo, et al. "Brain-Derived Neurotrophic Factor Maintains Exercise Capacity and Mitochondrial Function in the Skeletal Muscle Through Ampk-Pgc1α Signaling." *Circulation* 130, no. S2 (2014): http://circ.ahajournals.org/content/130/Suppl_2/A12182.short; Neeper, Shawne A., et al. "Physical Activity Increases Mrna for Brain-Derived Neurotrophic Factor and Nerve Growth Factor in Rat Brain." *Brain Research* 726, no. 1 (1996): 49–56.

15. Erickson, Kirk I., et al. "Exercise Training Increases Size of Hippocampus and Improves Memory." *Proceedings of the National Academy of Sciences* 108, no. 7 (2011): 3017–22. doi:10.1073/pnas.1015950108.

16. Ferris, Lee T., James S. Williams, and Chwan-Li Shen. "The Effect of Acute Exercise on Serum Brain-Derived Neurotrophic Factor Levels and Cognitive Function." *Medicine & Science in Sports & Exercise* 39 (2007): 728–34; Best, John R. "Effects of Physical Activity on Children's Executive Function: Contributions of Experimental Research on Aerobic Exercise." *Developmental Review* 30, no. 4 (2010): 331–51.

17. Wikgren, Jan, et al. "Selective Breeding for Endurance Running Capacity Affects Cognitive but Not Motor Learning in Rats." *Physiology & Behavior* 106, no. 2 (2012): 95. doi:10.1016/j.physbeh.2012.01.011.

18. Federation of American Societies for Experimental Biology (FASEB). "Road to Fountain of Youth Paved with Fast Food . . . and Sneakers? Exercise May Prevent or Delay Fundamental Process of Aging." *ScienceDaily.* April 28, 2014. www.sciencedaily.com/releases/2014/04/140428163639.htm.

19. Rönn, Tina, et al. "A Six Months Exercise Intervention Influences the Genome-wide DNA Methylation Pattern in Human Adipose Tissue." *PLoS Genetics* 9, no. 6 (2013): e1003572. doi:10.1371/journal.pgen.1003572.

20. Russomano, Thais. "GRAVITY: Learning about Life on Earth by Going into Space—an Interview with Joan Vernikos." *Aviation in Focus-Journal of Aeronautical Sciences* 4, no. 2 (2013): 5–9; Cotman, Carl W., and Nicole C. Berchtold. "Exercise: A Behavioral Intervention to Enhance Brain Health and Plasticity." *Trends in Neurosciences* 25, no. 6 (2002): 295–301; Hillman, Charles H., Kirk I. Erickson, and Arthur F. Kramer. "Be Smart, Exercise Your Heart: Exercise Effects on Brain and Cognition." *Nature Reviews Neuroscience* 9, no. 1 (2008): 58–65; Colcombe, Stanley J., et al. "Aerobic Exercise Training Increases Brain Volume in Aging Humans." *The Journals of Gerontology Series A: Biological Sciences and Medical Sciences* 61, no. 11 (2006): 1166–70.

21. Ferris et al., "The Effect of Acute Exercise"; Carro, Eva, et al. "Circulating Insulin-Like Growth Factor I Mediates Effects of Exercise on the Brain." *The Journal of Neuroscience* 20, no. 8 (2000): 2926–33; van Praag, Henriette.

"Exercise and the Brain: Something to Chew On." *Trends in Neurosciences* 32, no. 5 (2009): 283–90.

## Chapter 20: Twelve Tips to Beat It

1. Freiberger, Marianne. "Schrödinger's Equation—What Is It?" PlusMaths. org. August 2, 2012; Freiberger, Marianne. "Schrödinger's Equation—What Does It Mean?" PlusMaths.org. August 2, 2012.

2. "Erwin Schrödinger—Facts." Nobelprize.org.

3. Hameroff, S. "How Quantum Brain Biology Can Rescue Conscious Free Will." *Front Integr Neurosci* 6 (2012): 93.

4. Stapp, Henry P. "Quantum Collapse and the Emergence of Actuality from Potentiality." *Process Studies* 38, no. 2 (2009): 319–39.

5. My twenty-one-day brain detox can be found at http://perfectlyyou.com and http://21daybraindetox.com.

6. Pollan, *Food Rules*, 132.

7. The Daniel Fast omits meat, dairy, and other foods. Look up "Daniel Fast food list" online.

8. Salatin, *Folks, This Ain't Normal*, 255–56.

9. Jiménez-Monreal, A. M., et al. "Influence of Cooking Methods on Antioxidant Activity of Vegetables." *Journal of Food Science* 74, no. 3 (2009): H97–H103. http://www.naturaleater.com/Science-articles/133-cooking-methods-vegetable-antioxidants.pdf.

10. Everts, Sarah. "The Maillard Reaction Turns 100." *Chemical and Engineering News*. October 1, 2012. http://cen.acs.org/articles/90/i40/Maillard-Reaction-Turns-100.html; Goldberg, T. "Advanced Glycoxidation End Products in Commonly Consumed Foods." *J Am Diet Assoc* 104 (2004): 1287–91; Sutandyo, N. "Nutritional Carcinogenesis. Acta Med Indones-Indones." *J Intern Med* 42 (2010): 36–43; Parzefall, W. "Minireview on the Toxicity of Dietary Acrylamide." *Food and Chemical Toxicology* 46 (2008): 1360–64; Uribarri, J., et al. "Advanced Glycation End Products in Foods and a Practical Guide to Their Reduction in the Diet." *J Am Diet Assoc* 110 (2010): 911–16.

11. Sell, D. R., and V. M. Monnier. "Conversion of Arginine to Ornithine by Advanced Glycation in Aging Human Collagen and Lens Crystallins." *J. Biol. Chem.* 259 (2004): 54173–84; Mustata, G. T., et al. "Paradoxical Effects of Green Tea (Camellia Sinensis) and Antioxidant Vitamins in Experimental Diabetes: Improved Retinopathy and Renal Mitochondrial Defects but Deterioration of Collagen Matrix Glycoxidation and Crosslinking." *Diabetes* 54 (2005): 517–26.

12. Tareke, Eden, et al. "Analysis of Acrylamide, a Carcinogen Formed in Heated Foodstuffs, Department of Environmental Chemistry, Stockholm University, S-106 91 Stockholm, Sweden, and AnalyCen Nordic AB, Box 905, S-531 19 Lidktockh, Sweden." *J. Agric. Food Chem.* 50, no. 17 (2002): 4998–5006. doi:10.1021/jf020302f.

13. Cai, Weijing, et al. "Oral Advanced Glycation Endproducts (AGEs) Promote Insulin Resistance and Diabetes by Depleting the Antioxidant Defenses AGE

Receptor-1 and Sirtuin 1." *Proceedings of the National Academy of Sciences* 109, no. 39 (2012): 15888–93.

14. Kimura, Mieko, and Yoshinori Itokawa. "Cooking Losses of Minerals in Foods and Its Nutritional Significance." *Journal of Nutritional Science and Vitaminology* 36, no. 4, supplement I (1990): S25–S33. https://www.jstage.jst.go .jp/article/jnsv1973/36/4-SupplementI/36_4-SupplementI_S25/_article; Robinson, *Eating on the Wild Side.*

15. Zheng, W., and S. Lee. "Well-done Meat Intake, Heterocyclic Amine Exposure, and Cancer Risk." *Nutr Cancer.* 61, no. 4 (2009): 437–46; Goldberg, "Advanced Glycoxidation End Products"; Uribarri et al., "Advanced Glycation End Products in Foods"; Minger, *Death by Food Pyramid.*

16. Sugimura, Takashi, et al. "Heterocyclic Amines: Mutagens/Carcinogens Produced During Cooking of Meat and Fish." *Cancer Science* 95, no. 4 (2004): 290–99; Cantwell, Marie, et al. "Relative Validity of a Food Frequency Questionnaire with a Meat-Cooking and Heterocyclic Amine Module." *Cancer Epidemiology, Biomarkers and Prevention* 13, no. 2 (2004): 293–98; Minger, *Death by Food Pyramid,* 184; Anderson, Kristin. "Pancreatic Cancer Risk: Associations with Meat-Derived Carcinogen Intake." American Association of Cancer Research Meeting, Denver, CO: April 18–22, 2009; Zheng and Lee, "Well-done Meat Intake"; Sutandyo, N. "Nutritional Carcinogenesis." *Acta Med Indones-Indones J Intern Med* 42 (2010): 36–43. Uribarri et al., "Advanced Glycation End Products in Foods"; Minger, *Death by Food Pyramid.*

17. Andrews, Ryan. "All about Cooking & Carcinogens." *Precision Nutrition.* http://www.precisionnutrition.com/all-about-cooking-carcinogens; Uribarri et al., "Advanced Glycation End Products in Foods"; Melo, Armindo, et al. "Effect of Beer/Red Wine Marinades on the Formation of Heterocyclic Aromatic Amines in Pan-Fried Beef." *Journal of Agricultural and Food Chemistry* 56, no. 22 (2008): 10625–32; Minger, *Death by Food Pyramid,* 268.

18. See Fallon, *Nourishing Traditions*; Gibson, R. S., et al. "Improving the Bioavailability of Nutrients in Plant Foods at the Household Level." *Proceedings of the Nutrition Society* 65 (2006): 160–68; Gibson, R. S. "The Role of Diet- and Host-Related Factors in Nutrient Bioavailability and Thus in Nutrient-Based Dietary Requirement Estimates." *Food and Nutrition Bulletin* 28 (2007): S77–S100; Hotz, C., and R. S. Gibson. "Traditional Food-Processing and Preparation Practices to Enhance the Bioavailability of Micronutrients in Plant-Based Diets." *J Nutr* 137 (2007): 1097–1100; Sandberg, A. S. "Bioavailability of Minerals in Legumes." *British Journal of Nutrition* 88, no. S3 (2002): S281–S285.

19. Poulsen, Pia Brunn, et al. "More Environmentally Friendly Alternatives to PFOS-Compounds and PFOA." Environmental Project 1013 (2005): 2005; Posner, Stefan. "Perfluorinated Compounds: Occurrence and Uses in Products." *Polyfluorinated Chemicals and Transformation Products.* Berlin Heidelberg: Springer, 2012. 25–39; Begley, T. H., et al. "Perfluorochemicals: Potential Sources of and Migration from Food Packaging." *Food Additives and Contaminants* 22, no. 10 (2005): 1023–31.

20. Pollan, *Food Rules,* 132.

21. See Wansink, *Mindless Eating*.

22. Buettner, Dan. *The Blue Zone: Lessons for Living Longer from the People Who've Lived the Longest*. Washington, DC: National Geographic, 2008. Kindle Edition.

23. Kummerow and Kummerow, *Cholesterol Is Not the Culprit*, 49; Wansink, *Mindless Eating*.

24. Wansink, *Mindless Eating*.

25. Gustafson, *We the Eaters*, 189–90.

26. See Gokhale, Esther, and Susan Adams. *8 Steps to a Pain-Free Back: Natural Posture Solutions for Pain in the Back, Neck, Shoulder, Hip, Knee, and Foot*. Standford, CA: Pendo Press, 2008.

27. Barrès, Romain, et al. "Acute Exercise Remodels Promoter Methylation in Human Skeletal Muscle." *Cell Metabolism* 15, no. 3 (2012): 405. doi:10.1016/j.cmet.2012.01.001.

Dr. Caroline Leaf is a qualified communication pathologist with a bachelor's degree in logopaedics and both a master's and PhD in communication pathology, specializing in cognitive neuroscience and neuropsychology. She ran a clinical practice for twenty-five years, serving patients in health care, education, and the corporate world. Dr. Leaf is now an international and national conference speaker and author on topics relating to thinking, the mind and how it changes the brain, neuroplasticity, mental health, optimal brain performance, toxic stress, toxic thoughts, male/female brain differences, intellectual development and learning, controlling our thought lives, wisdom, and how to identify and use one's natural gifts. She and her husband, Mac, live with their four children in the United States.

# ALSO BY
# DR. CAROLINE LEAF

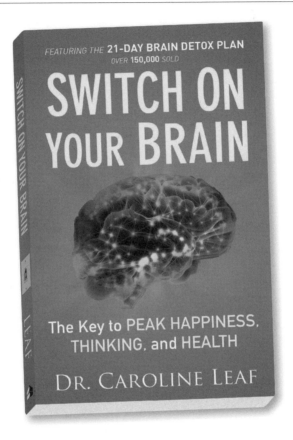

S upported by current scientific and medical research, Dr. Caroline Leaf gives you a prescription for better health and wholeness through correct thinking patterns. She exposes the "switch" in your brain that will enable you to live a happier, healthier, and more enjoyable life where you achieve your goals, get your thought life under control, and even become more intelligent. Her 21-Day Brain Detox Plan will guide you step-by-step through the process of replacing toxic thoughts with healthy ones.

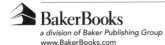

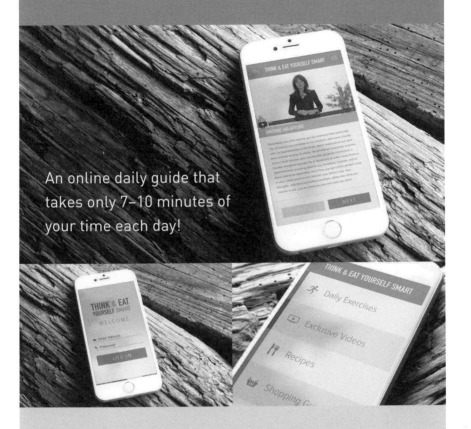